INTESTINAL ABSORPTION AND MALABSORPTION

Intestinal Absorption and Malabsorption

Editor:

T. Z. Csáky, M.D.
*Professor and Chairman
Department of Pharmacology
University of Kentucky
College of Medicine
Lexington, Kentucky*

Raven Press, Publishers • New York

© 1975 by Raven Press Books, Ltd. All rights reserved. This book is protected by copyright. No part of it may be duplicated or reproduced in any manner without written permission from the publisher.

Made in the United States of America

International Standard Book Number 0-89004-020-6
Library of Congress Catalog Card Number 74-80532

ISBN outside North and South America only: 0-7204-7538-4

Preface

The intestinal epithelium consists of morphologically and functionally differentiated cells performing both selective absorption and secretion of nutrients, inorganic (including water) and organic alike. Understanding the complex functions of the intestinal epithelium is not only of academic interest but is also helpful in elucidating the pathology of a number of diseases in which these functions are impaired, resulting in the breakdown of absorption and occasionally in a loss of nutrients into the lumen of the bowel. It is also clear that the malfunctions of the intestine cannot be understood without understanding the normal functions.

Research during the past decades has provided an increasing appreciation of the various functions of the intestinal epithelium. The findings suggested a need for bringing together experts in the various areas of intestinal absorption and malabsorption to discuss the present state of knowledge and exchange ideas. This was the reason for holding an international symposium entitled "Intestinal Absorption and Malabsorption" at the University of Kentucky in Lexington on May 28–30, 1974. The proceedings of this symposium are presented in this volume.

The actual presentations are published in full; the discussions following the presentations were edited and summarized in order to save space. An attempt was made to reproduce the essence of the discussions as fully and as accurately as possible; however, some omissions and even slight errors may have slipped into the final version due to either technical or human factors.

The editor acknowledges the excellent cooperation of each author in submitting manuscripts and reviewing the corresponding discussions.

It is hoped that this volume will be useful for those who wish to learn about the present state of knowledge of the physiological and pathological transport functions of the intestine.

T. Z. Csáky

Acknowledgments

The Symposium was sponsored by the Graduate School and the Medical Center, University of Kentucky. Special thanks are due to Dr. Wimberly C. Royster, Dean of the Graduate School, for financial aid and to Dr. Peter P. Bosomworth, Vice-President of the Medical Center, for offering both financial aid and the services of the office of Continuing Medical Education.

The generous financial aid provided by the Roche Laboratories, Division of Hoffmann-La Roche Inc., Nutley, New Jersey is acknowledged with thanks.

Many members of the University of Kentucky community provided their help in making the Symposium possible and successful. I should like to list a few persons who gave very generously of their time and energy: Dr. John G. Banwell who provided helpful counsel, suggestions and, together with Mrs. Banwell, acted as co-host for the participants; Mrs. Virginia Crutcher whose administrative and secretarial skill was greatly responsible for the smooth running of the Symposium; three doctoral students in pharmacology and in toxicology, Jeffrey L. Hill, Stuart T. Martin and Roger W. Valentine, were particularly helpful in making various arrangements. I would like to thank my wife for her patient understanding and generous help in arranging and hosting the Symposium and in editing the volume.

T. Z. C.

Contents

1   Epithelial Transport Phenomena
    H. H. Ussing

9   Energetics of Intestinal Transport
    D. S. Parsons

37 Role of Membrane-Bound Enzymes in Biological Transport
    William J. Waddell

45 Electrophysiology of Sodium Transport by Epithelial Cells of the Small Intestine
    William McD. Armstrong

67 Intestinal Transport of Monosaccharides
    V. Capraro, G. Esposito, and A. Faelli

77 Amino Acid Transport by the Small Intestine
    Stanley G. Schultz and Raymond A. Frizzell

95 Intestinal Transport of Peptides
    D. M. Matthews

113 Cation Effects on Intestinal Transport of Nonelectrolytes
    Peter F. Curran

127 Fifteen Years of Struggle with the Brush Border
    Robert K. Crane

143 Relationship Between Glycosidase Activity and Sugar Transport in the Intestine
    Donald F. Diedrich, Dan W. Hanke, and James O. Evans

155 The Intestinal Brush Border as an Organelle
    Robert G. Faust

177 Transcellular and Intercellular Intestinal Transport
    T. Z Csáky and Birgit Autenrieth

187 Comparative Biological Aspects of Intestinal Absorption
    K. C. Huang and T. S. T. Chen

197	The Effect of Unstirred Water Layers on Various Transport Processes in the Intestine *John M. Dietschy and Henrik Westergaard*
209	Action Mechanisms of Antiabsorptive and Hydragogue Drugs *W. Rummel, G. Nell, and R. Wanitschke*
229	Intestinal Absorption of Sugars in the Human *In Vivo* *John S. Fordtran*
237	The Role of the Intestinal Flora in Absorption: A Comparative Study Between Germ-free and Conventional Animals *H. A. Gordon*
253	Cholera-Toxin and Intestinal Transport *Thomas R. Hendrix*
273	The Influence of *Escherichia coli* and Other Bacterial Enterotoxins on Intestinal Fluid Transport *John G. Banwell*
285	Recent Advances in Tropical Sprue *José J. Corcino*
301	*Index*

Contributors

W. M. Armstrong
Department of Physiology
Indiana University School of Medicine
Indianapolis, Indiana 46202

Birgit Autenrieth
Department of Pharmacology
University of Kentucky
College of Medicine
Lexington, Kentucky 40506

John G. Banwell
University of Kentucky Medical Center
Department of Medicine
Division of Gastroenterology
Lexington, Kentucky 40506

V. Capraro
Istituto di Fisiologia Generale
Università di Milano
Milano, Italia

T. S. T. Chen
Department of Pharmacology
University of Louisville
School of Medicine
Louisville, Kentucky 40201

José J. Corcino
Tropical Malabsorption Unit
Departments of Medicine
Universities of Puerto Rico and Rochester
San Juan, Puerto Rico 00935

Robert K. Crane
Department of Physiology
College of Medicine and Dentistry of
  New Jersey
Rutgers Medical School
Piscataway, New Jersey 08854

T. Z. Csáky
Department of Pharmacology
University of Kentucky
College of Medicine
Lexington, Kentucky 40506

Peter F. Curran
Department of Physiology
Yale University School of Medicine
New Haven, Connecticut 06510

Donald F. Diedrich
Department of Pharmacology
University of Kentucky
College of Medicine
Lexington, Kentucky 40506

John M. Dietschy
Gastrointestinal-Liver Unit
Department of Medicine
University of Texas Southwestern Medical
  School
Dallas, Texas 75235

G. Esposito
Istituto di Fisiologia Generale
Università di Milano
Milano, Italia

James O. Evans
Department of Pharmacology
University of Kentucky
Lexington, Kentucky 40506

A. Faelli
Istituto di Fisiologia Generale
Università di Milano
Milano, Italia

Robert G. Faust
Department of Physiology
University of North Carolina
School of Medicine
Chapel Hill, North Carolina 27514

John S. Fordtran
University of Texas
Dallas, Texas 75235

Raymond A. Frizzell
Department of Physiology
University of Pittsburgh
School of Medicine
Pittsburgh, Pennsylvania 15261

CONTRIBUTORS

H. A. Gordon
Department of Pharmacology
College of Medicine
University of Kentucky
Lexington, Kentucky 40506

Dan W. Hanke
Department of Pharmacology
University of Kentucky
College of Medicine
Lexington, Kentucky 40506

Thomas R. Hendrix
Johns Hopkins University
Baltimore, Maryland 21205

K. C. Huang
Department of Pharmacology
University of Louisville
School of Medicine
Louisville, Kentucky 40201

D. M. Matthews
Department of Experimental Chemical Pathology
Vincent Square Laboratories of Westminster Hospital
124 Vauxhall Bridge Road
London SW1V 2RH, England

G. Nell
Institut für Pharmakologie und Toxikologie der Universität des Saarlandes
D-6650 Homburg, Germany

D. S. Parsons
Department of Biochemistry
University of Oxford
Oxford, England

W. Rummel
Institut für Pharmakologie und Toxikologie der Universität des Saarlandes
D-6650 Homburg, Germany

Stanley G. Schultz
Department of Physiology
University of Pittsburgh
School of Medicine
Pittsburgh, Pennsylvania 15261

H. H. Ussing
University of Copenhagen
Institute of Biological Chemistry A
Copenhagen, Denmark

William J. Waddell
Department of Pharmacology
University of Kentucky
College of Medicine
Lexington, Kentucky 40506

R. Wanitschke
Institut für Pharmakologie und Toxikologie der Universität des Saarlandes
D-6650 Homburg, Germany

Henrik Westergaard
Gastrointestinal-Liver Unit
Department of Medicine
University of Texas Southwestern Medical School
Dallas, Texas 75235

Intestinal Absorption and Malabsorption,
edited by T. Z. Csáky.
Raven Press, New York © 1975

Epithelial Transport Phenomena

H. H. Ussing

University of Copenhagen, Institute of Biological Chemistry A, Copenhagen, Denmark

I. INTRODUCTION

In order to obtain meaningful information concerning transport across composite structures such as epithelia, one should resort to simplified models, based on what are considered to be the most important parameters.

Over the years our group in Copenhagen has been mainly concerned with "model building," and I shall take my examples mostly from models that we have tested on the isolated frog skin. The viability and patience of this preparation have allowed us to do experiments that few other preparations would have tolerated. This, then, is my rationale for discussing frog skins in this volume.

In our own work three models of increasing complexity have succeeded each other. (a) The "black box" model yields via flux-ratio analysis information about active and passive transport (Ussing, 1949). The short-circuiting technique (Ussing and Zerahn, 1951) may be considered a special case of the flux-ratio approach. (b) The two-membrane model (Koefoed-Johnsen and Ussing, 1958) is based on the assumption of a continuous layer of cells, whose outward- and inward-facing membrane have different ionic selectivities and active transport mechanisms. (c) The third and most complex is the two-membrane model supplemented with extracellular (and cellular) shunt pathways (Ussing and Windhager, 1964) and a possible coupling between adjacent cell layers (Farquhar and Palade, 1964; Ussing and Windhager, 1964).

In the future we may have to include still more complications in our model. In the past I have discussed models (a) and (b) on many occasions. Here, I shall therefore deal mainly with certain unclear points relating to the third model. Finally, I shall discuss an intriguing new possibility, viz., that the endoplasmic reticulum system may play a role in the osmoregulation of the frog skin epithelium and, possibly, for the transepithelial ion transport (Voûte, Møllgaard, and Ussing, 1974).

II. INTERCELLULAR SHUNT PATHWAYS

The existence of intercellular shunt pathways in various epithelia is now well established, and there is every reason to believe that it is the tightness of the cell junctions that is the main factor in determining whether an epithelium belongs to the high- or low-resistance type. The literature has been reviewed recently (*cf.*, Ussing, Erlij, and Lassen, 1974).

III. TRANSCELLULAR SHUNT PATHWAYS

There is no doubt, however, that the resistance of the transcellular pathways may also exhibit substantial variations, even when we consider the same type of epithelium under different conditions. A good example of this is the drastic changes in permeability to water and small hydrophilic molecules that can be elicited by neurohypophyseal hormones in the amphibian skin and urinary bladder. For examples, see McKnight, Leaf, and Civan (1970) and Ussing (1973).

IV. EFFECT OF TRACE AMOUNTS OF Cu ON Cl PERMEABILITY

Another case, which we have studied recently (Koefoed-Johnsen, Lyon, and Ussing, 1973; Ussing and Koefoed-Johnsen, 1974), is the effect of traces of copper ions (10^{-5} M) on the outside of the isolated frog skin. Several years ago (Koefoed-Johnsen and Ussing, 1958) we found such concentrations of Cu to increase the frog skin potential by reducing drastically the chloride shunt. Since other investigators had failed to obtain this effect, the problem was reinvestigated. It then turned out that if the animals had been kept in a cold room for some time, the chloride permeability became rather low and it was unaffected by Cu. If the frogs had been kept at room temperature for a few days before the experiment, the Cl permeability became considerably higher, and it was drastically reduced after Cu-treatment. The sulfate and sucrose permeabilities (which may be assumed to be mainly intercellular) were unaffected by Cu, both in skins from cold- and warm-adapted frogs. The most likely explanation is that Cl follows the extracellular pathway just like sulfate and sucrose in skins from cold-adapted frogs, whereas, in skins from warm-adapted animals, chloride can pass through a cellular as well as an extracellular pathway. The cellular pathway can be closed by Cu-treatment.

V. COUPLING BETWEEN ADJACENT EPITHELIAL CELL LAYERS

Although this volume is largely devoted to intestinal epithelia, which typically have only one layer of cells, it may be permissible to discuss briefly the problems concerning the collaboration of the cells of different layers in multilayer epithelia like the frog skin.

Based upon experiments with microelectrodes, we advanced the hypothesis (Ussing and Windhager, 1964) that adjacent cell layers were coupled through rather high-resistance cell junctions. Junctions of the conducting type (Loewenstein and Kanno, 1964) were also observed by Farquhar and Palade (1964). The fact that lithium coming from the outside solution will pile up in all cell layers of the frog skin epithelium (Hansen and Zerahn, 1964; Leblanc, 1972) also speaks in favor of coupling between cell layers. The quantitative role of this coupling remained uncertain, however.

Smith (1971) working in our institute was able to demonstrate that, for the frog skin, the variation of impedance with frequency could be explained satisfactorily if one assumes two membranes in series, of which the outer one has a high resistance and a capacitance of about 2 $\mu F/cm^2$, whereas the inner one has a low resistance and a capacitance of some 50 $\mu F/cm^2$. This latter value is quite unreasonable for a single cell membrane, but could be explained if, for example, several cell layers were coupled. (Another highly hypothetical explanation will be mentioned later.) Although coupling between cell layers can explain many observations, other experiments speak against coupling as being of great quantitative importance, at least as far as the active sodium is concerned. Thus, if a hydrostatic pressure head of, say, 25-cm H_2O is applied on the inward-facing side of the isolated frog skin, the interspaces between the epithelial cells are expanded, and in many cases the connections between neighboring layers of cells may be drawn out to the extent of becoming very thin strands, longer than the cells themselves. Even under such conditions the short-circuit current usually remains constant (Voûte and Ussing, 1970). Actually as shown by my late collaborator Bernhard Andersen (unpublished) the strands between the cell layers may be forced to rip completely, so that the epithelium separates into a basal and distal part. Even in cases where the latter consisted of only one or two living cell layers (plus the cornified layer), the preparation produced normal circuit currents and potential. Thus the basal parts of the epithelium do not seem to contribute greatly to the normal transepithelial sodium transport. In this context it is also worth mentioning that only the outermost living cell layer reacts by swelling during short-circuiting (ingoing current) and shrinking under the influence of an outgoing current (Voûte and Ussing, 1968, 1970). It is this very cell layer that is held together with "tight seals." There is also very good kinetic evidence (Lindemann and Gebhardt, 1973; Martinez-Palomo, Erlij, and Bracho, 1971) that the selective membrane, governing the entry of sodium into the epithelium, is the outward-facing plasma membrane of this layer. The findng that the frog skin responds to ionic substitutions in a way that is in reasonably good agreement with the two-membrane hypothesis (Koefoed-Johnsen and Ussing, 1958) would then be due to the fact that one cell layer, connected with very tight junctions, dominates both the active sodium transport and the epithelial resistance. The model would then be formally identical to the one originally proposed by us (Koefoed-Johnsen and Ussing, 1958), but the active cell layer would be the outermost living cell layer, rather than the stratum germinativum.

VI. ENDOPLASMIC RETICULUM INVOLVEMENT IN ACTIVE SODIUM TRANSPORT

It has already been mentioned that the sodium-selective membrane must be the outward-facing boundary of the active cell layer. But where is the sodium pump located? According to our previous thinking, it ought to be placed in the cell membranes facing the interspaces of the epithelium. This may in fact be the main localization of the pump. Some very recent observations indicate, however, that part of the active sodium transport may be associated with the endoplasmic reticulum of the outermost living cell layer of the skin. In the experiments mentioned above (Voûte and Ussing, 1970) in which we studied the effect of a hydrostatic pressure head applied on the inward side of the isolated frog skin, we noticed the reversible appearance of vacuoles in the cells. In many cases the perinuclear space was blown up to a huge extent. This observation led to a study of the combined effects of hydrostatic pressure and short-circuiting (Voûte, Møllgaard, and Ussing, 1974).

When the hydrostatic pressure of the inside solution was raised by 20 to 80 cm of H_2O over and above that pressure on the outside, and if, at the same time, the skin was short-circuited, there was a characteristic change in the appearance of the outermost living cell layer of the epithelium. Light microscopically, one sees small light dots randomly distributed in the cytoplasm. The number of dots turned out to be closely correlated with the rate of active sodium transport through the skin. If the sodium on the outside of the skin was replaced with choline, the short-circuited current dropped to zero, and at the same time the light dots virtually disappear.

Electromicroscopically, the light dots turned out to be vacuoles or sacs about 1 μ in diameter bounded by a unit membrane and in intimate contact with tubules and sacs belonging to the endoplasmic reticulum. The endoplasmic reticulum as well as the perinuclear space were mostly abnormally expanded in these experiments with combined hydrostatic pressure and short-circuiting.

It should be pointed out that the "scalloped sacs" as we have named them, are also present in normal epithelium, even in the absence of short-circuiting. As far as the endoplasmic system is concerned, a general expansion can be seen during rapid sodium transport, for instance when a current double that necessary for short-circuiting is passed inward through the skin (cf. Voûte and Ussing, 1968, Fig. 9a). Saladino, Bentley, and Trump (1969), studying the effect of amphotericin B on the toad bladder, made the interesting observation that under the influence of the poison, there was an expansion of the endoplasmic system if sodium were present, but not in the absence of sodium. Thus there already exists some hints that the endoplasmic system may be involved in the handling of sodium. Perhaps one should also mention that the contractile vacuole of protozoans may be considered part of the endoplasmic system and that it seems to expel sodium (see Elliot, 1973).

Our present observation that the number of "scalloped sacs" is almost linearly correlated with the rate of sodium transport makes it very tempting to suggest a direct role in Na transport of these structures in particular and the endoplasmic system in general.

One may ask why the application of an outward-directed hydrostatic pressure gradient is usually necessary in order to make the "scalloped sacs" visible light microscopically. Possibly, the pressure impedes the emptying of the endoplasmic system. This would imply that the system opens constantly or intermittently on the inward-facing surface of the transporting cells. The effect would then be an enormous increase of the effective area of the inward-facing membrane. Such an arrangement might be part of the explanation of the enormous capacitance of this membrane (Smith, 1971).

Even if, for the sake of argument, we assume that there is active transport of sodium by way of endoplasmic system, there still is the question of whether it is an auxillary transport, which is only active during sodium overloading, or whether it is a main transport pathway.

In the latter case we are faced with an interesting problem, viz., although sodium must be delivered to the inside bathing solution together with a counter ion, nevertheless the short-circuit current is exactly equal to the net sodium transport. Thus, the counter ion must be recycled to the cell from the inside bathing solution. The counter ion cannot, during short-circuiting, come from the outside bathing solution, since that would reduce the number of positive charges associated with a given net sodium transport.

In this context it may be pertinent that the rate of sodium transport is positively correlated with the diffusibility of the bulk anion of the inside bathing solution, whereas anionic substitutions in the outside solution have little effect on the rate of sodium transport (Ussing, 1965; Huf, 1972).

A natural explanation would be if part of the cellular sodium were in fact located in the endoplasmic reticulum. Thus Zerahn (1969) has obtained kinetic data that can be interpreted to mean that the transport pool of sodium (i.e., cellular sodium with access to the pump) is much smaller than the total cellular amount of sodium.

It may also be mentioned that Natochin and Skulksky (1972), on the basis of inhibitor experiments, propose a localization of the sodium pump that is less accessible than the passive potassium diffusion path, when inhibitors are added to the inside bathing solution. Other arguments for and against the hypothesis of a participation of the endoplasmic system in active sodium transport could easily be added, but what we need now are more experiments. The hypothesis may be all wrong, but it would be a mistake not to study it carefully.

REFERENCES

Elliot, A. M. (Ed.) (1973): *Biology of tetrahymena,* Dowden, Huchinson and Ross, Stroudsburg, Penn.
Farquhar, M. G., and Palade, G. E. (1964): Functional organization of amphibian skin. Proc. Nat. Acad. Sci. *51:*569–577.
Hansen, H., and Zerahn, K. (1964): Concentration of lithium, sodium and potassium in epithelial cells of the isolated frog skin during active transport of lithium. Acta Physiol. Scand. *60:*189–196.
Huf, E. G. (1972): The role of Cl^- and other anions in active Na^+ transport in isolated frog skin. Acta Physiol. Scand. *84:*366–381.
Koefoed-Johnsen, V., Lyon, I., and Ussing, H. H. (1973): Effect of Cu ion on permeability properties of isolated frog skin (Rana temporaria). Abstr. XIV Scandavian Congress on Physiology and Pharmacology, Bergen, 1973. Acta Physiol. Scand. Suppl. 396:102.
Koefoed-Johnsen, V., and Ussing, H. H. (1958): The nature of the frog skin potential. Acta Physiol. Scand. *42:*298–308.
Koefoed-Johnsen, V., and Ussing, H. H. (1974): Transport pathways in frog skin and their modification by copper ion. In: *Secretory mechanisms of exocrine glands,* Alfred Benzon Symposium VII, Munksgaard, Copenhagen.
Leblanc, G. (1972): The mechanism of lithium accumulation in the isolated frog skin epithelium. Pflügers Arch. Ges. Physiol. *337:*1–18.
Lindemann, B., and Gebhardt, U. (1973): Delayed changes of Na-permeability in response to steps of $(Na)_o$ at the outer surface of frog skin and toad bladder. In: *Transport mechanisms in epithelia,* Alfred Benzon Symposium V, edited by H. H. Ussing and N. A. Thorn, Munksgaard, Copenhagen, pp. 115–130.
Loewenstein, W. R., and Kanno, Y. (1964): Studies on an epithelial (gland) cell junction. I. Modifications of surface membrane permeability. J. Cell Biol. *22:*565–586.
McKnight, A. D. C., Leaf, A., and Civan, M. M. (1970): Vasopressin: Evidence for the cellular site of the induced permeability change. Biochim. Biophys. Acta *222:*560–563.
Martinez-Palmo, A., Erlij, D., and Bracho, H. (1971): Localization of permeability barriers in the frog skin epithelium. J. Cell Biol. *50:*277–287.
Natochin, Y. V., and Skulsky, I. A. (1972): Dokl. Akad. Nauk SSSR (in Russian) *203:*1437–1440.
Saladino, A. J., Bentley, P. J., and Trump, B. F. (1969): Ion movements in cell injury. Am. J. Pathol. *54:*421–466.
Smith, P. (1971): The low-frequency electrical impedance of the isolated frog skin. Acta Physiol. Scand. *81:*355–366.
Ussing, H. H. (1949): The distinction by means of tracers between active transport and diffusion. Acta Physiol. Scand. *19:*43–56.
Ussing, H. H., and Zerahn, K. (1951): Active transport of sodium as the source of electric current in the short-circuited isolated frog skin. Acta Physiol. Scand. *23:*110–127.
Ussing, H. H., and Windhager, E. E. (1964): Nature of shunt path and active sodium transport path through frog skin epithelium. Acta Physiol. Scand. *61:*484–504.
Ussing, H. H. (1965): Relationship between osmotic reactions and active sodium transport in the frog skin epithelium. Acta Physiol. Scand. *63:*141–155.
Ussing, H. H. (1973): Effect of ADH on transport paths in toad skin. From: *Transport mechanisms in epithelia,* Alfred Benzon Symposium V, edited by H. H. Ussing and N. A. Thorn, Munksgaard, Copenhagen, pp. 11–19.
Ussing, H. H., Erlij, D., and Lassen, U. (1974): Transport pathways in biological membranes. Ann. Rev. Physiol. *36:*17–49.
Voûte, C. L., and Ussing, H. H. (1968): Some morphological aspects of active sodium transport. The epithelium of the frog skin. J. Cell. Biol. *36:*625–638.
Voûte, C. L., and Ussing, H. H. (1970): The morphological aspects of shunt-path in the epithelium of the frog skin (Rana temporaria). Exp. Cell Res. *61:*133–140.
Voûte, C. L., and Ussing, H. H. (1970): Quantitative relation between hydrostatic pres-

sure gradient, extracellular volume and active sodium transport in the epithelium of the frog skin (Rana temporaria). Exp. Cell Res. 62:375–383.

Voûte, C. L., Møllgaard, K., and Ussing, H. H. (1974): *in preparation*.

Zerahn, K. (1969): Nature and localization of the sodium pool during active transport in the isolated frog skin. Acta Physiol. Scand. 77:272–281.

DISCUSSION

ARMSTRONG was intrigued by the suggestion that the endoplasmic reticulum may be involved in the sodium transport. This may explain some of his own results in which he loaded muscle cells with sodium, then measured the total sodium versus the sodium activity in the cells. The increase of the activity following the loading was small whereas the absolute amount of sodium was considerably larger, indicating that part of the metal was sequestered and thus thermodynamically inactive. A similar phenomenon occurs when the gut mucosa is exposed to glucose: the entry of sodium into the cell increases but the amount of sodium in the cell is greater than the activity, as if some of the sodium would be in an inactive pool.

CURRAN asked about the possible role of the described phenomena in the transepithelial transport. In reply USSING has found it feasible to place the site of the pump on the surface of the cytoplasmic reticulum. This would mean that the transport takes place primarily into the interspaces as in the case of the known mechanism for the transport of fats and secretion of some hormones. One of the open questions in this regard concerns the presence of sodium-potassium-stimulated ATPase on the endoplasmic surface. Since it is rather difficult to separate the plasma membrane fraction from the endoplasmic membrane fraction, this question cannot be answered with certainty.

Intestinal Absorption and Malabsorption,
edited by T. Z. Csáky.
Raven Press, New York © 1975

Energetics of Intestinal Transport

D. S. Parsons

Department of Biochemistry, University of Oxford, Oxford, England

I. INTRODUCTION

The intestinal mucosa in its role as an organ of transport possesses specific energy requirements and exhibits a characteristic metabolism; but the intestine is also the portal of entry of energy foods into animals. Therefore, when discussing the energetics of intestinal transport, it should be borne in mind that a major role of the intestinal tract is to convert energy foods into fuels that are transported in the blood.

The absorption of energy foods by the intestinal mucosa is, generally speaking, inseparably associated with the processes of digestion. Whereas the energy foods are usually polymers, e.g., starch, dietary triglycerides, the fuels that are transported between the intestine and the various tissues are monomers and special reconstituted polymers, such as the chylomicrons. The energy foods that are consumed in the diet are not necessarily the fuels combusted in the tissues to provide the power necessary to drive cellular processes. This fact naturally raises questions as to the nature of the fuels combusted by the intestinal mucosa. For example, is only one type of fuel, e.g., glucose, combusted or can a variety of fuels be utilized? If so, is the pattern of fuels that is utilized constant or does the pattern vary with the nutritional state of the animal? What is the fuel of the fasting intestine?

Within the cell, the ultimate energy currency is the terminal pyrophosphate bond in ATP; this bond is generated by the combustion of tissue fuels, about 84 kJ (20 kcal) of energy food required per mole of ATP yielded by tissue metabolism. When considering the utilization of ATP by the intestinal mucosa from the point of view of the energetics of absorption, it is necessary to consider exactly where within the cells the ATP is utilized and for what purposes; such considerations naturally turn upon the way in which the epithelium is organized and upon the functioning of the various membranes upon which the epithelial transport activity depends.

Membrane transport driven directly by ATP hydrolysis may charge up a store of potential energy that can be used to power other membrane transport systems. *In vivo,* membrane transport and hence epithelial transport must to some extent be energized by the cardiovascular system, the functioning of which depends upon the hydrolysis of ATP.

II. GASTROINTESTINAL TRACT—THE PORTAL OF ENTRY OF ENERGY FOODS

In carnivorous and omnivorous animals, including human beings, and in the suckling young of ruminants and herbivores, the site of entry of energy into the body is, of course, the small intestine, especially the more oral sections, e.g., jejunum; in adult ruminants and in the herbivores, the major sites of entry of energy into the body are the rumen and the cecum and large intestine, respectively. It is in these organs of microbial and protozoal fermentation that the energy foods of the diet are converted into the volatile fatty acids that represent the form in which energy is assimilated by the intestinal tract for onward transfer in these species (see, for example, Annison and Lewis, 1959).

The magnitude of the total energy load translocated across the intestinal tract is of interest. In the case of an adult human, for example, with an intake of 10.5 MJ (2,500 kcal) per day, this will amount over a year to 3.8 GJ (9×10^6 kcal) moving across the mucosa of the small intestine. The metabolism of the intestinal mucosa will amount to about 24 liters of O_2 per day equivalent to 480 kJ per day, equivalent to about 175 MJ per year. It therefore appears that $\frac{1}{20}$ (5%) of the energy handled by the mucosa is sufficient to sustain the intermediary metabolism of the tissue.[1] In practice, when computing the expense of assimilation of energy foods by an animal, the energy cost of gastrointestinal mobility, of secretion of digestive juices, and of sustaining the mesenteric circulation should also be added to the cost of metabolism.

When considering the flow of the derivatives of energy foods through the mucosal epithelium, it is of interest to know to what extent this flow is separated from the path of fuel that is combusted by the tissue in the course of tissue metabolism. In other words are fuels derived from the diet contained in compartments that are distinct from those compartments containing the fuels required to sustain the tissue metabolism? In general terms it is not yet possible to answer this question adequately because the organization of the intestinal cells is not yet fully understood (see also Sec. VI).

III. CONTINUOUS ENERGY EXPENDITURE OF ANIMALS

In animal tissues, energy expenditure is a continuing process, although the rate may not necessarily be constant. The energy expended by tissues may be

---

[1] This estimate is calculated on the basis that the rate of respiration of the small intestinal mucosa is 10 µl per mg dry wt per hr (see, e.g., Bronk and Parsons, 1966), that the dry weight of the mucosa of the adult human intestine is 100 g, and that the heat equivalent of oxygen is 20 kJ per liter (Royal Society, 1971). The energy requirements of the fed and fasting intestine are assumed to be approximately equal. If the energy requirements are lower during fasting, then the "efficiency" of the processes of energy translation from the diet into the blood will be correspondingly increased.

divided into two components. These are (a) basal requirements and (b) additional requirements of work.

Basal requirements of energy are those necessary to support the organization and operation of fundamental cellular processes. These processes include the ionic pumping underlying the stabilization of cell volume, membrane synthesis, and protein synthesis, which itself may represent a major energy requirement in rapidly growing tissues, such as the small intestine. It appears that the processes of ion pumping may account for more than 50% of the basal energy requirements of some tissues and the turnover of tissue proteins may account for some 15% of basal requirements (Whittam, 1964; Milligan, 1971).

The work requirements of animals include, firstly, mechanical events such as those induced by the movements of skeletal (locomotory) muscles and the generation of tension in the walls of hollow viscera such as those enclosing the gastrointestinal tract; secondly, the energy expended in inducing and maintaining the bulk movement of water and solutes across epithelial layers such as the mucosae of the gastrointestinal tract, of the digestive glands, and of the renal tubule.

IV. EPISODIC ENERGY INPUT

A. Episodic Input

In contrast to the expenditure of energy, which in the tissues is a continuing process, the input of energy into the whole animal is discontinuous. Two important consequences arise from the fact that the input of energy foods is intermittent. Firstly, the processes of intestinal digestion and absorption are intermittent. For any particular region of the intestine, it is therefore possible to specify various metabolic "states," e.g., preabsorptive,

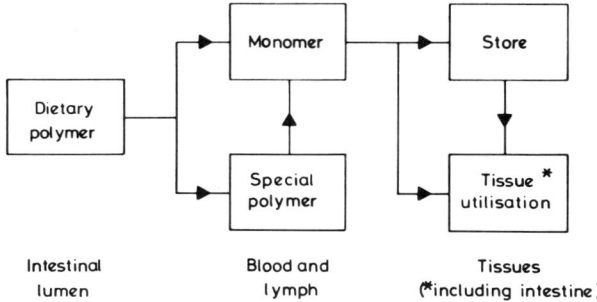

FIG. 1. Diagram showing flow of fuels in animals. Fuels such as glucose or precursors of fuel and amino acids are transported from the intestine as monomers. Lipids containing long-chain fatty acids are transported from the intestine in the form of special polymers, the chylomicra.

absorptive, and so on, each of which may have characteristic energy requirements that are met by the combustion of specific fuels. Secondly, because energy input is episodic even though the requirements of tissues are continuous, there must exist in animals (a) systems for storing and releasing fuels of metabolism, (b) transportation of fuel between the intestine and these stores, and (c) an additional transport of the fuel that is released from these stores to the tissues. These tissues include those of the intestine (Fig. 1).

B. Rate of Energy Input in Different Species

The length of time devoted to energy input varies remarkably among different species; some data on this subject are given in Table 1. Generally speaking, carnivorous animals occupy a very small fraction of their life ingesting energy foods (less than 1%). In contrast, herbivorous animals may spend up to 20% of their life eating. In human subjects the time spent eating is extremely variable and depends upon racial, social, and occupational factors; however the average adult appears to spend approximately 5% of his

TABLE 1. *Species variation in rates of consumption of energy foods*

	Bodyweight (kg)	Period of food intake (min/day)	Percent of day spent consuming food	Energy consumption (MJ/24 hr)	Rate of input of energy (kJ/kg bodyweight/min)
Carnivores					
Lion	250	17	1.1	38.6	9.2
Leopard	75	12	0.9	12.9	14.2
Fox	5.5	8	0.5	1.7	39.8
Omnivores					
Boar	200	40	2.8	20.3	2.6
Badger	9	31	2.1	5.4	19.7
Herbivores					
Zebra	340	405	28.1	14.6	0.13
Pony	125	414	28.9	15.2	0.29
Sheep	70	155	13.0	6.6	0.63
Hare	5	234	16.2	1.3	1.1
Human					
Professor resident in Oxford college	80	110	7.6	12.1	1.4
Male graduate student:					
Weekday	70	40	2.7	10.5	3.7
Sunday		80	5.6	11.3	2.0

Note that a fox ingests energy foods at nearly 30 times the rate of an Oxford professor who in turn consumes joules at about twice the rate of a sheep. Data from Parsons (1973). See also Fabry (1969).

time eating, although between different subjects, apparently members of the same occupational group, there appears to be much variation in how this time is allocated during the day.

The data presented in Table 1 raise the question of what is the duration of intestinal absorption in the various species. There is remarkably little data available on this subject for the length of time during which absorption is occuring may not be simply related to the length of the eating time; for example, the ingested food is stored and processed before being absorbed by the small intestine. Because of the sequential nature of the events that constitute digestion and absorption, at any particular time different parts of the intestinal tract may be in differing nutritional states. Thus consider a short segment of the mid small intestine of a fasting animal. When the animal starts to eat, the intestinal segment may be regarded to be a fasting intestine until gastric emptying begins. At this time the products of absorption of the energy foods begin to enter the blood as monomers and as special polymers (chylomicra). These will continue to be available in the blood to the segment of intestine until the intestinal contents descend to it, when any remaining energy foods become available from the lumen. After the intestinal contents have been propelled onward in the aboral direction so that the segment is again empty, fuel becomes again available to the segment only from the blood.

We may therefore conclude that both eating and absorption are episodic phenomena, although under natural conditions the actual duration of the absorptive phase of any particular portion of the intestine is not known; nevertheless, it must be determined by gastrointestinal motility. Metabolic fuel is continually available to a segment of the intestine from the blood in one form or another; metabolic fuel in the form of energy foods and their digestive products is available only intermittently at the luminal and basal surfaces of the absorbing epithelium.

C. Energy Stores

Because energy input is episodic, whereas the expenditure is continuous, systems for storing and transporting energy are present in animals. The nature of the fuels combusted in the tissues depends upon the nutritional status of the animal; in addition some tissues exhibit unique fuel requirements. For example, the central nervous system (CNS) has a continuing requirement for glucose and mammalian red cells depend upon the availability of glucose for maintaining a stable cell volume; the dependence of Na transport in rat jejunum on glucose will be discussed below (Sec. VI).

During the absorptive phase and the immediate postabsorptive phase nutrients are stored in the tissues and glucose is extensively utilized as fuel. In the later postabsorptive and fasting states amino acids are mobilized and utilized in the liver to supply the blood glucose by the glucogenic pathway. The ketones and fatty acids (NEFA) mobilized from the peripheral stores

TABLE 2. *Influence of nutritional status on rates of transport (mM per hour) of major fuels and their precursors in the circulation of human subjects*

	Time after feeding		
	12–18 hr	48–96 hr	4–6 weeks[a]
Fuel			
Glucose[b]	31	41	11
Free fatty acids	25	50	50
Ketone bodies	10	29	29
Precursors			
Amino acids	12.5	21	8
Glycerol	4	7	11

[a] Obese subjects.
[b] Neglects about 5 mM glucose per hour derived from Cori (lactate) cycle. Estimates based on data of Havel (1972).

become the predominant tissue fuels in late fasting and in starvation. In Table 2 data are given on the rates of transport of some major fuels and their precursors in the circulation of human subjects in different nutritional states. In herbivorous animals, including ruminants, the carbohydrates of the feed are converted by microbial (bacterial and protozoal) fermentations into volatile fatty acids (VFA) which form a major form of fuel transport in these species (see Sec. II *supra*). In the rabbit cecal mucosa there is evidence that VFA may be metabolized to ketone bodies which may then be utilized by other tissues (see Henning and Hird, 1927a,b).

V. ENERGY EXPENDITURE BY THE INTESTINE

As in the case of other tissues, the energy requirements of the intestine can be considered under two headings: basal requirements and work requirements.

The basal requirements for fuel by the fasting, nonabsorbing intestine represent the requirements necessary to provide the energy to sustain the ion pumping essential to maintain the individual epithelial cells at a stable volume and to support the synthesis of macromolecules in connection with the growth and differentiation of the cells of the epithelium. For the small intestine, as opposed to the colon, the rate of turnover of the epithelium is high.

The work requirements for energy by the absorbing epithelium are the requirements for solute and water translocation across the membranes of epithelium and the energy requirements for the delivery and the clearance of substrate to and from the epithelium.

Computations of the energy requirements for the overall processes of transport in complex organs such as the intestinal mucosa, the digestive glands, or the kidney are surely meaningless exercises until data are available on the magnitude and direction of the electrochemical gradient across each of the steps through which every substrate must move during the overall process of translocation. The sum of work done for each substrate that is moving must also be taken.

A major difficulty is the complex morphology of the absorbing epithelium, although, unlike frog skin, it is but one cell thick. For example, in the steady state of absorption under *in vivo* conditions the gradient of concentration or of voltage across the basal ("output") plasma membranes of the epithelial cells cannot be expected to be uniform. For example, according to current models of epithelial functioning (Diamond, 1971), the electrochemical potential gradient at the luminal end of the intercellular spaces (b-b) as shown in Fig. 2 cannot be expected to be the same as that obtaining at the vascular end of the space (c-c, Fig. 2) or indeed across the plasma membrane in the region of the basement membrane. This at once means that calculation of the thermodynamic efficiency of absorption is not a very profitable exercise.

Clearly, if the concentrations at the input and at the output are used as the basis of the calculations, a very misleading impression is obtained. As an ex-

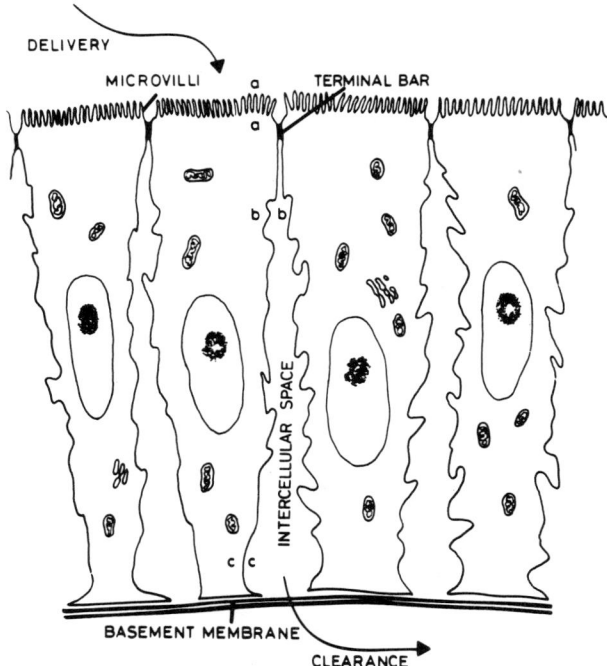

FIG. 2. Diagram showing interrelations of intestinal epithelial cells. a-a, Brush border membrane. b-b, Basolateral membrane at luminal end of the intercellular space. c-c, Basolateral membrane at vascular end of intercellular space. Substrate translocated through the epithelium is cleared from the intercellular space across the basement membrane into the mesenteric vascular system.

ample, suppose that in an experiment *in vivo* a segment of intestine is absorbing an isotonic solution of NaCl. Let the concentrations in the lumen be (mM/kg H_2O), Na, 120; Cl, 95; and of HCO_3, 25, and suppose the fluid secreted from the epithelium into the blood (10 mv + ve) is Na, 130; Cl, 100; and HCO_3, 30. Treating the organ as a "black box" (see Lifson and Visscher, 1944; Johnson and Knudsen, 1965) and considering only the Na, the epithelium seems to be doing very little work for an enormous expenditure of energy with a machine efficiency of possibly less than 1%. However, if one is prepared to take the lid off the "black box," it appears that the activity of the Na ions visible to probing electrodes is low within the cells, around 10 in the case of frog intestinal epithelial cells (Lee and Armstrong 1972).

Neglecting the complexities caused by the intercellular space mentioned above and of ergastoplasmic membranes, it would therefore seem that the Na is pumped out of the cell across the "output" faces up a concentration gradient of at least 10:130 and against a voltage of around 40 mV, a task which requires the expenditure of a significant amount of energy (see below, Sec. VII D). Of course at the input face, it appears that the Na leaks into the cell down a respectable electrochemical gradient, but at the moment it may not be justified to subtract the energy thus dissipated when considering the overall efficiency of Na pumping; but this is a nice point for it is conceivable that the influx of Na could be used to synthesize a fuel such as ATP that is immediately available to drive transport.

As regards the efficiency of Na pumping across individual membranes such as those of erythrocytes and nerve, this is thought to be reasonably high when considered in terms of the number of moles of Na pumped per mole of ATP cleaved, figures of the order of 60% being quoted (Whittam, 1964). The discrepancy between the apparent input-output efficiency of the whole system (approximately 1%) and the apparent efficiency of the individual steps within the system may be related to entropy effects in the sense that the pumping of Na and K seems to be associated with the establishment of local large electrochemical potential gradients that are dissipated when transport ceases or metabolism is arrested. But here we are entering deep theoretical waters which I would prefer to avoid.

Other aspects of energy utilization associated with absorption have already been referred to: I will not consider these in detail here, although they are of very great importance.

The delivery of foodstuffs along the interior of the intestinal canal to the site of absorption is clearly of importance. This transport may indeed be rate limiting to the transfer of substrate from the stomach into the blood. Such transport in the oral-aboral direction along the intestinal lumen is driven by the mechanical actions of the intestinal musculature; the immediate fuel for the contraction of this muscle is naturally ATP.

The clearance of absorbed substrates away from the intestinal epithelium is a function of the cardiovascular system. A continuing circulation of the blood in the minute vessels in the mesenteric vascular bed maintains a low concentration of substrate in the extracellular fluids of the epithelium, including presumably that in intercellular spaces; such effects are ultimately achieved by the energy expended by the heart in maintaining the circulation. In this instance, the immediate source of fuel is again ATP. In the absence of the vascular circulation the absorbed substrate often appears to be concentrated in the tissue wall; values of the ratio of concentration of the substrate in the tissue to that in the medium are frequently greater than one in experiments based on the classical techniques for studying absorption *in vitro* (see, for example, Fisher and Parsons, 1953a,b). From our own work, it appears that during absorption with the circulation intact, accumulation of substrate occurs to a much lesser extent. This could imply a marked difference in the energy cost, in terms of tissue metabolism, of absorption between *in vivo* and *in vitro* conditions (see Sec. VIII).

TABLE 3. *Net yield of high-energy phosphate as ATP from different sources*

Substrate	Moles ATP per mole substrate metabolized
Glucose (i) aerobic	38
(ii) anaerobic	3
Acetoacetic acid	22
Propionate	18
Butyrate	27
Stearic acid	146
100 g protein	23

The energy requirements of transport will be discussed from two points of view: first, the nature of the fuels combusted by the intestine and then the consequences of, as a result of membrane transport driven by ATP hydrolysis, a store of electrochemical potential energy being generated across a membrane and this energy being used to power other transport systems. For a comparison of the different fuels, the yield of ATP per mole of substrate metabolized is given in Table 3.

VI. METABOLIC FUELS OF THE INTESTINE

From what has been said earlier, it is clear that the metabolic fuel of the intestine is likely to vary according to whether the intestine is in the absorbing state or whether it is fasted and, if so, for how long.

Considering first the case of the absorbing intestine, there seem to be marked differences in the nature of the fuel required to sustain salt absorption in different species and again in different parts of the intestinal tract.

In the rat, for example, glucose has a marked stimulatory effect on fluid transport, largely, but perhaps not entirely due to a stimulation of NaCl transport. Nearly 25 years ago when Fisher and I demonstrated the so-called "active transport" of glucose and galactose by rat intestine *in vitro,* we also noticed that fluid transport occurred at a high rate when glucose was present in the lumen but only at a much lower rate in the presence of galactose (see Fisher and Parsons, 1953b, p. 227). Later Lifson and I showed it was possible to induce fluid transport with glucose supplied from the serosal side only (Lifson and Parsons, 1957). However, in order to do this, the glucose had to be present in very high concentrations (150mM).

TABLE 4. *Capacity of different substrates and inhibitors to sustain fluid absorption by rat intestine in vitro*

Substrate	Relative rates of fluid absorption		
	Jejunum	Ileum	Colon
None	27 ± 3	69 ± 6	50 ± 6
Glucose	100 ± 6	100 ± 6	100 ± 6
Anoxia + glucose	34 ± 4	2 ± 2	4 ± 3
Mannose	—	—	91 ± 7
Fructose	38(2)	—	71 ± 15
Pyruvate	3(3)	60 ± 5	72 ± 13
Acetate	0(2)	—	90 ± 7
Butyrate	2(2)	—	92 ± 9
Succinate	—	—	52 ± 7
Citrate	20 ± 2	75 ± 10	40 ± 7
Fluoroacetate + glucose	87 ± 12	53 ± 13	26 ± 5

Values are of means ± SE of the rate of fluid absorption relative to that with glucose = 100. Unless indicated in parentheses, each value is based on the mean of 4 to 25 observations. Substrate concentrations in range 10 to 28 mM. Data of Parsons (1967).

The effects of various substrates on fluid transport in different regions of the rat intestine are shown in Table 4.

It is found, in practice, that the rates of fluid transport in the absence of added substrate vary according to the treatment of the animals before the experiment, e.g., previously well-fed animals have appreciable rates of fluid transport; thus there seems to be some evidence that the tissue is able to draw upon endogenous fuel stores.

In the frog intestine we find that tissue from well-nourished animals can be sustained in good physiological condition for periods of up to more than 3 hr *in vitro* with no added substrate; however, butyrate is an excellent substrate for these animals.

In the chick intestine *in vitro* my colleague Karrer (1968) has shown that in the absence of exogenous substrate, glucose is secreted into the serosal fluid at rates that are relatively high in the intestine from fed birds and low in that from fasted birds. He also finds that fructose supports fluid absorption by chick intestine *in vitro*. Incidentally, in the chicken intestine it seems that fructose uptake from the lumen is markedly reduced when choline is substituted for the Na in the lumen and that the fructose is not converted to glucose but gives rise to a secretion of lactate in the serosal fluid (see Table 5).

The question of aerobic glycolysis by the intestine is of interest. It has been known for a long time that under aerobic conditions rat intestine produces lactate *in vitro;* indeed, in the early experiments of Fisher and Parsons it was found that a substantial amount of glucose absorbed from the mucosal fluid did not appear in the serosal fluid and the discrepancy was not accounted for by the large amounts of glucose which accumulated in the wall under *in vitro* conditions (see, e.g., Fisher and Parsons, 1953a). Wilson later found that the lactate formed would largely account for the glucose that disappeared (see, e.g., Wilson, 1956).

We have recently reinvestigated this question using rat jejunum *in vitro* which is perfused through the mesenteric vascular bed with an artificial blood containing corpuscles. Such a preparation, foreshadowed by Fisher and Parsons (1953b, p. 231), is technically very much more difficult to maintain than a similar sort of preparation of Anuran intestine such as that described by Parsons and Prichard (1968) and by Boyd, Cheeseman, and Parsons (1973). Nevertheless Peter Hanson in my laboratory has succeeded in maintaining the vascular circulation of the jejunum of the rat for almost 2 hr. His findings with respect to lactate formation are shown in Table 6. The findings clearly show that when glucose is presented to the tissue via the mesenteric circulation there is a dramatic fall both in the rate of utilization of glucose and also in the fraction of the metabolized glucose that is converted to lactate. On the other hand, there is undoubtedly a continuing formation of lactate under conditions of aerobic perfusion and the absolute amount of glucose that is converted to other metabolites than lactate is relatively unchanged.

The fact that the rate of glucose utilization and of lactate production *in vitro* is high in the absence of vascular perfusion need not mean that the recirculated preparation is inadequately oxygenated, although it is one explanation already mentioned. As in the absence of a vascular circulation, glucose accumulates in the intestinal wall, and it may prove that a local accumulation stimulates glucose utilization and lactate production. The effects on utilization and lactate production of changing the concentrations of glucose into the arterial inflow to the perfused preparation are clearly of interest here.

It therefore appears from the data presently available that very little is known about the rates of utilization of the various physiological fuels that are available to the intestine from the blood or from the luminal contents.

It appears that glucose, mannose (see Duerdoth, Newey, Sandford, and Smyth, 1965), fructose (in the chick), and substrates such as pyruvate and butyrate can stimulate fluid and Na transport when present in the intestinal lumen and that rat jejunum *in vitro* seems to depend upon glucose as a fuel

TABLE 5. *The rate of secretion of fluid, fructose, lactate, and glucose into serosal fluids by chick jejunum recirculated in vitro at different grades of fasting*

	Fasting Time					
	0		24 hr		48 hr	
	No substrate	+ fructose	No substrate	+ fructose	No substrate	+ fructose
Water	4.4 ± 0.4 (6)	10.5 ± 0.8 (6)	2.9 ± 0.3 (5)	11.2 ± 0.5 (6)	2.3 ± 0.3 (6)	11.5 ± 0.5 (6)
Fructose	—	83.4 ± 7.1 (6)	—	60.6 ± 1.9 (6)	—	70.4 ± 8.2 (6)
Lactate	112 ± 8 (6)	315 ± 30 (6)	46.3 ± 4.7 (5)	409 ± 24 (6)	38.9 ± 5.4 (5)	424 ± 26 (6)
Glucose	41 ± 9 (6)	32.7 ± 5.4 (6)	2.0 ± 0.2 (5)	0.8 ± 0.3 (6)	1.5 ± 0.6 (6)	1.2 ± 0.3 (6)

The luminal fluid was Krebs-Ringer bicarbonate saline containing 0.5 g fructose 100 ml. Duration of experiment: 1 hr (data of Karrer, 1968). Values are of means ± SE of mean (no. of observations). Units are ml or μM per hr per g fat-free dry weight of whole wall.

TABLE 6. *Glucose utilization and lactate production by rat jejunum in vitro*

Preparation	Glucose utilization (μmoles)	Lactate production (μmoles)	Glucose conversion to metabolites other than lactate (μmoles)	Proportion of metabolized glucose converted to lactate (%)
Recirculated	736 ± 50	1,288 ± 115	92 ± 18	87 ± 3
Vascular perfused	222 ± 20	144 ± 28	150 ± 28	34 ± 9

Data from four animals measured over 1 hr, means ± SE of mean, units: μmoles g dry weight^{-1} hr^{-1}. In the recirculated preparation the arrangement is similar to that of Fisher and Parsons (1953a, b) but a single medium of Krebs-Ringer-bicarbonate containing 10 mM glucose is circulated through the lumen and over the serosal surface of the segment at 35 ml min^{-1}. In the perfused preparation the vascular perfusate (Krebs-Ringer-bicarbonate, 40% bovine erythrocytes and 3% bovine serum albumin with 10mM glucose) is recirculated at 1.5 ml min^{-1}. The lumen fluid (Krebs-Ringer-bicarbonate, no added glucose) is recirculated at 2 ml min^{-1}. All media 37° C and gassed with 95% O_2 and 5% CO_2. Unpublished data of P. J. Hanson.

to support fluid absorption. There appears no information on the utilization of long chain fatty acids by the intestine.

With substrate present in the lumen, the intestine is absorbing, i.e., is "fed." What are the fuels of the fasted intestine? Again little is known about this, although it appears that at least the initial rate of glucose utilization *in vitro* by intestine from fasted rats is considerably less than for fed rats (see Shakespeare, Srivastava, and Hübscher, 1969). On the principle that during fasting ketone bodies and fatty acids become increasingly important as tissue fuel, the metabolism of these substrates by the intestinal mucosa appears to merit investigation.

In this connection, what are the functions of the fasting intestine? Does it continue to function as an endocrine organ? Does it secrete? The guinea pig small intestine appears to go through phases of secretion of fluid that may be related to the maintenance of the fluidity of contents of the cecum and large intestine of this herbivore.

A question that is related to the nature of fuels combusted by the absorbing intestine is whether a potential fuel that is being *absorbed* (e.g., glucose) is confined to a pool inside the cells that is separate from that of the glucose that is *metabolized*. Many current models of the sugar-absorbing intestinal mucosal cell assume that absorbed substrate is uniformly distributed throughout the cell; but this may not be so. Thus, intestinal mucosal cells contain many organelles that may not all be equally penetrated by, e.g., glucose. This question is one of the points that we are endeavoring to investigate with our preparations of perfused intestine from the rat and frog.

VII. IMMEDIATE ENERGY SOURCES

A. Direct Utilization of ATP

The combustion of fuels in the course of intermediate metabolism yields ATP which is, of course, the prime immediate source of energy (see Table 3). Where in the absorbing cells is this ATP used for the purposes of membrane transport? The answer, so far as the transport of Na and K is concerned, is unquestionably in the basolateral plasma membrane. This has been particularly well demonstrated by the experiments of Fujita, Ohta, Kawai, Matsui, and Nakao (1972) and others (see Douglas, Kerley, and Isselbacher 1972). This conclusion fits in well with other evidence that supports what can be regarded as the classical (Ussing) model for Na pumping across epithelia. But are there other ATP-consuming systems in the plasma membranes of the intestinal mucosal cells, and in particular are such systems present in the brush border membranes? An unambiguous answer to this question requires the use of brush border membranes uncontaminated by residual basolateral membranes and also by the core material of the microvilli which may be contractile protein (see Parsons and Boyd, 1972). At present there is some evidence for the presence of a Ca^{2+}-activated ATPase in the microvillus membrane (Forstner, Sabesin, and Isselbacher, 1968); the matter is clearly of importance and will doubtlessly be clarified.

Finally, as anyone who has worked with Na-K activated ATPases knows, there is in every preparation, residual Mg-dependent ATPase activity; this is certainly true of purified brush border membranes, but whether such activity represents a facet of some membrane-transporting system or is a manifestation of some nonspecific activity is presently not clear. The complete characterization of systems for the hydrolysis of ATP by "pure" plasma membranes, especially brush border membranes, evidently merits more investigation.

B. Indirect Utilization of ATP

It has already been pointed out that membrane transport driven directly by ATP hydrolysis may charge up a store of electrochemical potential energy, e.g., as a gradient of concentration across a membrane; the discharge of this store may then be used to power other membrane transport systems. A notable feature of this concept is that ATP hydrolysis need not occur at every cellular location where an energy-consuming membrane transport process is operating. The potential energy of the store, released as downhill flux of stored substrate across a membrane, could, in theory, be captured by some other membrane transport system or be used to synthesize ATP. Certainly in red cell membranes, an inward flux of Na has been shown to yield ATP synthesis (see Whittam and Wheeler, 1970). The role of Na ions, in particular, as such a store has been the subject of much speculation and experimentation, and the field has been extensively reviewed (see, for example, Schultz and Curran, 1970).

C. Some History

I wish to draw attention to the work of that pioneer experimenter in the field of intestinal absorption, E. Waymouth Reid (see, for example, Reid, 1900; Cathcart and Garry, 1948; Parsons, 1968). This distinguished experimenter demonstrated very clearly the importance of NaCl on absorption. In very carefully controlled experiments Reid (1902) showed that in the dog

TABLE 7. Data of E. Waymouth Reid, first published in 1902, showing stimulating effects of NaCl on glucose absorption

	Fluid absorption (ml)	Glucose absorption (mg)
NaCl present	13.8 ± 1.3	237 ± 21
NaCl absent	17.5 ± 1.0	207 ± 20
Difference	−3.7 ± 0.8[b]	30 ± 12[a]

[a] $p < 0.05$.
[b] $p = 0.001$.

Note that the addition of salt to intestinal contents reduces the net absorption of fluid. NaCl concentration, 0.4 or 0.6 g/100 ml. Initial concentration of glucose, 2 g/100 ml. Dog intestine. Paired experiments on each of 11 jejunal and ileal segments of 50 cm. Absorption measured over 15 min. Values are of means ± SE of mean.

intestine the absorption of glucose from a solution containing 2 g/100 ml initially was stimulated by the addition of 0.2 or 0.6 g/100 ml NaCl. A solution containing 0.2 g/100 ml glucose is hypotonic and fluid absorption naturally occurs more rapidly from it than when salt is added, yet in spite of this the glucose is absorbed more rapidly with salt present (Table 7). Reid attributed his findings to the fact that NaCl exerted its effect "by specific cell action, possibly involving chemical excitation" which seems to be as clear a statement as any that could be made today to explain the mode of action of Na. The experiments of Reid also show a feature that was not described again for 50 years, namely the existence of a linear relationship between the rate of fluid transport and the rate of glucose absorption from the intestinal tract (Fig. 3) (see Fullerton and Parsons, 1956).

D. Possible Candidates for Ion Gradients As Driving Force for Transmembrane Fluxes

In attempting to assess the maximum potential energy that could be realized from a store having the form of a gradient of electrochemical potential of an

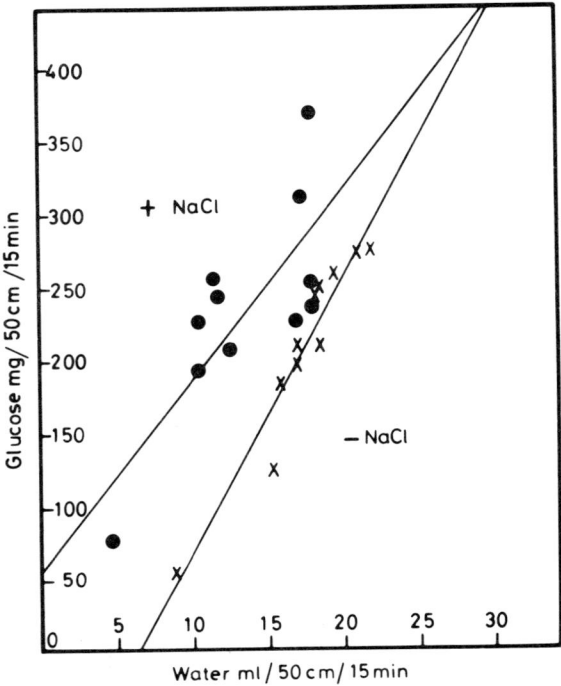

FIG. 3. Data of E. Waymouth Reid (1902) showing relationships between water and glucose absorption in the dog intestine. Initial glucose concentration 2 g/100 ml. See also Table 7. In the absence of NaCl: Glucose absorbed (mg) = 18.52 ± 2.08 (water absorbed ml) − 116 ± 37 (11). For significance of slope, p is less than 0.0001; for intercept, p = 0.01. Mean apparent concentration of glucose in exit stream, 1.85 ± 0.21 g/100 ml. In the presence of NaCl: Glucose absorbed (mg) = 12.92 ± 3.37 (water absorbed, ml) + 58.5 ± 48.6 (11). For significance of slope, p is less than 0.01; intercept is not significantly different from zero. Mean apparent concentration of glucose in exit stream, 1.29 ± 0.34 g/100 ml.

ionic species across a membrane, account must be taken of the membrane potential in the steady state, as well as the gradient of ionic activities. A neglect of this in the past has caused confusion. However, there are formidable technical difficulties in estimating the relevant values of the electromotive force (emf), not the least of which in epithelia, such as the intestine, follows from the presence of shunt paths of low resistance in the direction normal to the plane of the epithelium (Schultz, 1973). Another complication is that the individual cells of the epithelium may be connected by electrical pathways of low resistance.

Lee and Armstrong (1972) and Armstrong, Byrd, and Hamang (1973) have investigated the case for Na as a store of potential energy to drive monosaccharide fluxes in anuran small intestine.

I would like to draw attention to the possibility of other ions, in addition to Na, as candidates for transmembrane energy stores that might be used

TABLE 8. Possible candidates for supply of energy via downhill ionic gradients

Ion	Molar concentrations		Ratio of concentrations	Voltage gradient favorable?	Chemical gradient (a)	Maximum potential energy (J mole^{-1})	
	outside	inside				Electrochemical gradient (b)	Relative to Na (c)
Na$^+$	1.5×10^{-1}	10^{-2}	15	yes	7,000	10,800	100
K$^+$	5×10^{-3}	1.5×10^{-1}	30	no	8,800	4,900	45
H$^+$	4×10^{-8}	4×10^{-7}	10	no	5,900	2,100	19
H$^+$	4×10^{-8}	4×10^{-9}	10	yes	5,900	9,800	91
Ca^{2+}	1×10^{-3}	10^{-7}	10^4	yes, yes	23,700	31,500	292
Cl$^-$	10^{-1}	10^{-2}	10	no	5,900	2,100	19

Energy released (or absorbed) at 37° by ions that are of physiological significance and are moving through a boundary across which differences of concentration and voltage exist. In column (a) is given the maximum theoretical potential energy dissipated (or absorbed) by the ion moving down (or up) the concentration gradient specified. The energy values given in column (b) are derived on the supposition that in the steady state of flux there exists a membrane potential, 40 mV, interior negative. In column (c) the data in column (b) are given relative to Na = 100.

Note that if the fractional efficiency of the pump is e_1, ($e_1 < 1$), then the real metabolic cost of solute pumping, e.g., of extruding Na ions, is C/e where C is the theoretical requirement. Similarly, the maximum energy that could be extracted by a mechanism coupled to the downhill fluxes is C · e_2, where e_2 is the fractional efficiency of the coupling mechanism. ($e_2 < 1$). Thus suppose that to pump a certain quantity of an ion out of a cell 100 J are required. Then with $e_1 = 0.66$, 150 J will have to be supplied to the pump. In the steady state the ion will be leaking back into the cell at the same rate that it is pumped out. With $e_2 = 0.3$, 30 J will be captured so that the real cost of maintaining the steady state will be 150−30 = 120 Js.

to power transmembrane fluxes. Some suggestions are shown in Table 8, the calculations being based on the assumptions that (a) the relevant membrane potential is 40 mV (inside -ve) (Lee and Armstrong, 1972) and (b) inside the cell, the ion is uniformly distributed within a well-stirred compartment (see also Sec. V and Fig. 2). The data in Table 8 can be regarded as a calculation of the energy that would have to be expended to pump 1 mole of the ion out of (or into) the cell. Thus, although the segregation of Ca, for example, might be used as a subtantial store of potential energy, it would be correspondingly expensive to charge up such a store.

The basis of speculation of this sort is to promote experimentation and the acquisition of new facts and it is to be hoped that someone will look for alterations in the fluxes of, for example, Ca and/or protons during the transport of amino acids and monosaccharides. It must also be borne in mind that energy from one store might be drawn upon to charge up another store, e.g., an influx of Na ("downhill") may charge up a "store" of Ca ions (out of the cell and "uphill"), as seems to occur in some tissues (see Whittam and Wheeler, 1970).

In such systems the effects of the efficiency of the coupling of energy transduction is of great importance. Thus, suppose the efficiency of Na transport driven by ATP hydrolysis is 50%, then, if the theoretical energy required to pump Na out of some compartment is 100 J, ATP equivalent to 200 J will have to be hydrolyzed. If, with Na leaking back into the cell in the steady state, there is some form of energy transduction (e.g., coupling to another flux) with an efficiency of, say, 50%, then of the 100 J dissipated by the Na entering at this step, 50 could be captured for useful work. The net work done is then $100 + 50 = 150$ J at a cost very close to 200 J of ATP hydrolyzed, i.e., with an apparent machine efficiency of around 75% (see also Table 8).

In conclusion, the fact has to be pointed out that electrochemical potential gradients of ions, e.g., Na, may be shown to exist across membranes. Although this is a necessary condition, it is not sufficient to prove that, e.g., sugar pumping depends upon a direct interaction of Na with the sugar transport system. The effects may be secondary to some other action of Na, e.g., an action inside the cellular compartment into which sugar transport is occurring, or to an action upon the movement of some other substance upon which movement the sugar movement itself primarily depends.

E. Energy of Hydrolysis of Energetic Foodstuffs

It has been pointed out elsewhere that although the standard free energy of hydrolysis of maltose or lactose is low, that of sucrose and of small peptides is relatively high (Parsons, 1972). Thus there may be an energetic advantage in assimilating small peptides and also sucrose directly into the brush border membrane. The possibility exists that the free energy of hydrolysis of such oligomers, if captured by some mechanism, could be used for the forward propulsion of the constituent monomers and that the oligopeptidases and the sucrose present in brush border membranes may have some role in transport.

VIII. ENERGETICS OF EXIT FROM THE MUCOSAL EPITHELIUM

A. Influence of Circulation

When considering the energetics of absorption, attention is usually devoted entirely to the processes discussed in the preceding sections, namely, the exergonic and endergonic chemical processes occurring within the mucosal cells and those associated with metabolism and with membrane function. It has already been mentioned that *in vivo* the potential energy of the blood perfusing the mesenteric microcirculation is continually used as a source of power to assist epithelial transport (Sec. V). The source of the energy sustaining the circulation derives from the combustion of fuel in the cardiac muscle fibers.

Consider now the effects upon epithelial transport of a flow of fluid in the mesenteric vascular bed. In the presence of an adequate mesenteric vascular perfusion, products of absorption do not significantly accumulate in the extracellular tissue fluid present in the intercellular spaces and in the submucosal tissue adjacent to the mucosal cells, i.e., the local extracellular accumulation of substrate is kept to a minimum. In contrast, when intestinal absorption of amino acids and of sugars is studied using classical *in vitro* preparations, i.e., with no mesenteric perfusion, substrate accumulation within the wall may occur to a marked extent (see Fisher and Parsons, 1963a,b; Agar, Hird, and Sidhu, 1954, for early observations on this extensively investigated subject).

One result of such an accumulation is that the extracellular environment of the intestinal mucosal cells in the tissue wall is determined almost entirely by the activities of the absorbing cells and scarcely at all by the nature of the medium bathing the serosal surface of the isolated segments (see Lifson and Parsons, 1957).

B. Methods

In an attempt to throw some light on the properties of the processes underlying the exit of monosaccharides and amino acids from the mucosal epithelium of the small intestine, my colleagues and I have recently investigated absorption of these substances in a development of an earlier preparation for the vascular perfusion of the mesenteric bed of the anuran intestine (Parsons and Prichard, 1968). The chief modification to the original preparation is the continual collection and sampling of the portal venous effluent; over 90%, usually more than 96%, of the arterial inflow was recovered.

An outline of the procedure used is given by Boyd, Cheeseman, and Parsons (1973); it should be noted that the separate circulations through the intestinal lumen and the vascular bed pass only once through the tissue, i.e., there is no recirculation.

Instead of undertaking experiments in which transport rates are measured in steady-state conditions, we have used what is essentially a perturbation technique. In this the mucosal epithelium is loaded up, usually from the lumen with an appropriate substrate, e.g., monosaccharide or amino acid. The lumen fluid is rapidly replaced by substrate-free Ringers solution and the appearance of the substrate from the tissue (unloading) is monitored in both the lumen and vascular circuits (see Fig. 4). We have used amino acids and

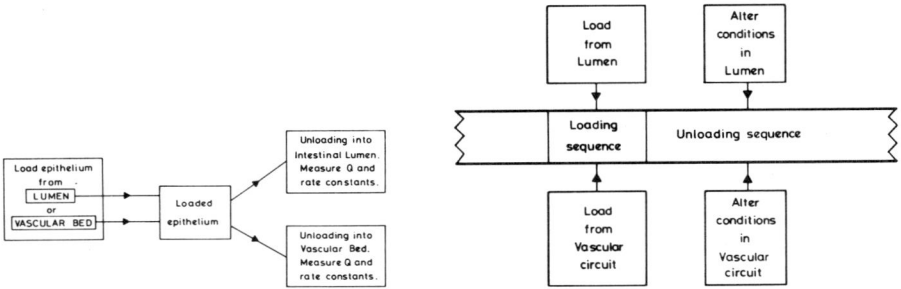

FIG. 4. Procedure for investigating efflux of previously absorbed substrate from intestinal mucosal epithelium using a preparation perfused *in vitro* through the mesenteric vascular bed. (Left) General procedure. (Right) Diagram showing that the epithelium may be loaded with substrate from either the vascular or the luminal side and that during the unloading sequence, the effects of changing the conditions in either the lumen or in the circuits may be followed.

hexoses as substrates, both unlabeled and labeled with tracer. With this approach it is found that the substrate is discharged from the epithelium into both the lumen and the vascular circulation and that, by making additions to or by changing the composition of the appropriate fluid, it proves possible to investigate the factors that influence the unloading into either circuit (Fig. 4 right).

C. Unloading into the Vascular Circulation

An interesting feature of the appearance of substrate in the vascular circulation when the tissue is unloading is that the quantity appearing at any time is determined by a double exponential function (Fig. 5). Thus if Q is the total quantity of substrate that has appeared in the vascular circulation after time then

$$Q = A(1 - \exp - k_1 t) + B(1 - \exp - k_2 t)$$

where A and B are constants and k_1 and k_2 rate constants with dimensions of time $^{-1}$.

The physical meaning of this sort of relationship is really quite simple; it means that substrate appearing in the vascular effluent appears to be derived from two pools, each with different capacities and drained at different rates.

Our data indicate that one pool (pool A) is larger and drains at a faster rate, the other (pool B) is smaller and drains at a slower rate. For 3-O

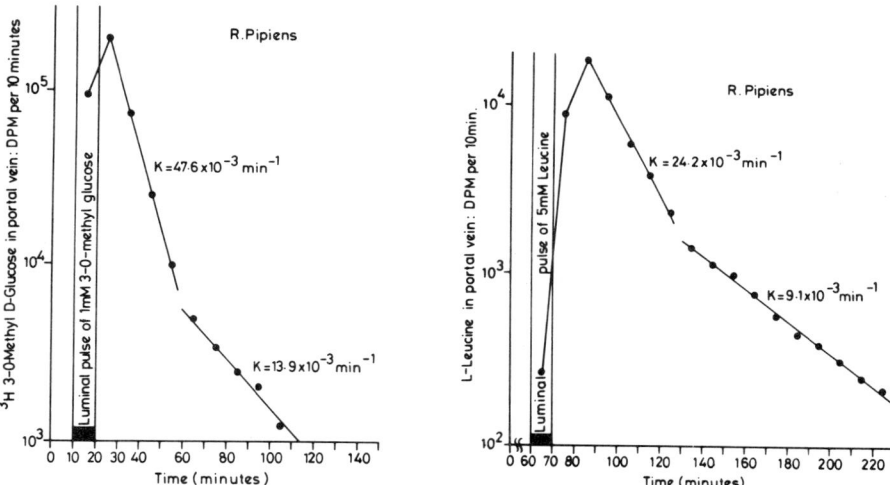

FIG. 5. The form of the "washout" (unloading) of substrate into the vascular effluent in portal vein of R. pipiens. Note logarithmic scale of ordinate and "fast" and "slow" rate constants. (Left) Substrate is ^{3}H-3-O-methyl-D-glucose. (Right) Substrate is ^{14}C-L-leucine. In this experiment the subsequent use of "cold" (i.e., unlabeled) L-leucine yielded identical values for the rate constants, the amino acid being measured by an enzymic method. (Unpublished data of C. A. R. Boyd.)

methyl glucose (3-O-MeG), pool A accounts for about 85% of the substrate that appears on the vascular effluent and pool B for the remaining 15%. The amino acids leucine and α-aminoisobutyric acid behave in a similar way in that the appearance in the vascular fluid is determined by discharge from two pools. For the very diffusible substance urea, however, there may be only one pool, i.e., if there is a second pool, it is very small.

An interesting feature of the unloading process is that the rate of vascular perfusion determines the value of the fast rate constant, k_1 (Fig. 6). It is also found that the fraction of pool B that is drained in unit time into the vascular bed (k_2) is unaffected by the flow rate. It also seems that at zero rates of vascular perfusion, the two rate constants (k_1 and k_2) become identical (Fig. 6); this means that under classical *in vitro* conditions, i.e., no vascular

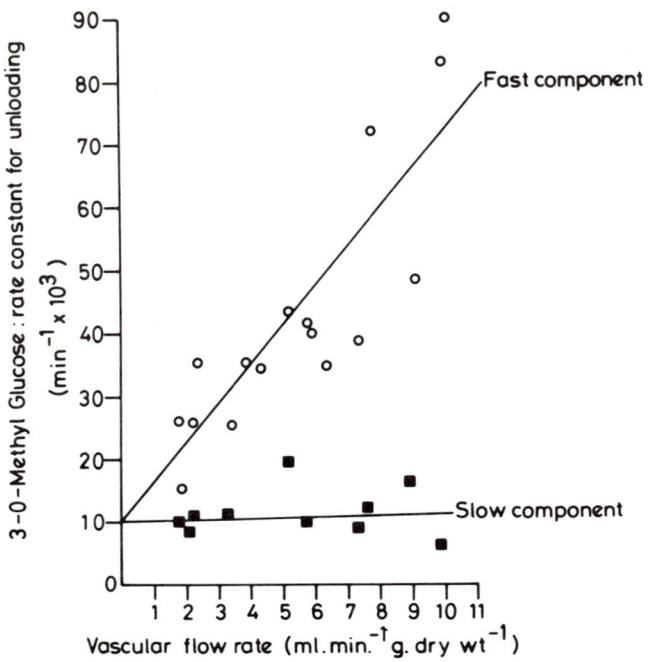

FIG. 6. The effects of the rate of perfusion of the mesenteric vascular bed upon the magnitude of the rate constants of the efflux into the circulation of previously absorbed 3-O-methyl-D-glucose. See text for further details. Values of k_1 are corrected. (Unpublished data of C. A. R. Boyd.)

perfusion, $Q = (A + B) \exp - k_2 t$, and the substrate appears to be derived from a single pool.

What other factors in addition to the extent of vascular perfusion affect the unloading from the tissue? In our experiments butyrate is provided as substrate in the vascular circulation. The addition of glucose to the vascular infusate, butyrate also being present, has interesting effects on the unloading of 3-O-MeG into the vascular effluent. At a concentration of 10 mM in the arterial inflow, glucose has two effects, which are both exerted on pool A. It increases the rate at which the pool drains, i.e., k_1 is increased but also the total quantity of 3-O-MeG that appears in the vascular effluent is also increased (Fig. 7). In other words, with glucose present in the vascular fluid, pool A is apparently made larger.

The simplest explanation of the increase in rate of clearance from the tissue into the vascular effluent is that exit of 3-O-MeGl from the tissue is stimulated by glucose; this could follow either because of a countertransport effect or because exit of 3-O-MeG is energized by some metabolic process for which glucose is a substrate.

We have not at present attempted to distinguish between these possibilities

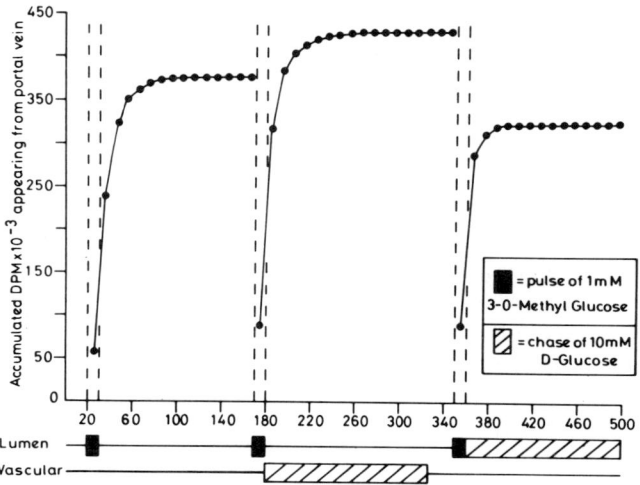

FIG. 7. Effects of glucose on the efflux into the mesenteric circulation of ^{3}H-3-O-methyl glucose previously absorbed from the lumen. Note that, compared with the control, glucose present in the vascular system stimulates the unloading of the substrate, but when glucose is present in the lumen, less substrate is unloaded into the circulation. (Unpublished data of C. A. R. Boyd.)

but provisionally prefer the counterexchange hypothesis on the grounds that metabolizable substrate is already provided in the form of butyrate. It is to be noted that either possibility has implications with respect to energy exchanges during the exit of 3-O-MeG from the mucosa into the blood.

The quantity of substrate (3-O-MeG) loaded up into the tissue ("absorbed") is always the same; the apparently paradoxical observation that the quantity discharged from the epithelium into the vascular system is greater with glucose present has the implication that the size of the pool of substrate is greater with glucose present in the vascular circulation. It has to be remembered that in fact the epithelium discharges substrate during the unloading phase into the lumen (where it can be reabsorbed) as well as into the vascular bed (Sec. VIIID); indeed substrate molecules absorbed into the epithelial cells at the proximal end of the segment could pass many times to and fro between the cells and the luminal contents before finally emerging either in the fluid flowing from the lumen or from the portal vein. With glucose present in the vascular inflow the exit of 3-O-MeG into the lumen fluids is reduced. Thus it seems that glucose enters the tissue from the circulation and either reduces backflux of substrate (3-O-MeG) from the tissue into the lumen or stimulates reuptake, thereby leaving more available to be discharged into the circulation. This explanation implies that intracellular glucose and 3-O-MeG share a common transport system for transport between the lumen and cells.

It is well known that phloridzin is remarkably effective in inhibiting the entry of certain hexoses from the intestinal lumen into epithelium. When present in the fluid perfused through the mesenteric vascular bed, phloridzin has no effect on the exit of 3-O-MeG; on the other hand, the aglycone, phloretin, when present in the arterial inflow at concentrations of 10^{-4} M has the effect of reducing the rate constant of exit, k_1.

Our findings in these experiments indicate that the exit of 3-O-MeG into the vascular system from the intestinal wall occurs from two compartments; these we tentatively identify as (a) the epithelium and the mucosal extracellular fluid in the intestinal lumen, and (b) the remaining tissue fluid of the intestinal wall. The rate of exit from the first compartment is markedly influenced by the rate of vascular perfusion of the tissue; it is stimulated by the presence of glucose in the vascular inflow and the rate of exit is somewhat inhibited by phloretin. The exit of about 15% of the absorbed substrate occurs into the vascular system from the second compartment and this exit is not flow limited.

Diffusion in a restricted or porous medium could be rate limiting to this component of the exit process. From a knowledge of the rate constant, it is possible to make an estimate of the apparent diffusion coefficient and it appears that the effective diffusion coefficient is considerably less than 1% of that in free solution.

D. Unloading into the Luminal Fluid

After the tissue has been loaded with substrate, the fluid pumped through the lumen is changed to one that is substrate free. Examination of this fluid after it has passed through the preparation during the subsequent period of unloading reveals that the total quantity of substrate in the effluent from the lumen is accountable in terms of three components. One, very rapidly exhausted, appears to represent unabsorbed substrate initially present in the fluid flowing freely through the lumen. The second, which clears more slowly, appears to represent the substrate present in a phase of the extracellular space that is relatively small and from which movement is more restricted. This might represent an unstirred layer of fluid for example. The third phase appears to represent an exit from the tissue itself. The addition of glucose to the fluid present in the intestinal lumen during the phase of unloading stimulates the efflux back into the lumen of previously absorbed substrate. This effect is entirely analogous to the effect produced by the presence of glucose in the vascular inflow, where the efflux of previously loaded substrate was also stimulated, in this case, into the circulation.

The effects of the presence of phloridzin in the intestinal luminal contents during the unloading phase of 3-O-MeG are interesting. The gross effect is to increase the amount of previously absorbed substrate that appears in the fluid flowing from the lumen, with a corresponding reduction in that appearing in the vascular outflow. But this effect is largely due to the inhibitory effects of phloridzin on absorption of residual 3-O-MeG present in the restricted extracellular compartment in the lumen. In the absence of phloridzin it is absorption from this phase that contributes to the pool that is unloaded into the circulation. In the presence of phloridzin in the lumen more substrate remains behind in this phase to be washed out from the lumen. With regard to the third phase of washout of substrate into the lumen, this is inhibited by phloridzin. In other words, it seems that the exit of previously absorbed 3-O-MeG across the brush border into the lumen occurs by some process that is blocked by phloridzin when this is present in the lumen. We have already concluded that movement of 3-O-MeG between the tissue into the intestinal lumen occurs by some system that is influenced by glucose in the tissue (see Sec. VIIIC).

E. Pool Size

It is possible to obtain estimates of the size of the transport pool A (Sec. VIIIC, *supra*). It is found that the minimum size of the transport pool for 3-O-MeG (1 mM in lumen) is 17 ± 6 (11) nmoles, a value considerably smaller than that for leucine. The pool for L-leucine (1 mM in lumen) is estimated as approximately 500 nmoles. The estimates for the concentration of absorbed substrate within the pool will depend upon the volume of tissue in which the substrate is distributed. Of course, we have no knowledge of this, but we estimate that if 3-O-MeG is distributed throughout the whole of the tissue water (about 500 μl), the concentration of the sugar in that compartment will be considerably less than that in the lumen, yet above that in the vascular effluent.

Thus, in these experiments, the presence of the circulation enables a translocation to occur from the lumen without a massive accumulation of substrate in the intestinal wall. In addition the presence of glucose in the circulation augments the exit of previously absorbed monosaccharide into the vascular outflow.

By using phloridzin it is also possible to discover the volume of the slowly exchanging compartment in the intestinal lumen. Knowing the dimensions of the segment of intestine used, it is possible to estimate the thickness of the compartment. For this it is assumed that the compartment represents a layer of fluid adjacent to the mucosa ("unstirred layer"). The estimates of the thickness obtained naturally depend upon the rate of flow of fluid through the lumen, but, generally speaking, values found are of the order of 100–150 μm, a thickness similar to that estimated to obtain in certain mammalian intestinal systems (see, for example, Winne, 1973).

IX. CONCLUSIONS

The intestine is the portal of entry of energy foods; whereas energy expenditure by animal bodies is continuous, the input of energy to the body and intestinal absorption is discontinuous.

The nature of the fuels combusted in tissue metabolism, i.e., glucose, ketones, fatty acids, depends upon the absorptive state. For example, the fuels of fasting tissues are ketones and fatty acids. Little is known of either the functioning of the fasting intestine or the nature of its fuel, but the fasting metabolism requires an uptake of fuel across the blood-facing membranes of the epithelium, for there is no evidence for the existence of significant stores of fuel, e.g., glycogen, fat, in the cells. Although fatty acids may serve as fuel, in certain intestines, e.g., rat jejunum, salt transport requires glucose. What is the partition between the substrates that are combusted and those combustible substrates that are transported across the absorbing intestine? For example, is the glucose that is metabolized kept in a separate compartment from that which is translated across the cells from the intestinal lumen into the blood? As yet we have no answer to this question.

The ultimate fuel of the cell is ATP, the hydrolysis of which may directly or indirectly drive membrane transport. Membrane transport processes driven directly by ATP hydrolysis may charge up a store of electrochemical potential energy, e.g., as a gradient of concentration across a membrane. This store may then be used to power other membrane transport systems. Theoretically the hydrolysis of polymer foodstuffs might provide energy for the transport of the monomeric constituents of the polymer.

In our experiments the intestinal epithelium is loaded with a suitable substrate, such as an amino acid or a monosaccharide, and the subsequent unloading of the previously absorbed substrate into the vascular bed and into the intestinal lumen is examined. It is found that the mesenteric circulation has a great influence on the transfer of absorbed substrate into the fluid in the vascular bed. The potential energy of the fluid in the circulation is therefore of considerable significance in the energetics of absorption. It also appears that the entry of glucose into the tissue energizes the exit of another monosaccharide, already present within the cell. These findings therefore raise questions of energy exchanges at the blood-facing membranes of the epithelium.

ACKNOWLEDGMENTS

I am very grateful to Dr. Richard Boyd, Dr. Chris Cheeseman, Peter Hanson, and Hetty Volman-Mitchell for much stimulating discussion and for allowing me to quote from their experimental findings. I am also indebted to the Medical Research Council which has supported much of our work.

REFERENCES

Agar, W. T., Hird, F. J. R., and Sidhu, G. S. (1954): The uptake of amino acids by the intestine. Biochim. Biophys. Acta 14:80–84.
Annison, D. F., and Lewis, D. (1959): *Metabolism in the rumen,* Methuen, London.

Armstrong, W. McD., Byrd, B. J., and Hamang, P. M. (1973): The Na^+ gradient and D-galactose accumulation in epithelial cells of bullfrog small intestine. Biochim. Biophys. Acta *330:*237–241.
Boyd, C. A. R., Cheeseman, C. I., and Parsons, D. S. (1973): Transport and metabolism of peptides and amino acids by frog intestine perfused through the vascular bed *in vitro.* J. Physiol. *234:*10–11.
Bronk, J. R., and Parsons, D. S. (1965): The polarographic determination of the respiration of the small intestine of the rat. Biochim. Biophys. Acta *107:*397–404.
Cathcart, E. P., and Garry, R. C. (1948): Edward Waymouth Reid, 1862–1948. Obituary Notices of Fellows of the Royal Society *6:*213–218.
Diamond, J. M. (1971): Water-solute coupling and ion selectivity in epithelia. Phil. Trans. Royal Soc. *B262:*141–151.
Douglas, A. P., Kerley, R., and Isselbacher K. J. (1972): Preparation and characterization of the lateral and basal plasma membranes of the rat intestinal epithelial cell. Biochem. J. *128:*1329–1338.
Duerdoth, J. K., Newey, H., Sandford, P. A., and Smyth, D. H. (1965): Stimulation of intestinal fluid transfer by mannose and fructose. J. Physiol. *176:*23p–24p.
Fabry, p. (1969): *Feeding pattern and nutritional adaptations,* Butterworth, London.
Fisher, R. B., and Parsons, D. S. (1953a): Glucose movements across the wall of the rat small intestine. J. Physiol. *119:*210–223.
Fisher, R. B., and Parsons, D. S. (1953b): Galactose absorption from the surviving small intestine of the rat. J. Physiol. *119:*224–232.
Forstner, G. G., Sabesin, S. M., and Isselbacher, K. J. (1968): Rat intestinal microvillus membranes. Biochem. J. *106:*381–390.
Fujita, M., Ohta, H., Kawai, K., Matsui, H., and Nakao, M. (1972): Differential isolation of microvillus and basolateral plasma membranes from intestinal mucosa. Biochim. Biophys. Acta *274:*336–347.
Fullerton, P. M., and Parsons, D. S. (1956): The absorption of sugars and water from rat intestine *in vivo.* Quart. J. Exp. Physiol. *41:*387–397.
Henning, S. J., and Hird, F. J. R. (1972a): Ketogenesis from butyrate and acetate by the caecum and colon of rabbits. Biochem. J. *130:*785–790.
Henning, S. J., and Hird, F. J. R. (1972b): Transport of acetate and butyrate in the hind gut of rabbits. Biochem. J. *130:*791–796.
Johnson, H. A., and Knudsen, K. D. (1965): Renal efficiency and information theory. Nature *206:*930–931.
Karrer, O. (1968): Observations on absorption of sugars by animal intestine. D. Phil. Thesis, University of Oxford.
Lee, C. O., and Armstrong, W. McD. (1972): Activities of sodium and potassium ions in epithelial cells of small intestine. Science *175:*1261–1264.
Lifson, N., and Parsons, D. S. (1957): Support of water absorption by rat jejunum *in vitro* by glucose in serosal fluid. Proc. Soc. Exp. Biol. Med. *95:*532–534.
Lifson, N., and Visscher, M. B. (1944): Osmosis in living systems. In: *Medical physics,* edited by O. Glasser, Year Book Publishers, Chicago.
Milligan, L. P. (1971): Energetic efficiency and metabolic transformations. Fed. Proc. *30:*1454–1465.
Parsons, D. S. (1967): Salt and water absorption by the intestinal tract. Brit. Med. Bull. *23:*252–257.
Parsons, D. S. (1968): Methods for investigation of intestinal absorption. In: *Handbook of physiology,* Sec. 6, Vol. 3, American Physiological Society, Washington, D.C., Chap. 64, p. 1177–1216.
Parsons, D. S. (1972): Summary. In: *Transport across the intestine: A glaxo symposium,* edited by W. L. Burland and P. D. Samuel. Churchill-Livingstone, London, Chap. 24.
Parsons, D. S. (1973): Energy foods. In: *Nutritional problems in a changing world,* edited by D. Hollingsworth and M. Russell, Applied Science Publishers, London, Chap. 15.
Parsons, D. S., and Boyd, C. A. R. (1972): Transport across the intestinal mucosal cell: Hierarchies of function. Int. Rev. Cytol. *32:*209–255.

Parsons, D. S., and Prichard, J. S. (1968): A preparation of perfused small intestine for the study of absorption in amphibia. J. Physiol. *198:*405–434.
Shakespeare, P., Srivastava, L. M., and Hübscher, G. (1969): Glucose metabolism in the mucosa of the small intestine. Biochem. J. *111:*63–67.
Reid, E. W. (1900): On intestinal absorption, especially on the absorption of serum, peptone, and glucose. Phil. Trans. Royal Soc. *B102:*211–297.
Reid, E. W. (1902): Intestinal absorption of solutions. J. Physiol. *28:*242–256.
Royal Society (1972): Report of the Subcommittee on Metrication of the British National Committee for Nutritional Sciences. Royal Soc. London.
Schultz, S. G. (1973): Shunt pathway, sodium transport and the electrical potential pathway across rabbit ileum. In: *Transport mechanisms in epithelia,* edited by H. H. Ussing and N. A. Thorn, Munksgaard, Copenhagen.
Schultz, S. G., and Curran, P. F. (1970): Coupled transport of sodium and organic solutes. Physiol. Rev. *50:*567.
Whittam, R. (1964): The interdependence of metabolism and active transport. In: *The cellular functions of membrane transport,* edited by J. F. Hoffman, Prentice-Hall, Englewood Cliffs, N.J., p. 139.
Whittam, R., and Wheeler, K. P. (1970): Transport across cell membranes. Ann. Rev. Physiol. *32:*21–60.
Wilson, T. H. (1956): The role of lactic acid production in glucose absorption from the intestine. J. Biol. Chem. *222:*751–763.
Winne, D. (1973): Unstirred layer, source of biased Michaelis constant in membrane transport. Biochim. Biophys. Acta *298:*27–31.

DISCUSSION

CURRAN asked about the two components of the exit, whether they may represent two pools washing out at different rates. PARSONS answered yes: the slow component probably represents the wash-out from the extracellular space, perhaps muscle, etc. The other component probably represents the wash-out from the intracellular pool. It is interesting that the size of the latter pool may vary, e.g., with a 3-O-methyl glucose it is very small, $1/50$ to $1/10$ of the pool's size with amino acids.

Intestinal Absorption and Malabsorption,
edited by T. Z. Csáky.
Raven Press, New York © 1975

Role of Membrane-Bound Enzymes in Biological Transport

William J. Waddell

Department of Pharmacology, College of Medicine, University of Kentucky, Lexington, Kentucky 40506

Many drugs that are weak acids or bases distribute across biological membranes in a predictable manner. The unbound, unionized drug freely crosses the membrane to reach the same concentration on each side; the extent of ionization of the drug on each side of the membrane is a function of the dissociation constant of the drug and the pH value of the water. In studies of the distribution of such compounds across the cells lining the gastrointestinal tract the agreement between predicted and experimentally observed values is quite good for the stomach (Hogben, 1960).

On the other hand, the absorption of most weak acids and bases from the intestine is in the direction predicted by the pH gradient, although the quantitative extent frequently does not agree with the calculated ratio. It was apparent that either some modification in the theory was necessary or that unexplained events were compromising the calculated distribution. Hogben (1960) proposed that there is a microenvironment on the mucosal surface of the intestinal epithelium that has a pH value of about 5.3 which remains relatively constant in spite of larger changes in the pH value of the bulk mucosal fluid. This possible explanation has never appealed to me personally because of the need to invoke different rates of diffusion for the two species of the drug between the microlayer and its adjacent bulk phases. To postulate that a microenvironment could account for such a distribution artifact would be analogous to the intracellular pH of epithelial cells affecting the distribution across the cell. No discordant distribution has been reported for any epithelial layer except the intestine.

There are a few other even more perplexing discrepancies between predicted and observed distribution ratios across the intestinal epithelium. Wilson (1954) found that lactate produced by the intestine appeared in higher concentration on the side with the lower pH value; this is completely opposite from the predicted distribution. Conversely, lactate added to the perfusing solutions was not transferred against a pH gradient. A careful analysis of the transfer of cholic acid and taurocholic acid across the intestinal wall indicated that a sizeable percentage of the distribution was due to nonionic diffusion and pH equilibrium, but the bulk of the transport was active, presumably for the ionic species (Dietschy, Salomon, and Siperstein, 1966).

The paradoxical distribution of 5,5-dimethyl-2,4-oxazolidinedione (DMO) across the intestinal wall (Dietschy and Carter, 1965) compels consideration of a mechanism other than passive, nonionic distribution. This synthetic compound has been widely used for the estimation of intracellular pH (Waddell and Bates, 1969) and in all other studies appears to distribute passively according to the pH gradient. Across the wall of the intestine, however, it moved against the pH gradient, against the concentration gradient, and against the net water flow (Dietschy and Carter, 1965). Since the equilibrium by nonionic diffusion is usually very rapid, the capacity of the active transport process must have been very large to maintain this gradient in the reverse direction. Since the pH value of the serosal and mucosal fluids changed during these experiments, some people saw micro pH gradients as explanations for the process.

Another possible explanation is suggested by recent experiments on intercellular flow of water and solutes. Figure 1 depicts the accumulation of DMO inside the epithelial cell due to a high intracellular pH. A transcellular flow of solvent through a leaky serosal membrane could transfer DMO to the serosal fluid. Subsequent return of water to the mucosal fluid through the intercellular junctions with the exclusion of DMO would furnish a transport mechanism.

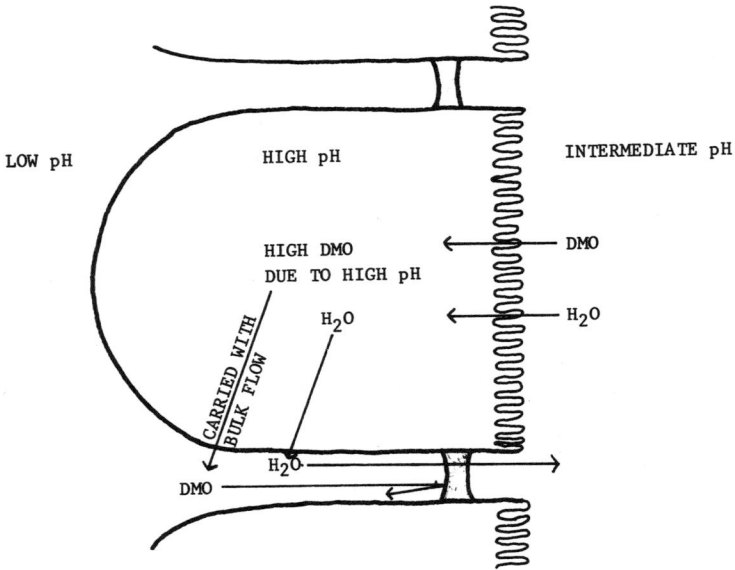

FIG. 1. Diagrammatic representation of an intestinal epithelial cell which accumulates DMO due to a high intracellular pH and appears to transport the substance to the serosal fluid. Leakage of DMO through the serosal membrane from bulk flow of water and impermeability of cell junction account for the high serosal concentration. Mucosal surface is to the right and serosal is to the left.

This mechanism is consistent with at least two observations: (a) an accumulation of DMO in intestinal epithelial cells (Waddell, 1972b) and (b) an apparent impermeability of the intercellular junction to anions of the approximate size of DMO (Schultz, Frizzell, and Nellans, 1974).

Validation of any proposed mechanism to explain the anomalous distribution of DMO obviously will require detailed knowledge of microgradients of pH across the intestinal wall and probably knowledge of how these gradients are generated. In the absence of experimental evidence concerning these pH gradients and their generation I should like to propose some possible mechanisms. Furthermore, such pH gradients might be important in the transfer of other, less obvious solutes.

The active generation of a pH gradient across an epithelial cell requires the polarization of water into hydronium and hydroxyl ions with separation of the two products across an anisotropic barrier. It seems that the most reasonable location of this barrier would be either the mucosal or serosal cell membrane. Knowledge of the intracellular pH and the pH value of the serosal and mucosal fluids would establish which of these two membranes is the anisotropic barrier. Such studies have been done on at least one epithelial cell; the intracellular pH of the turtle bladder epithelium is higher than that of the serosal solution, whereas the mucosal fluid pH is several pH units below that of the serosal fluid (Fig. 2) (Steinmetz, 1969). Assuming that this

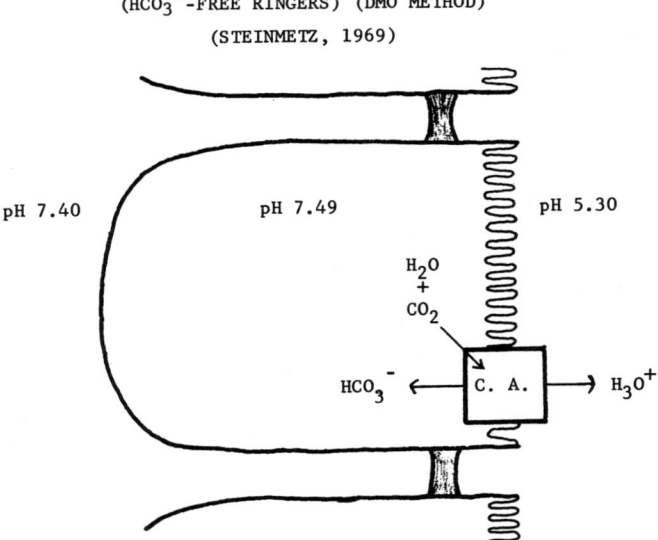

FIG. 2. Diagram of pH gradients across the turtle bladder epithelial cell. Carbonic anhydrase (C.A.) appears to be involved in generating the acid secretion into the mucosal fluid (right side).

intracellular pH is representative of the bulk cytoplasmic fluid, then the mucosal membrane must be the anisotropic barrier. The primary gradient is between mucosal fluid and cytoplasmic water; passive diffusion between cytoplasmic water and serosal fluid would account for this small gradient.

Inhibition of carbonic anhydrase (C.A.) markedly reduced the rate of acidification of the mucosal fluid (Steinmetz, 1969); this makes it tempting to suggest that carbonic anhydrase is the machine which generates the pH gradient. If this enzyme is anisotropically oriented on the mucosal membrane, then discharge of the products of its catalysis to opposite sides of the membrane could explain this generation of a proton gradient. Detailed drawings and discussion of such an orientation of carbonic anhydrase on membranes of epithelial cells have already been presented (Waddell, 1972a). However, in the turtle bladder, at least, complete inhibition of carbonic anhydrase does not destroy the pH gradient; therefore, some other mechanism must be found to effect the primary polarization. Carbonic anhydrase appears only to accelerate the process or perhaps to participate secondarily.

The $Na^+ - K^+$ ATPase is known to be membrane bound and is an even better candidate for the proton pump (Waddell, 1972a). The liberation on the outside of the cell of the proton produced in the hydrolysis of ATP would be an obvious mechanism to assist the cell in disposing of acid produced during the oxidation of substrates. It is indeed unfortunate that the proton that is produced in this hydrolysis is so frequently neglected by biologists. Energetically, one cannot forget this proton because -7.0 kcal of the total of -8.3 kcal of energy available per mole of ATP hydrolyzed is from the energy of ionization of this proton (Rutman and George, 1961). Figure 3 depicts an intestinal epithelial cell with ATPase anisotropically located across the serosal membrane. This is exactly the orientation which is currently in such wide vogue for the enzyme that functions as a Na^+ pump. The only addition is the proton (hydronium ion) which is produced. It is shown being released on the outside of the membrane with the Na^+ ion. The ATPase would consequently function as a proton pump just as effectively as it does as a sodium pump. Accordingly, the intracellular pH would be higher than that of the serosal fluid and that of the mucosal fluid would be intermediate between the two.

The metabolic activities of the mitochondrion and carbonic anhydrase are, of course, closely coupled with those of this pump. The CO_2 produced from the oxidation of substrates (CHO) in the mitochondrion in turn produces protons when the CO_2 is hydrated. These protons supply a source for those needed in the production of ATP from ADP and orthophosphate.

In this scheme carbonic anhydrase has not been placed on the membrane for several reasons. (a) There is little direct evidence to indicate that it is membrane bound. (b) The experiments, cited above, with the turtle bladder make it difficult to be the sole polarizing mechanism. (c) Lastly, an intracellular nonoriented position makes the explanation easier for the alternately

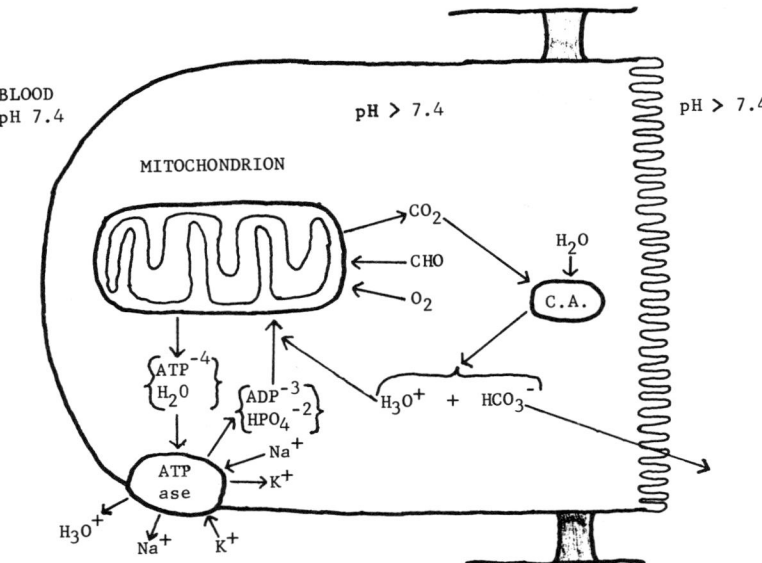

FIG. 3. Scheme illustrating the role of membrane-bound ATPase in pumping Na^+ and H_3O^+ ions into the serosal fluid. The mitochondrion and carbonic anhydrase (C.A.) are coupled with this pump through the generation and consumption of protons. Serosal fluid is to the left.

acid and alkaline pH value of the mucosal fluid which is seen in the intestinal lumen. The fluid in the jejunal contents is frequently acidic; this would be consistent with the scheme shown if loss of protons from the cell into the serosal fluid was not sufficient to balance their production in the cell. Passive equilibrium of the pH gradient between cell interior and mucosal fluid can result in muscosal fluid pH values that are either alkaline or acidic. The intracellular pH value would determine the pH value of the mucosal fluid.

Finally, a third enzyme might be considered for its effect on micro pH gradients. Adenyl cyclase is membrane bound, perhaps to both the serosal and mucosal membranes, and is known to be associated with metabolic events that are influenced by pH changes. For example, in renal tubular cells addition of parathyroid hormone increases cyclic AMP and the production of glucose (Rasmussen, 1970). However, the production of glucose can be increased to an even greater extent, in the absence of parathyroid hormone or an increase in cyclic AMP, merely by lowering the pH value of the medium. One wonders if the effect of parathyroid hormone on cyclic AMP effects the increase in glucose production or whether parathyroid hormone or cylic AMP lowers the intracellular pH which then increases glucose production.

Adenyl cyclase catalyses the molecular rearrangement of ATP into cyclic AMP and pyrophosphate without hydrolysis. The two high energy bonds of ATP remain; one is in the cyclic AMP and the other in pyrophosphate. This catalysis neither consumes nor yields a proton. However, the cyclic AMP catalyzes a cascade of events which hydrolyzes ATP in the phosphorylation of proteins, etc. This could be expected to cause an intracellular acidification; the proton is released in these hydrolyses of ATP. However, whether the stimulation of adenyl cyclase results in net intracellular acidification depends on the summation of all the reactions.

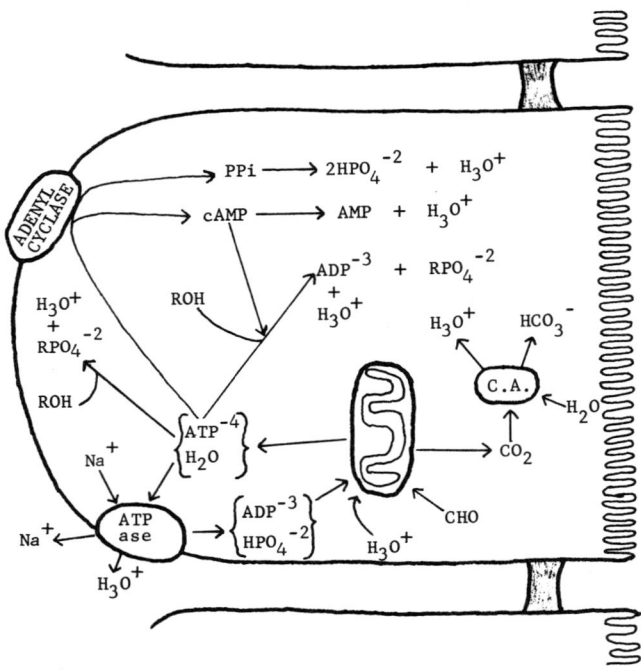

FIG. 4. Representation of an intestinal epithelial cell and the stoichiometric coupling of the reactions of ATPase, adenyl cyclase, and carbonic anhydrase (C.A.). See text for explanation. Mucosal fluid is to the right.

Figure 4 combines the reactions catalyzed by each of the three enzymes we have considered. The stoichiometry of each reaction includes the frequently omitted proton. This clearly illustrates the interdependence of these reactions on the proton. Another pivotal substance is ATP; its net production or consumption is affected by many reactions. The fact should be kept in mind, however, that the production and consumption of ATP is inextricably coupled with the consumption and production of protons. The effect of these protons on the intracellular pH and transcellular pH gradients in epithelial cells is at present unknown; however, the possible significance is such as to warrant careful investigation.

ACKNOWLEDGMENTS

The assistance of Carolyn Marlowe in the preparation of the manuscript is gratefully acknowledged.

REFERENCES

Dietschy, J. M., and Carter, N. W. (1965): Active transport of 5,5-dimethyl-2,4-oxazolidinedione. Science *150:*1294–1296.
Dietschy, J. M., Salomon, H. S., and Siperstein, M. D. (1966): Bile acid metabolism. I. Studies on the mechanisms of intestinal transport. J. Clin. Invest. *45:*832–846.
Hogben, C. A. M. (1960): The first common pathway. Fed. Proc. *19:*864–869.
Rasmussen, H. (1970): Cell communication, calcium ion, and cyclic adenosine monophosphate. Science *170:*404–412.
Rutman, R. J., and George, P. (1961): Hydrogen ion effects in high-energy phosphate reactions. Proc. N.A.S. *47:*1094–1109.
Schultz, S. G., Frizzell, R. A., and Nellans, H. N. (1974): Ion transport by mammalian small intestine. Ann. Rev. Physiol. *36:*51–91.
Steinmetz, P. R. (1969): Acid-base relations in epithelium of turtle bladder: site of active step in acidification and role of metabolic CO_2. J. Clin. Invest. *48:*1258–1265.
Waddell, W. J., and Bates, R. G. (1969): Intracellular pH. Physiol. Rev. *49:*285–329.
Waddell, W. J. (1972a): Subcellular and molecular aspects of intracellular pH. Chest (suppl.) *61:*56S–59S.
Waddell, W. J. (1972b): The role of carbonic anhydrase in the control of intracellular pH. In: *Hemoglobin and red cell structure and function*, edited by G. J. Brewer, Plenum Press, New York.
Wilson, T. H. (1954): Concentration gradients of lactate, hydrogen and some other ions across the intestine *in vivo*. Biochem. J. *56:*521–527.

DISCUSSION

PARSONS inquired whether, if protons are secreted into both the serosal space and into the lumen, should, according to Waddell's model, ATPase be required on both membranes?

WADDELL responded that he proposes a primary mechanism for the extrusion of protons on the basolateral membrane. The appearance of acid or alkali in the lumen requires a reversible system. For this reason he proposes that the luminal proton secretion is connected to carbonic anhydrase. One of the difficulties in these studies stems from the uncertainty in quantitating bicarbonate because it is not known whether the bicarbonate ion or the carbonic acid is transferred. This cannot be answered without more exact knowledge of the intracellular pH.

DOBSON noted that he and Stevens described an active transport of DMO in the rumen epithelium. Thus, because the concentration of the drug within any intermediary layer would be a steady-state concentration, it would be improper to draw conclusions from this regarding the intracellular pH. WADDELL agreed with this.

DIETSCHY pointed out that his work and that of others indicate that the cell membranes are more polar than they were suspected to be; consequently ionic species can penetrate. With bile acids of varying pK_a he could develop a permeability coefficient for the ionic species and a separate one for the nonionic species. Then one can calculate and carefully titrate the unidirectional flux of such a complex system through the intestine. Interestingly, the titration curve could be exactly predicted from the equation using a finite permeability for the ionized as well as the nonionized species, based upon the pH condition of each phases. This may be accepted as evidence that there is probably no significant physiological shift in the pH as the molecule approaches the interface.

WADDELL assumes that, if the membrane is permeable to the ionized form of a weak acid, it must be very poorly so. If there is a transfer of the ionized form of a compound across the membrane which is nearly as great as that of the unionized form, there could be no pH gradient. This is exactly what Mitchell proposed. The mechanism of the action of the uncouplers is that both species, namely the one with the proton and the one without the proton, penetrate the membrane with equal facility. This would therefore destroy the pH gradient. He is bothered about the calculation on the transfer of the ion. One has to be very careful whether the actual ion passes across or whether it was combined with the proton when it passed the membrane.

DOBSON returned to their experiments with the rumen epithelium. They analyzed the conditions necessary for transport. This tissue in the short-circuited form actually transports weak bases in one direction and weak acids in the opposite direction. They assume that the driving force was not the pH gradient but the electrochemical gradient of the hydrogen ion taking into account the potential. It turns out that for pumping to occur two qualifications have to be fulfilled: a gradient of the electrochemical activity of the hydrogen ion between the inside and outside of the cell, and, secondly, a difference in the ratio of permeability for the charged and uncharged form on either side. WADDELL stressed that in these studies one has to be well aware of the contribution of the transfer through the cell and between the cells. The potential difference alone across the entire membrane may not be strictly representative of what is passing through the cell; the intercellular route through the tight junction may also be a contributing factor.

Intestinal Absorption and Malabsorption,
edited by T. Z. Csáky.
Raven Press, New York © 1975

Electrophysiology of Sodium Transport By Epithelial Cells of the Small Intestine

W. McD. Armstrong

Department of Physiology, Indiana University School of Medicine, Indianapolis, Indiana 46202

I. INTRODUCTION

Epithelial cells of the small intestine, like many other epithelial cells, have the ability to effect net Na^+ transfer in a mucosal $\rightarrow$ serosal ($m \rightarrow s$) direction. In several animal species, net $m \rightarrow s$ Na^+ transport has been found to occur in the absence of chemical and electrochemical gradients (Clarkson and Toole, 1964; Schultz and Zalusky, 1964; Barry, Smyth, and Wright, 1965; Taylor, Wright, Schultz, and Curran, 1968; Quay and Armstrong, 1969) and is generally believed to involve direct, metabolically linked, active transport of Na^+ ions (Schultz and Curran, 1968). Although, in certain respects, the concept of active Na^+ transport by the small intestine still awaits rigorous proof (Curran, 1968; Schultz and Curran, 1968), it has been included as a working hypothesis in the great majority of recent studies on intestinal transport of Na^+ *per se* and on the interactions that exist between the net transport of Na^+ and that of sugars and amino acids by this tissue (Schultz and Curran, 1970; Kimmich, 1973). Its existence as a component of net $m \rightarrow s$ Na^+ transfer in the intestine will be assumed herein.

The present discussion is not intended to be a comprehensive review of intestinal Na^+ transport. It is concerned mainly with the impact of recent electrophysiological studies on the development of current ideas concerning the nature of net Na^+ transfer by this tissue, and the electrical correlates of such transfer, the transmural potential difference (E_{Tr}) and short circuit current (I_{sc}). Since this admittedly restricted approach reflects the author's major area of personal involvement in the study of the complex and fascinating problem of intestinal transport, it is perhaps understandable that much of the discussion is based on studies conducted in his laboratory. It seems appropriate to point out at the outset that these studies were performed with the amphibian (*Rana catesbeiana*) rather than the mammalian small intestine. In normal sodium chloride Ringer solutions the electrophysiology of the isolated bullfrog small intestine is complicated by the fact that this tissue has the capacity for net $m \rightarrow s$ transfer of Cl^-, as well as Na^+, under short-circuit conditions (Quay and Armstrong, 1969; Armstrong, Suh, and Gerencser, 1972). However, when Cl^- is completely replaced by sulfate ions, with appropriate addition of an "inert" solute such as mannitol to maintain approximate isosmolality, the electrophysiological behavior of the isolated small intestine of the bullfrog parallels, in many respects, that of the isolated mammalian small intestine. These similarities include the maintenance of a serosal positive E_{Tr} under open circuit conditions and a quantitative equivalence between net Na⁺ transport and I_{sc} (Quay and Armstrong, 1969), a similar response of E_{Tr}, I_{sc}, and the mucosal membrane potential (E_m) to actively transported sugars and amino acids (Quay and Armstrong, 1969, 1969a; White and Armstrong, 1970, 1971) and a similar pattern of sensitivity to metabolic inhibitors including the cardiac glycoside ouabain (Gerencser and Armstrong, 1972). In addition, the isolated bullfrog small intestine possesses a remarkable temporal stability with respect to its electrophysiological properties. This readily permits the performance of *in vitro* experiments over a time period of 6 to 8 hr.

II. THE ROLE OF EXTRACELLULAR IONIC CONDUCTANCE IN INTESTINAL ELECTROPHYSIOLOGY

A. A Model for Na⁺ Transport in the Small Intestine

As a point of departure, the model for intestinal Na⁺ transport, shown in Fig. 1, may be considered. In its original form (Schultz and Zalusky, 1964a) this model gained widespread acceptance as a scheme which drew together a number of important observations within a self-consistent framework and led to experimentally testable predictions. With appropriate modifications it continues to provide a useful basis for studies of intestinal Na⁺ transport and related phenomena in mammalian species and in the frog under the experimental conditions discussed above.

The detailed implications of the model illustrated in Fig. 1 have been extensively discussed (see e.g., Schultz and Curran, 1970; Kimmich, 1973). Therefore, only those of its features that are of particular interest in the present context will be briefly recapitulated. One of these is the location of the active component of $m \rightarrow s$ Na⁺ transport (the Na⁺ pump) in the serosal, or lateral/serosal, membrane of the absorptive cell. This is suggested by the usual steady-state concentration distribution of Na⁺ in *in vitro* studies, i.e., a low intracellular Na⁺ concentration relative to those of the bathing media permits an energetically downhill inward movement of Na⁺ across the lumenal membrane but, when combined with a serosal positive E_{Tr}, appears to require an uphill or active extrusion of Na⁺ from the cell to the serosal medium. Conversely, a serosal or lateral/serosal Na⁺ pump could account satisfactorily for the observed serosal positive E_{Tr} which is normally associated with net Na⁺ transport in this tissue.[1]

---

[1] Contrary to a somewhat persistent oral tradition, Schultz and Zalusky (1964a) did not stipulate an *electrogenic* pump mechanism for their original model. Much later, as

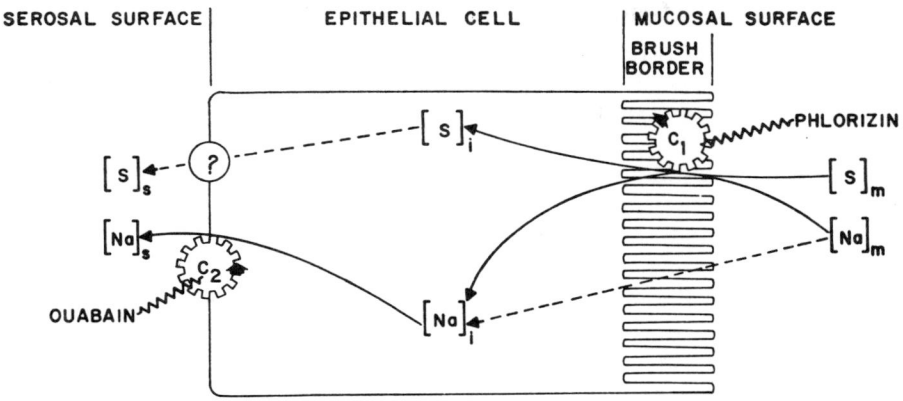

FIG. 1. A model for Na$^+$ transport and for interaction between Na$^+$ and sugar transport in the small intestine (from Schultz and Zalusky, 1964a, reproduced with permission).

Further support for a lateral or lateral/serosal Na$^+$ pump emerged from the observation (Sawada and Asano, 1963; Schultz and Zalusky, 1964) that ouabain, a potent Na$^+$ pump inhibitor in a number of cell species, affects net Na$^+$ transport only when it is present in the medium bathing the serosal surface of the isolated rat or rabbit small intestine. Later, this was shown to hold also for the isolated bullfrog small intestine (Gerencser and Armstrong, 1972). In addition, the studies of Gilles-Baillien and Schoffeniels (1965) and of Wright (1966) on the electrical potential profile across isolated intestinal mucosa from the Greek tortoise indicated that this consists of two potential steps, one (E_m) being the measured potential difference between the mucosal medium and the cell interior, the other (E_s) being the corresponding potential difference between the cell interior and the serosal medium. Both E_m and E_s are oriented in such a way that the cell interior is electrically negative with respect to the appropriate bathing solution, E_s being normally a few millivolts larger than E_m and E_{Tr} being equal to the difference between them. Thus, the electrochemical potential gradient is normally downhill from the mucosal solution to the cell interior and uphill from the cell interior to the serosal solution.

As indicated in Fig. 1, the model readily lends itself to an interpretation of the enhancement of net Na$^+$ transport by actively transported sugars and amino acids, when these solutes are added to the mucosal medium (Schultz and Zalusky, 1964a, 1965), if coupled entry of Na$^+$ and the organic solute

---

discussed elsewhere in this review, Rose and Schultz (1971) did consider a possible contribution of metabolically dependent electromotive forces to E_{Tr} but pointed out that such a contribution could arise either from an electrogenic Na$^+$ pump or from diffusion potentials and/or streaming potentials generated in the lateral spaces between the epithelial cells by an electrically neutral ion pump (see also Machen and Diamond, 1969).

across the brush border membrane is assumed (as, for example, in the bifunctional carrier hypothesis of Crane, 1962). Much evidence for such coupled entry of Na⁺ and organic solutes into the absorptive cells of the small intestine now exists (Schultz and Curran, 1970).

B. Low-Resistance Extracellular Ionic Pathways—Coupling between E_m and E_{Tr}

In its original form the model illustrated in Fig. 1 was concerned exclusively with *transcellular* movement across the epithelial cell layer. This continued to be the major center of interest for several years, although the existence of low-resistance extracellular ionic "shunts" similar to those proposed for frog skin (Ussing and Windhager, 1964) and for renal tubules (Boulpaep, 1967) was strongly indicated by the work of Smyth and Wright (1966) on streaming potentials in the rat small intestine and that of Clarkson (1967) on salt and water fluxes in this tissue and could, in fact, be inferred from the observation of Schultz and Zalusky (1964) that the unidirectional serosal to mucosal Na⁺ flux (J_{sm}) in the isolated rabbit ileum was unaffected by ouabain (Frizzell and Schultz, 1972). Direct evidence for the existence of such shunt pathways emerged from the studies of White and Armstrong (1970, 1971) and of Rose and Schultz (1970, 1971) on the response of the membrane potentials of intestinal epithelial cells to actively transported sugars and amino acids. It is well known that actively transported sugars and amino acids, when added to the mucosal medium, elicit parallel increases in E_{Tr} and I_{sc} across the isolated small intestine (Schultz and Curran, 1970; Kimmich, 1973). Early studies (Gilles-Baillien and Schoffeniels, 1965; Wright, 1966) of the effects of these solutes on E_m, E_s, and E_{Tr} in isolated mucosa from the small intestine of the Greek tortoise and in the hamster jejunum indicated that the increase in E_{Tr} induced by the organic solute was due exclusively to an increase in E_s, E_m being unaffected. In addition, phlorizin, a powerful inhibitor of intestinal sugar transport, when added to the mucosal medium, abolished the glucose induced increase in E_{Tr} by inhibiting the increase in E_s found in the presence of glucose alone (Wright, 1966). These observations are readily interpreted in terms of the model shown in Fig. 1, which does not imply any direct electrical coupling between E_m and E_s and therefore permits a change to occur in one of these parameters without any necessary change in the other. One such interpretation (Barry, 1967) is that enhancement of E_{Tr} by sugars and amino acids involves a direct stimulation of an electrogenic Na⁺ pump in the lateral/serosal membrane of the epithelial cell. A suggested mechanism for this stimulus invokes an increased intracellular Na⁺ pool due to sugar or amino acid coupled Na⁺ influx through the luminal membrane into the cells. Such influx has been shown to occur (Schultz, Curran, Chez, and Fuisz, 1967; Goldner, Schultz, and Curran, 1969), but attempts to demonstrate by direct measurement that actively transported sugars and amino acids cause a significant increase in steady-state intracellular Na⁺ concentrations have been rather consistently unsuccessful (Schultz, Fuisz, and Curran, 1967; Csaky and Esposito, 1969; Koopman and Schultz, 1969; Armstrong, Musselman, and Reitzug, 1970).

Aside from this, several aspects of the electrical response of the isolated small intestine to actively transported sugars and amino acids were not too easily accounted for in terms of the above hypothesis. Among these was the rapidity of the increase in E_{Tr} following exposure of the mucosal surface of the epithelial cells to these solutes which had in fact been tentatively interpreted as indicative of a surface event at the luminal rather than the lateral or serosal face of the absorptive cells (Schultz and Zalusky, 1964a; Smith, 1964; Lyon and Crane, 1966; Hoshi and Komatsu, 1970). The rapidity with which phlorizin abolished sugar-induced increases in E_{Tr} (Schultz and Zalusky, 1964a; Wright, 1966; Gerencser and Armstrong, 1972) suggested a similar interpretation and, finally, the pattern of amino acid transfer by the tortoise small intestine (Gilles-Baillien and Schoffeniels, 1966) appeared to differ significantly from that found in the mammalian small intestine (Schultz and Curran, 1970), suggesting that the response of E_m and E_s to actively transported amino acids might not be the same in the tortoise as in other animal species.

Direct investigation of the effect of actively transported sugars and amino acids (added to the mucosal medium) on E_m and E_s in the bullfrog small intestine (White and Armstrong, 1970, 1971) and the rabbit ileum (Rose and Schultz, 1970, 1971) indicated that, in these tissues, the primary electrical response to the transported solute is a *decrease* in E_m (Fig. 2).[2] This decrease is not observed in the absence of Na⁺ or in the presence of solutes

---

[2] Recently, this finding has been challenged in at least two publications in which it is claimed that, as stated earlier by Wright (1966) for tortoise and hamster intestine, the increase in E_{Tr} elicited by actively transported sugars in the small intestine of the rat is due solely to an increase in E_s. The first of these studies (Lyon and Sheerin, 1971) appears to be subject to the same criticisms as those advanced by Rose and Schultz (1971) in discussing Wright's (1966) data. The measured values of E_m are low (9 to 10 mV for the jejunum and the ileum in the absence or in the presence of 20 mM mucosal glucose) compared to those reported by Rose and Schultz (1971) and White and Armstrong (1971) in the absence of transported solutes (about 36 mV and 44 mV, respectively) and little indication is given that any rigorous criteria for acceptability were applied to individual impalements. Thus one cannot exclude the possbility that, in Lyon and Sheerin's measurements, many of the impaled cells were damaged and, in consequence, their mucosal membranes were leaky. This would explain the apparent insensitivity of E_m to mucosal glucose. Since E_{Tr} is an averaged signal from a very large number of cells, one would not expect it to be noticeably affected by the presence of a small number of leaky cells.

Similar findings concerning the effects of actively transported sugars and amino acids on E_m and E_s in epithelial cells of stripped sacs of rat jejunum were reported by Barry and Eggenton (1972). Once again the average membrane potentials recorded by these authors were disconcertingly low (about 10 mV for E_m and 11 to 20 mV for E_s). Also Barry and Eggenton concluded that any sharp increase in negativity of their recordings which "remained stable for more than 15 sec" constituted an acceptable penetration. In the present author's experience such a criterion for acceptability of intestinal membrane potentials is far from adequate.

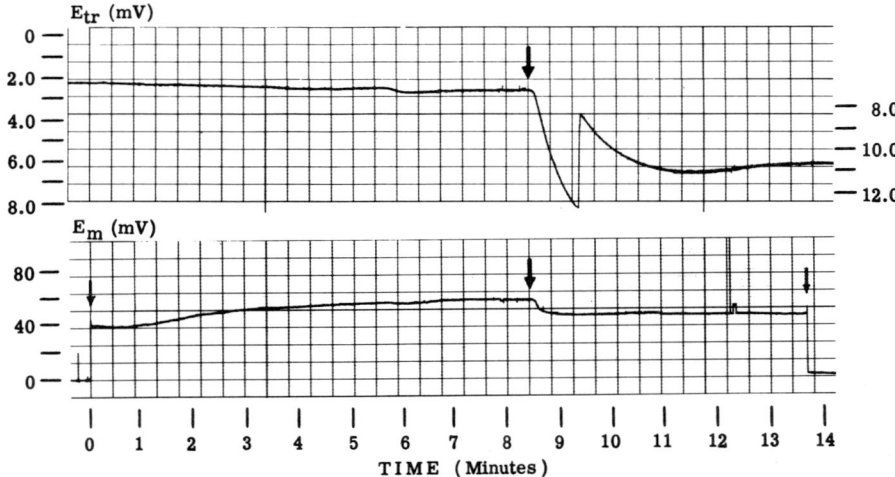

FIG. 2. Effect of 65-mM D-galactose on E_{Tr} (upper tracing) and E_m (lower tracing) in bullfrog small intestinal epithelia in sodium sulfate Ringer solution. Arrows on right- and left-hand sides of the lower tracing indicate times of insertion and retraction of the microelectrode. Central arrow in both tracings marks time at which substrate-free medium (mucosal and serosal) was replaced by a medium containing galactose. Note that shortly after the addition of sugar the zero setting of the E_{Tr} recording was adjusted to keep tracing on the recording paper (from White and Armstrong, 1971, reproduced with permission).

such as D-valine, mannitol, fructose (Rose and Schultz, 1971), or sorbose (White and Armstrong, 1971) whose mucosal influx is independent of Na^+. Since it is known (Curran et al., 1967; Goldner et al., 1969) that the movement of actively transported sugars and amino acids across the brush border or epithelial cells is associated with an increase in Na^+ influx it seems reasonable to suppose that the decrease in E_m elicited by these solutes is the result of sugar- or amino acid-induced electrogenic Na^+ movement from the mucosal medium to the cell interior.

In the absence of coupling between E_m and E_s, and assuming no direct action of actively transported solutes on the serosal membrane of the epithelial cells, one would expect quantitative equivalence between the decrease in E_m (ΔE_m) and the concomitant increase in E_{Tr} (ΔE_{Tr}). However, in many instances, $\Delta E_m > \Delta E_{Tr}$ at a high level of statistical significance (White and Armstrong, 1971; Rose and Schultz, 1971) indicating that, in addition to a decrease in E_m, actively transported sugars and amino acids, induce a concomitant, smaller decrease in E_s. This is readily explained if one assumes that E_m and E_s are electrically coupled so that a change in one of these parameters is necessarily associated with a corresponding change in the other.

A simple model for electrical coupling between E_m and E_s in intestinal epithelia is shown as an equivalent electrical circuit in Fig. 3. In this figure V_m and V_s represent the intrinsic electromotive forces across the mucosal and serosal (or lateral/serosal) membranes of the epithelial cell, R_1 and R_2

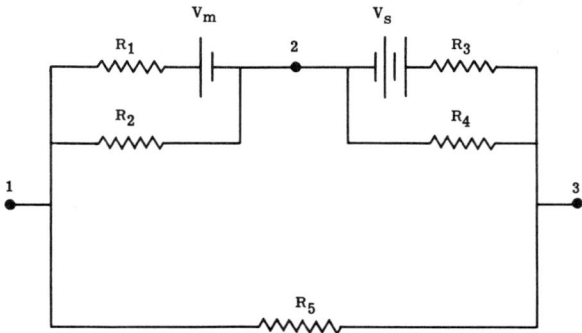

FIG. 3. Equivalent electrical circuit illustrating the relationship between E_m, E_s, and E_{Tr} across an epithelial cell of the small intestine.

are the internal resistances of these batteries, and R_3 and R_4 are shunt resistances across the mucosal and serosal membranes respectively. R_5 represents the resistance of a transepithelial extracellular shunt pathway for ions. The points designated 1, 2, and 3 in Fig. 3 represent the positions of recording electrodes placed in the mucosal solution, the cell interior, and the serosal solution, respectively. For the purposes of this discussion it will be assumed that all emf's are referred to the electrode at point 1, which is at ground (zero) potential. It is also assumed that the solutions bathing the mucosal and serosal surfaces of the epithelial cells are identical.

The circuit illustrated in Fig. 3 leads in a straightforward way to a number of predictions that are consistent with the electrical findings reported by White and Armstrong (1971). Taking into account the orientation of V_m and V_s with respect to the reference point, and solving the circuit for E_m and E_{Tr} one obtains

$$E_m = -[V_m R_m (R_3 R_s + R_5) + R_1 R_m V_s R_s]/R_t, \quad (1)$$

and
$$E_{Tr} = R_5 (V_s R_s - V_m R_m)/R_t, \quad (2)$$

where $R_m = R_2/(R_1 + R_2)$, $R_s = R_4/(R_3 + R_4)$, and $R_t = R_1 R_m + R_3 R_s + R_5$.

It is at once apparent from Eq. (2) that if R_5 is very high compared to the other resistive elements in Fig. 3 (i.e., $R_5 \to \infty$ and $R_5/R_t \to 1$), then $E_{Tr} = V_s R_s - V_m R_m = E_s - E_m$ and E_m and E_s are essentially uncoupled. This is analogous to the situation represented by Fig. 1. At the other extreme, when $R_5 \to 0$, $E_{Tr} \to 0$ and the epithelial cell becomes electrically symmetrical.[3]

---

[3] This is of course the situation with isolated epithelial cells of the small intestine (Kimmich, 1970; Reiser and Christiansen, 1971) and should, in the present author's opinion, be carefully considered when comparing the transport properties of isolated cells to those of intact epithelial sheets (Kimmich, 1970a; Kimmich and Randles, 1973, 1973a; Tucker and Kimmich, 1973; Gall, Butler, Tepperman, and Hamilton, 1974).

As pointed out by Rose and Schultz (1971), the ability of epithelial tissues like the gall bladder, renal proximal tubules, and the small intestine, which have relatively low transepithelial resistances, to maintain relatively large transmembrane potential differences (35 to 80 mV) indicates that, in these systems, extracellular shunt pathways contribute very significantly to total transepithelial conductance. In other words, in these tissues total transepithelial resistance seems to be governed largely by R_5 which may be assumed to be small compared to the other resistive elements shown in Fig. 3.

In the small intestine this accords well with the observation (Schultz and Zalusky, 1964a, 1965; Quay and Armstrong, 1969a) that E_{Tr} and I_{sc} are equally increased by actively transported sugars and amino acids (i.e., total transmural resistance is not markedly affected by these solutes). If the total transepithelial resistance is in fact predominantly a function of R_5, and if R_5 is not greatly changed by these solutes, any other resistance change that occurs under these conditions (e.g., the change in R_m which is a necessary consequence of the mechanism postulated above for the depolarizing effects of actively transported sugars and amino acids on E_m) may not significantly affect total transmural resistance. Similarly the response of E_m and E_{Tr} to actively transported sugars and amino acids reported by White and Armstrong (1971) and by Rose and Schultz (1971), i.e., $\Delta E_m > E_{Tr}$, can be qualitatively predicted if a small but finite value for R_5 relative to $R_3 R_s$, is assumed. From Eqs. (1) and (2) it is easily deduced that, for a change in E_{Tr} which is the consequence of a change in E_m alone,

$$\Delta E_{Tr}/\Delta E_m = 1/(1 + R_3 R_s/R_5), \qquad (3)$$

i.e., the degree to which ΔE_{Tr} is attenuated relative to ΔE_m depends directly on the ratio $R_3 R_s/R_5$.

Thus, the concept of an extracellular shunt pathway leads to a simple equivalent circuit (Fig. 3), which satisfactorily explains, in a qualitative way, the observed electrical responses of the isolated rabbit ileum and the bullfrog small intestine to actively transported sugars and amino acids. White and Armstrong (1971) considered that the decrease in E_m together with an associated but smaller decrease in E_s (which is reflected in an increase in E_{Tr} smaller than the observed decrease in E_m) were sufficient to explain their observations. However, the results of Rose and Schultz (1971) and Frizzell and Schultz (1972) suggest that, in the rabbit ileum at least, the quantitative relationship between ΔE_m and ΔE_{Tr}, may, under certain conditions, require the generation, by these solutes, of an additional emf. This could be either a direct increase in E_s due to stimulation of an electrogenic Na^+ extrusion mechanism in the lateral/serosal membrane or a diffusion and/or streaming potential due to electroneutral Na^+ extrusion into the lateral intercellular spaces (Machen and Diamond, 1969). The evidence for this is as follows. Rose and Schultz (1971) found that in tissues poisoned with KCN, iodoacetate, and ouabain, L-alanine elicited a decrease in E_m.[4] However, under these conditions there was little change in E_{Tr}, which had already declined to near zero values. The average value for $\Delta E_{Tr}/\Delta E_m$ found in poisoned tissues was 0.06 compared to a value of 0.3 in nonpoisoned tissues. According to Eq. (3), this could result from a decrease in R_5, but since total transepithelial resistance was increased in poisoned tissues this explanation was considered unlikely, and Rose and Schultz concluded that the relative lack of response of E_{Tr} to L-alanine in poisoned tissue was due to inhibition, under these conditions, of a lateral/serosal Na^+ extrusion which in nonpoisoned conditions gives rise to an increase in E_{Tr} as discussed above. An alternative explanation, based on Eq. (3), i.e., that the lack of response of E_{Tr} to L-alanine could be due to an increase in R_3R_s in the presence of inhibitors was dismissed by Rose and Schultz because of a lack of evidence but cannot, in the present author's opinion, be rigorously excluded as a possible interpretation of these results.

The results of Frizzell and Schultz (1972) are of more compelling import in relation to the shunt pathway, and its effects on the electrical parameters of the isolated small intestine. In this study mucosal influxes of Na^+, K^+, and Cl^- were measured under transmural voltage clamp by the method of Schultz et al. (1967). The results indicated that the partial ionic shunt conductance of these ions accounted for at least 82% of the total tissue conductance. Further the calculated shunt permeability ratio $P_K/P_{Na}/P_{Cl}$ was found to be 1.14/1.00/0.55. Frizzell and Schultz concluded that their results were consistent with ionic permeation through aqueous channels lined with electronegative neutral polar groups rather than fixed anionic charges.[5]

These results suggest that, if the change in E_{Tr} induced by actively transported sugars and amino acids were due solely to an effect on E_m, the predicted values of $\Delta E_{Tr}/\Delta E_m$ would be 0.16 instead of 0.3 as found by Rose and Schultz (1971). Thus the data of Frizzell and Schultz lend further support to the idea that an increase in E_s may be an additional factor in the overall electrical changes induced by these solutes.

The probable anatomic location of the shunt pathway has also been discussed by Frizzell and Schultz (1972). White and Armstrong (1971) and Rose and Schultz (1971) considered two possible pathways, one being the extracellular region comprising the so-called tight junctions between adjacent epithelial cells and the lateral intercellular spaces. The other, as suggested by Clarkson (1967), consists of areas of denudation formed by epithelial cell exfoliation. Although a contribution from denuded areas to the overall properties of the transepithelial shunt pathway in the small intestine cannot

---

[4] Although the absolute value of E_m in the presence of inhibitors was lower than the value found under control conditions, ΔE_m was of a similar magnitude in both situations.

[5] Recently Munck and Schultz (1974) using the same technique have reached essentially similar conclusions concerning the shunt pathway in the isolated rat jejunum.

be ruled out, Frizzell and Schultz (1972) advance convincing arguments for regarding the tight junction-intercellular space complex and, specifically, the tight junction itself as the principal rate-limiting barrier to transepithelial flows of ions. Among the supporting evidence for this viewpoint cited by these authors is the fact that, anatomically and electrophysiologically, the small intestine closely resembles a number of other tissues such as the gall bladder and the proximal renal tubules, which possess tight junctions and lateral intercellular spaces but do not exhibit spontaneous cell exfoliation, and the results of microscopic studies of the permeation of epithelia by visible tracers such as hemoglobin (Farquhar and Palade, 1963) and horseradish peroxidase (Bentzel, Tourville, Parsa, and Tomasi, 1971). In addition the data of Loeschke, Bentzel, and Csaky (1970) on asymmetric water flow in the frog intestine might be interpreted as supporting this view (see also the review by T. Z. Csaky elsewhere in this volume).

C. Effect of Changes in R_5 on E_m and E_{Tr}: The Orientation of V_m and V_s in Epithelial Cells of Small Intestine:

A short but penetrating analysis by Schultz (1972) of the equivalent circuit shown in Fig. 3 uncovered an important effect of R_5 on the relationship between the intrinsic electromotive force across the mucosal membrane of epithelial cells (V_m) and the corresponding *measured* membrane potential (E_m). When cell emf's are taken with respect to the mucosal solution as a zero reference point, four combinations of V_m and V_s are theoretically possible (Fig. 4). Of these, two only, a and b, will be considered in this analysis.

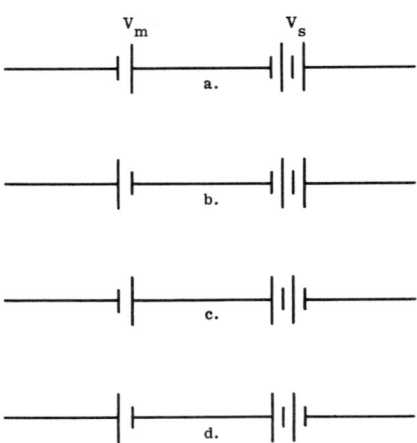

FIG. 4. Possible orientations of V_m and V_s with respect to a mucosal solution reference at zero (ground) potential.

Combination a is the orientation generally believed to occur in high-resistance epithelia such as amphibian skin (Whittembury, 1964; Cereijido and Curran, 1965) and toad bladder (Frazier, 1962). Combination b corresponds to the orientation suggested for low-resistance epithelia such as the small intestine (Gilles-Baillien and Schoffeniels, 1965; Wright, 1966; Rose and Schultz, 1971; White and Armstrong, 1971). Inserting V_m as oriented in Fig. 4a into the circuit shown in Fig. 3 and solving for E_m and E_{Tr}, one obtains

$$E_m = [V_m R_m (R_3 R_s + R_5) - V_s R_s R_1 R_m]/Rt, \quad (4)$$
and
$$E_{Tr} = R_5 (V_m R_m + V_s R_s)/Rt. \quad (5)$$

Equations (4) and (5) are exactly analogous to Eqs. (1) and (2) which were derived on the assumption that V_m is oriented as shown in Fig. 4b.

In the absence of electrical coupling between V_m and V_s (i.e., if $R_5 \to \infty$), E_m will always reflect the orientation of $V_m R_m$ and, for the situation shown in Fig. 4a, the measured electrical profile across the cell will have the form illustrated in Fig. 5a. When $R_5 < \infty$, E_m can have the same or the opposite polarity to $V_m R_m$, depending on the relative magnitudes of the resistive elements shown in Fig. 3. Formally, this can be demonstrated as follows. Rearranging Eq. (4), one obtains

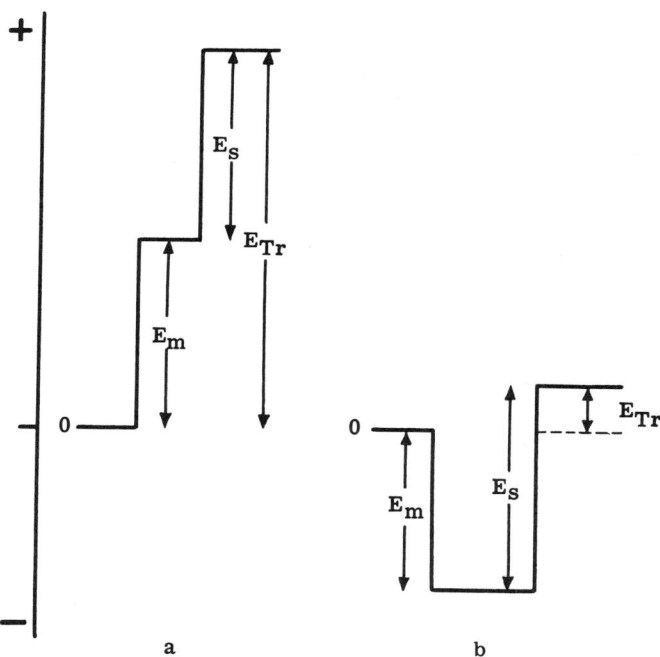

FIG. 5. Measured electrical potential profiles (with respect to grounded mucosal solution—0) across an epithelial cell in which V_m and V_s are oriented as shown in Fig. 4a; (a) R_5 large; (b) R_5 relatively small (from Schultz, 1972, reproduced with permission).

$$\frac{E_m R_t}{R_1 R_m} = \frac{V_m R_m (R_3 R_s + R_5)}{R_1 R_m} - V_s R_s, \tag{6}$$

from which it is apparent that

$$E_m > 0 \text{ when } V_s R_s < [(R_3 R_s + R_5)/R_1 R_m] V_m R_m, \tag{7}$$
$$E_m < 0 \text{ when } V_s R_s > [(R_3 R_s + R_5)/R_1 R_m] V_m R_m. \tag{8}$$

Inequalities (7) and (8) will give rise to the electrical potential profiles shown in Fig. 5a and b, respectively.

The salient conclusions that emerge from this analysis are, first, that the observation that E_m, in low-resistance epithelia such as the small intestine, is so oriented that the cell interior is negative with respect to the mucosal solution does not *per se* yield any information about the magnitude or orientation of V_m (or $V_m R_m$). Second, it is apparent from (7) and (8) above that the transition from $E_m < 0$ to $E_m > 0$ can be mediated by a decrease in R_5 alone, all other parameters of the system remaining constant (Schultz, 1972).

Further analysis of the circuit shown in Fig. 3 reveals, that, in certain circumstances, the effect of changes in R_5 on the magnitude of E_m can be used to obtain information concerning the orientation of $V_m R_m$ in the isolated small intestine. If all other parameters remain constant, and V_m is oriented (with respect to the mucosal solution) as shown in Fig. 4a, it is evident from Eq. (6) that if E_m is oriented so that the cell interior is negative with respect to the mucosal solution in a given control situation (as it normally is in the small intestine) then decreasing R_5 should result in the cell interior becoming more negative with respect to the mucosal solution (i.e., E_m should become more negative). Conversely, an increase in R_5 should result in decreased negativity of the cell interior with respect to the mucosal solution (i.e., E_m, if negative, should decline toward zero). On the other hand, if V_m and V_s are oriented as shown in Fig. 4b, one obtains from Eq. (1)

$$\frac{E_m R_t}{R_1 R_m} = - \frac{V_m R_m (R_3 R_s + R_5)}{R_1 R_m} - V_s R_s. \tag{9}$$

Unlike Eq. (6) which permits E_m to have either of the orientations shown in Fig. 5a and b depending on the magnitude of R_5, Eq. (9) requires that E_m have the orientation shown in Fig. 5b for all finite values of R_5 (i.e., $E_m < 0$). More important in the present context is the fact that for a change in R_5 only, Eq. (9) unlike Eq. (6) permits E_m to become more negative if R_5 is increased and vice versa. It should be noted that both Eq. (2) and Eq. (5) predict an increase in E_{Tr} when R_5 is increased and vice versa.

In the light of this analysis we have recently performed a series of experiments designed to examine the response of E_m in the isolated bullfrog small intestine to changes in R_5 (Armstrong, Byrd, Cohen, Cohen, and Hamang, *in prep.*). In these experiments, sheets of isolated intestine were mounted between identical sodium sulfate Ringer solutions in the perfusion chamber described by White and Armstrong (1971). This chamber was slightly modified to permit more rapid changes of the perfusion medium. The media used were identical in ionic composition to that described by Quay and Armstrong (1969). However, since it has been reported that the shunt resistances across the frog skin epithelium, the renal proximal tubules, and the rabbit ileum are inversely related to the osmolality of the bathing medium (Ussing and Windhager, 1964; Windhager, Boulpaep, and Giebisch, 1966; Rose and Schultz, 1971), an attempt was made to vary R_5 by adjusting the amount of mannitol added to the media used in these experiments. One of these media (259 ± 2 mosm/kg H_2O) was hyperosmotic compared to that described by Quay and Armstrong (1969) which had a mean osmolality of 208 ± 1 mosm. The second (151 ± 1 mosm) was hypo-osmotic compared to this medium. E_{Tr} was monitored continuously throughout the experiment, displayed on the

TABLE 1. Effect of medium osmolality on E_{Tr} and E_m in the isolated bullfrog small intestine (mean values $\pm$ SE)

Change	n	ΔE_{Tr}[a]	ΔE_m[a]
Hyper $\rightarrow$ Hypo	15	1.7 ± 0.3	-4.2 ± 1.2
Hypo $\rightarrow$ Hyper	21	-1.8 ± 0.2	4.7 ± 0.9

[a] A positive value for ΔE_{Tr} means that E_{Tr} became more positive with respect to the mucosal solution and vice versa. A positive ΔE_m means that the cell interior became less negative with respect to the mucosal solution and vice versa.

screen of a Hewlett-Packard Model 132AV dual beam oscilloscope and simultaneously recorded on one channel of a Brush Mark 240 strip chart recorder. E_m was measured with high-resistance microelectrodes as described by White and Armstrong (1971), displayed on a Fairchild Model 7050 multimeter, and recorded on a second channel of the Brush recorder. Following successful impalement and measurement of the steady-state E_m in one of these media, the tissue was perfused with the other medium with the microelectrode still in place and E_m and E_{Tr} were recorded until a new steady state was reached. This frequently required 20 to 30 min. To avoid possible complications due to the generation of emf's in the shunt pathway, both the mucosal and serosal perfusion media were changed simultaneously.

Table 1 is a summary of the results obtained. It is seen that on changing from the hyperosmotic to the hypo-osmotic medium both E_{Tr} and E_m increased significantly ($p < 0.05$). Similarly, on changing from the hypo-osmotic to the hyperosmotic medium equal and opposite changes in E_{Tr} and E_m were recorded. If one assumes that the electrophysiological responses of the tissue to a change in the osmolality of the bathing medium are mediated by a resulting increase in R_5, these data indicate that the normal, inside negative, E_m in epithelial cells of the small intestine reflects the true orientation of V_m across the mucosal membrane.[6]

IIII. SODIUM AND POTASSIUM ION ACTIVITIES IN EPITHELIAL CELLS OF THE SMALL INTESTINE

A. Intracellular Ionic Activities and Coupled Transport of Sugar and Na⁺

Lee and Armstrong (1972) reported direct measurements with cation-selective microelectrodes of intracellular Na⁺ and K⁺ activities in epithelial cells of the isolated bullfrog small intestine maintained at 25°C in a sodium sulfate Ringer solution (Quay and Armstrong, 1969). The technique used in making these measurements is described in detail elsewhere (Lee and Armstrong, 1974). Under control conditions the average sodium activity (a_{Na}^i) was 14.4 ± 3.1 (SD) mM. Under identical conditions the average sodium concentration (C_{Na}) of these cells was found by chemical analysis to be 27 ± 7 mM/kg cell water (Armstrong et al., 1970). These results indicate that in epithelial cells of the small intestine, as in most cell species so far studied (Lev and Armstrong, *in press*), a relatively large fraction of the intracellular Na⁺ is not present in an osmotically active form in the cytoplasm surrounding the cation-selective microelectrode (this fraction has been estimated by Lee and Armstrong to contain about one-half of the total cell Na⁺). By contrast, the average K⁺ activity (a_K^i) was found to be 85.4 ± 6.0 mM, the corresponding K⁺ concentration (C_K) being 86 ± 7 mM/kg cell water. This again is in general agreement with the results reported for other types of cells (Lev and Armstrong, *in press*) and indicates that most of the cell K⁺ is in "free" or osmotically active solution. In fact the apparent activity coefficient for K⁺ (a_K^i/C_K) is higher than one would predict on the assumption that the mean activity coefficient of the cytoplasm is identical to that of the bathing solution. A similar finding had previously been reported by McLaughlin and Hinke (1966) for depressor muscle fibers of the giant barnacle, *Balanus nubilus,* and had been interpreted by these authors as indicating the presence of a significant fraction of nonsolvent water in these fibers (see also Hinke, 1970). A similar interpretation seems likely in the case of epithelial cells of the small intestine (Lee and Armstrong, 1972).

These results, and particularly those relating to Na⁺ activity, are of interest in connection with the coupling of intestinal Na⁺ transport to the active accumulation across the brush border of sugars and amino acids. Ion gradient hypotheses, i.e., the idea that the free energy available from the dissipation

---

[6] Preliminary results from experiments in which the effect of medium osmolality on intracellular Na⁺ and K⁺ concentrations was measured indicate that, under the conditions discussed above, the changes in these parameters would not account for the observed changes in E_m (Table 1).

of the transmembrane electrochemical potential gradient for an ion can be used to drive the uphill movement, across the same membrane, of a second ion or a nonelectrolyte, have been much invoked in recent studies of coupled transport phenomena (see e.g., Heinz, 1972). In particular, the Na$^+$-gradient hypothesis for accumulative transfer of sugars across the brush border of epithelial cells of small intestine (Crane, 1962, 1965) has been widely supported and also vigorously criticized (Schultz and Curran, 1970; Kimmich, 1973). In essence, this hypothesis postulates that the energy for sugar accumulation across the brush border of epithelial cells is entirely derived from the concomitant downhill movement, in the same direction, of Na$^+$ ions. In this hypothesis, one role of the lateral/serosal Na$^+$ pump (Schultz and Zalusky, 1964) is the conservation of the Na$^+$ electrochemical potential gradient across the brush border through the maintenance of a low intracellular Na$^+$ concentration. A similar hypothesis has been widely invoked to account for the effect of mucosal Na$^+$ on the accumulation of neutral amino acids (Schultz and Curran, 1970).

It is obvious that a necessary, although not sufficient, criterion for this hypothesis (and, in fact, the argument applies with equal force to all ion-gradient hypotheses) is that enough energy should be available from the Na$^+$ electrochemical potential gradient under given conditions to account for the steady-state cell/lumen concentration gradient of sugar, or other solute, achieved under the same conditions. The direct measurement of Na$^+$ and K$^+$ activities in epithelial cells permits a more rigorous evaluation of this criterion than was previously possible.

Armstrong, Byrd, and Hamang (1973a, b) utilized this approach to evaluate transmucosal Na$^+$ chemical and electrochemical gradients ($\Delta\mu_{Na}$ and $\Delta\bar{\mu}_{Na}$), and the corresponding K$^+$ electrochemical gradient ($\Delta\bar{\mu}_K$) in epithelial cells of the bullfrog small intestine maintained at 25°C in an oxygenated sodium sulfate Ringer solution containing 102.4 mM Na$^+$ and 5 mM K$^+$. These gradients were compared with the reversible work ($\Delta\mu_{Gal}$) required to achieve a steady-state intracellular concentration of D-galactose from the same solution containing 2 mM of this sugar. In these studies the Na$^+$ and K$^+$ activities of the bathing medium and the cell interior (a_{Na}^0, a_{Na}^i, a_K^0, and a_K^i), E_m, and the steady-state intracellular galactose concentration (C_i) were determined under steady-state conditions (see Armstrong et al., 1973b for experimental details) and were used to calculate $\Delta\mu_{Gal}$, $\Delta\mu_{Na}$, $\Delta\bar{\mu}_{Na}$, and $\Delta\bar{\mu}_K$ as shown in Table 2.

The results shown in Table 2 indicate that, assuming a Na$^+$/sugar coupling ratio of unity (as found by Goldner et al., 1969, for Na$^+$ coupled transport in the isolated rabbit ileum) for Na$^+$-dependent galactose influx in the bullfrog small intestine, $\Delta\mu_{Na}$ alone is insufficient to account for the value of C_i attained in these experiments (7.8 mM). The energy deficit involved may in fact be greater than Table 2 indicates since, in this study, C_i was computed on the assumption that all the epithelial cell water is available as a solvent for galactose. Lee and Armstrong's (1972) results suggest that about 15% of the cell water is unavailable as a solvent for intracellular ions. Hence the value of 7.8 mM for C_i used in computing $\Delta\mu_{Gal}$ as shown in Table 2 may be an underestimate. $\Delta\bar{\mu}_{Na}$ (Table 2) could provide sufficient energy for galactose accumulation but, for a 1/1 Na$^+$/galactose coupling ratio, would require an efficiency of about 50%. If, as has been suggested (Schultz and Curran, 1970), $\Delta\bar{\mu}_{Na}$ and $\Delta\bar{\mu}_K$ can function as a joint source of energy for sugar accumulation, the required efficiency under these conditions would be about 30%. It is of course apparent that if the Na$^+$/galactose coupling ratio in the bullfrog small intestine is greater than unity, the required efficiencies would be correspondingly less.

TABLE 2. *Comparison of the reversible work ($\Delta\mu_{Gal}$) required to achieve a steady-state cell/medium galactose concentration in epithelial cells of the bullfrog small intestine with the maximum reversible work obtainable from the chemical ($\Delta\mu_{Na}$) and electrochemical ($\Delta\bar{\mu}_{Na}$) transmucosal Na$^+$ gradients and the corresponding K$^+$ electrochemical gradient ($\Delta\bar{\mu}_K$) under the same conditions*

$\Delta\mu_{Gal}$	RT ln C_i/C_o	3,400
$\Delta\mu_{Na}$	RT ln a^i_{Na}/a^o_{Na}	2,700
$\Delta\bar{\mu}_{Na}$	$\Delta\mu_{Na} + E_mF$	5,800
$\Delta\bar{\mu}_K$	RT ln $a^i_K/a^o_K - E_mF$	5,700

Values are in joules/mole galactose or joules/equ. Na$^+$ or K$^+$ transferred across the mucosal membrane. Average E_m in these experiments was 32 mV (data from Armstrong, Byrd, and Hamang, 1973b).

Very few direct estimates of the thermodynamic efficiency of coupled transport processes are available at present; Geck, Heinz, and Pfeiffer (1972) investigated the efficiency of coupling between Na$^+$ and α-amino-isobutyrate influxes in Ehrlich ascites cells and concluded that the maximum efficiency attainable for this process was about 8%. However, a recent re-examination of the question by Heinz and Geck (1974) in which allowance is made for the fraction of Na$^+$ influx that is not coupled to α-aminosobutyrate influx leads to the conclusion that the maximum attainable efficiency is much higher than this.

Clearly, further studies of ionic activity gradients and coupling efficiencies in the same tissue under the same conditions are needed to clarify the question of the energetic feasibility of ion gradient hypotheses in general. However, it seems reasonable to conclude from the data of Table 2 that, at present, the Na$^+$ gradient hypothesis for intestinal sugar accumulation cannot be rejected on energetic grounds.

B. Effect of an Actively Transported Solute on Intracellular Na⁺ and K⁺ Activities

As already discussed, several investigations of the effect of actively transported sugars and amino acids on the intracellular Na⁺ concentration of epithelial cells of the small intestine rather consistently failed to detect any significant change in this parameter following exposure of the mucosal surface of the cells to these solutes. Specifically, Csaky and Esposito (1969) and Armstrong et al. (1970) failed to observe any significant effect of the actively transported sugar analogue 3-O-methyl glucose on C_{Na} in mucosal cells of the isolated bullfrog small intestine following immersion in sodium sulfate Ringer solutions. Because of the uncertainties inherent in estimating C_{Na} by conventional methods (see Lev and Armstrong, *in press*, for a discussion of this question) it seemed possible that this approach might fail to uncover relatively small but real changes in cell Na⁺ following exposure of the cells to transported solutes. For this reason Lee and Armstrong (1972) examined the effect of 26 mM 3-O-methyl glucose on $a_{Na}{}^i$ and $a_K{}^i$. In these experiments $a_{Na}{}^i$ and $a_K{}^i$ were determined during perfusion of flat sheets of small intestine by a sodium sulfate Ringer solution (White and Armstrong, 1971). Following this, the cells were perfused with a solution similar to the control medium but in which 26 mmole/l 3-O methyl glucose were substituted for an equivalent amount of mannitol. E_{Tr} was monitored continuously throughout the experiment and, when it reached a new steady state following exposure of the tissue to 3-O-methyl glucose, activity measurements were resumed. The results were as follows. Under control conditions $a_{Na}{}^i$ was 14.9 ± 1.4 (SE) mM and $a_K{}^i$ was 85.0 ± 4.0 mM. Following exposure to 3-O-methyl glucose $a_{Na}{}^i$ was 12.1 ± 1.4 mM and $a_K{}^i$ was 64.4 ± 4.5 mM.

The marked decrease in $a_K{}^i$ is consistent with the observation (Csaky and Esposito, 1969; Armstrong et al., 1970) that C_K is significantly reduced under similar conditions and can be ascribed to the same cause, dilution of osmotically active cytoplasmic K⁺ by osmotic entry of water into the cells. Less expected is the observation that there is a small but highly significant ($p < 0.001$) decrease in $a_{Na}{}^i$ following exposure of the cells to 3-O-methyl glucose. Although Na⁺ influx from the lumen to the cell is increased in the presence of 3-O-methyl glucose (Goldner et al., 1969), the absence of any increase in $a_{Na}{}^i$ under these conditions is not too surprising in view of the concomitant increase in cell water (Csaky and Esposito, 1969; Armstrong et al., 1970). Recalling that I_{sc}, as well as E_{Tr}, is increased by 3-O-methyl glucose (Schultz and Zalusky, 1964; Quay and Armstrong, 1969), it is pertinent to ask how (if one assumes that the fraction of cell Na⁺ which is detectible by cation-selective microelectrodes is implicated in lateral/serosal Na⁺ pumping) this increase in I_{sc}, which involves an increase in Na⁺-pump activity, can be reconciled with a *decrease* in $a_{Na}{}^i$.

A tentative answer to this question can be formulated in terms of the energetics of net Na⁺ transport from the interior of the epithelial cell to the serosal solution. Under open circuit conditions, the work associated with the reversible transfer of 1 g equiv. of Na⁺ is given by

$$w = RT \ln (a_{Na}^{0}/a_{Na}^{i}) + E_s F. \qquad (10)$$

If it is assumed that the cellular supply of metabolic energy and the efficiency with which it is coupled to the Na⁺ pump are unaffected by 3-O-methyl glucose, the known decrease in E_s in the presence of this solute (White and Armstrong, 1971) would permit the maintenance of a lower steady state a_{Na}^{i} under open circuit conditions since the other parameters of Eq. (10) are unchanged. It seems reasonable to conclude that the increased Na⁺ current observed when the tissue is brought to the short circuit condition in the presence of 3-O-methyl glucose simply reflects the increased rate of lateral/serosal Na⁺ pumping required to maintain a lower a_{Na}^{i} in the face of a sugar induced increase in mucosal Na⁺ influx.

SUMMARY

Some recent electrophysiological studies of the interaction between the transport of Na⁺ and that of sugars and amino acids by epithelial cells of the small intestine are described. These studies demonstrated the existence of electrical coupling between the mucosal and serosal membrane potentials in this tissue and led to the concept of a relatively low-resistance extracellular transepithelial ionic "shunt" pathway (tentatively identified with the tight junction-lateral intercellular space complex) as a major determinant of its ion transport and electrical properties. A simple electrical equivalent circuit for intestinal mucosa, which embodies the extracellular shunt concept, is presented and discussed. The model predicts that the magnitude of the shunt resistance (relative to the other resistive elements in the epithelial cell layer) and changes in its magnitude can significantly modify the measured electrical parameters of the mucosal cell layer. Experiments which support this prediction are described.

The measurement with cation-selective microelectrodes of intracellular Na⁺ and K⁺ activities in epithelial cells of the isolated bullfrog small intestine is described. These measurements show that in these cells, as in other cell species, a large proportion of the intracellular Na⁺ is not detectable by a microelectrode inserted into the cytoplasm. The use of intra- and extracellular ionic activity measurements in assessing the energetic adequacy of the Na⁺ gradient hypothesis for active sugar transport is discussed together with the effect of the actively transported sugar analogue 3-O-methyl glucose on intracellular Na⁺ and its relationship to the stimulatory effect of this solute on transmural P.D. and short circuit current.

ACKNOWLEDGMENT

The support received from the U.S. Public Health Service (Grants AM 12715 and HE 06308) in the studies from the author's laboratory described herein is gratefully acknowledged.

REFERENCES

Armstrong, W. McD., Byrd, B. J., and Hamang, P. M. (1973a): Energetic adequacy of Na$^+$ gradients for sugar accumulation in epithelial cells of small intestine. Biophys. Soc. Abstr. p. 137a.
Armstrong, W. McD., Byrd, B. J., and Hamang, P. M. (1973b): The Na$^+$ gradient and D-galactose accumulation in epithelial cells of bullfrog small intestine. Biochim. Biophys. Acta *330*:237–241.
Armstrong, W. McD., Musselman, D. L., and Reitzug, H. C. (1970): Sodium, potassium and water content of isolated bullfrog small intestinal epithelia. Am. J. Physiol. *219*:1023–1026.
Armstrong, W. McD., Suh, T. K., and Gerencser, G. A. (1972): Stimulation by anoxia of active chloride transfer in isolated bullfrog small intestine. Biochim. Biophys. Acta *255*:647–662.
Barry, R. J. C. (1967): Electrical changes in relation to transport. Brit. Med. Bull. *23*:266–269.
Barry, R. J. C., and Eggenton, J. (1972): Membrane potentials of epithelial cells in rat small intestine. J. Physiol. *227*:201–216.
Barry, R. J. C., Smyth, D. H., and Wright, E. M. (1965): Short circuit current and solute transfer by rat jejunum. J. Physiol. *181*:410–431.
Bentzel, C. J., Tourville, D. R., Parsa, B., and Tomasi, T. B., Jr. (1971): Bidirectional transport of horseradish peroxidase in proximal tubule of Necturus kidney. J. Cell. Biol. *48*:197–202.
Boulpaep, E. L. (1967): Ion permeability of the peritubular and luminal membrane of the renal tubular cell. In *Symposium über Transport und Funktion Intercellulärer Elecktolyte*, edited by F. Kruck, Urban und Schwartzenberg, Munich, Germany, p. 98.
Cereijido, M., and Curran, P. F. (1965): Intracellular electrical potentials in frog skin. J. Gen. Physiol. *48*:543–557.
Clarkson, T. W. (1967): The transport of salt and water across isolated rat ileum: evidence for at least two distinct pathways. J. Gen. Physiol. *50*:695–727.
Clarkson, T. W., and Toole, S. R. (1964): Measurement of short circuit current and ion transport across the ileum. Am. J. Physiol. *206*:658–668.
Crane, R. K. (1962): Hypothesis for mechanism of intestinal active transport. Fed. Proc. *21*:891–895.
Crane, R. K. (1965): Na$^+$ dependent transport in the intestine and other tissues. Fed. Proc. *24*:1000–1005.
Csaky, T. Z., and Esposito, G. (1969): Osmotic swelling of intestinal epithelial cells during active sugar transport. Am. J. Physiol. *217*:753–755.
Curran, P. F. (1968): Coupling between transport processes in intestine. Physiologist *11*:3–23.
Farquhar, M. G., and Palade, G. E. (1963): Junctional complexes in various epithelia. J. Cell. Biol. *17*:375–412.
Frazier, H. S. (1962): The electrical potential profile of the isolated toad bladder. J. Gen. Physiol. *45*:515–528.
Frizzell, R. A., and Schultz, S. G. (1972): Ionic conductances of extracellular shunt pathway in rabbit ileum. J. Gen. Physiol. *59*:318–346.
Gall, D. G., Butler, D. G., Tepperman, F., and Hamilton, J. R. (1974): Sodium ion transport in isolated epithelial cells. The effect of actively transported sugars on sodium ion efflux. Biochim. Biophys. Acta *339*:291–302.

Geck, P., Heinz, E., and Pfeiffer, B. (1972): The degree and the efficiency of coupling between the influxes of Na⁺ and α-aminoisobutyrate in Ehrlich cells. Biochim. Biophys. Acta 288:486–491.

Gerencser, G. A., and Armstrong, W. McD. (1972): Sodium transfer in bullfrog small intestine—stimulation by exogenous ATP. Biochim. Biophys. Acta 255:663–674.

Gilles-Baillien, M., and Schoffeniels, E. (1965): Site of action of L-alanine and D-glucose on the potential difference across the intestine. Arch. Int. Physiol. Biochim. 73:355–357.

Gilles-Baillien, M., and Schoffeniels, E. (1966): Metabolic fate of L-alanine actively transported across the tortoise intestine. Life Sci. 5:2253–2255.

Goldner, A. M., Schultz, S. G., and Curran, P. F. (1969): Sodium and sugar fluxes across the mucosal border of rabbit ileum. J. Gen. Physiol. 53:362–383.

Heinz, E., editor (1972): *Na⁺-Linked transport of organic solutes,* Springer-Verlag, New York.

Heinz, E., and Geck, P. (1974): The efficiency of energetic coupling between Na⁺ flow and amino acid transport in Ehrlich cells—a revised assessment. Biochim. Biophys. Acta 339:426–431.

Hinke, J. A. M. (1970): Solvent water for electrolytes in the muscle fiber of the giant barnacle. J. Gen. Physiol. 56:521–541.

Hoshi, T., and Komatsu, Y. (1970): Effects of anoxia and metabolic inhibitors on the sugar-evoked potential and demonstration of sugar-outflow potential in toad intestine. Tohuko J. Exp. Med. 100:47–60.

Kimmich, G. A. (1970): Preparation and properties of mucosal epithelial cells isolated from small intestine of the chicken. Biochemistry 9:3659–3668.

Kimmich, G. A. (1970a): Active sugar accumulation by isolated intestinal epithelial cells. A new model for sodium-dependent metabolite transport. Biochemistry 9:3669–3677.

Kimmich, G. A. (1973): Coupling between Na⁺ and sugar transport in small intestine. Biochim. Biophys. Acta 300:31–78.

Kimmich, G. A., and Randles, J. (1973): Effect of K⁺ and K⁺ gradients on accumulation of sugar by isolated intestinal epithelial cells. J. Membrane Biol. 12:23–46.

Kimmich, G. A., and Randles, J. (1973a): Interaction between Na⁺-dependent transport systems for sugars and amino acids. Evidence against a role for the sodium gradient. J. Membrane Biol. 12:47–68.

Koopman, W., and Schultz, S. G. (1969): The effects of sugars and amino acids on mucosal Na⁺ and K⁺ concentrations in rabbit ileum. Biochim. Biophys. Acta 173:338–340.

McLaughlin, S. G. A., and Hinke, J. A. M. (1966): Sodium and water binding in single striated muscle fibers of the giant barnacle. Can. J. Physiol. Pharmacol. 44:837–848.

Lee, C. O., and Armstrong, W. McD. (1972): Activities of sodium and potassium ions in epithelial cells of small intestine. Science 175:1261–1264.

Lee, C. O., and Armstrong, W. McD. (1974): State and distribution of potassium and sodium ions in frog skeletal muscle. J. Membrane Biol. 15:331–362.

Lev, A. A., and Armstrong, W. McD. (*in press*): Ionic activities in cells. In: *Current Topics in Membranes and Transport,* edited by F. Bronner and A. Kleinzeller, Vol. 6, Academic Press, New York.

Loeschke, K, Bentzel, C. J., and Csaky, T. Z. (1970): Asymmetry of osmotic flow in frog intestine: functional and structural correlation. Am. J. Physiol. 218:1723–1731.

Lyon, I., and Crane, R. K. (1966): Studies on transmural potentials *in vitro* in relation to intestinal absorption. I. Apparent Michaelis constants for Na⁺ dependent sugar transport. Biochim. Biophys. Acta 112:278–291.

Lyon, I., and Sheerin, H. E. (1971): Studies on transmural potentials *in vitro* in relation to intestinal absorption. VI. The effect of sugars on electrical potential profiles in jejunum and ileum. Biochim. Biophys. Acta 249:1–14.

Machen, T. E., and Diamond, J. M. (1969): An estimate of the salt concentration in the lateral intercellular spaces of rabbit gall bladder during maximal fluid transport. J. Membrane Biol. 1:194–213.

Munck, B. G., and Schultz, S. G. (1974): Properties of the passive conductance pathway across *in vitro* rat jejunum. J. Membrane Biol. *16:*163–174.
Quay, J. F., and Armstrong, W. McD. (1969): Sodium and chloride transport by isolated bullfrog small intestine. Am. J. Physiol. *217:*694–702.
Quay, J. F., and Armstrong, W. McD. (1969a): Enhancement of net sodium transport in isolated bullfrog intestine by sugars and amino acids. Proc. Soc. Exp. Biol. Med. *131:*46–51.
Reiser, S., and Christiansen, P. A. (1971): Inhibition of amino acid uptake by ATP in isolated intestinal epithelial cells. Biochim. Biophys. Acta *233:*480–484.
Rose, R. C., and Schultz, S. G. (1970): Sugar and amino acid effects on the electric potential profile across rabbit ileum. Biochim. Biophys. Acta *211:*376–378.
Rose, R. C., and Schultz, S. G. (1971): Studies on the electrical potential profile across rabbit ileum. Effects of sugars and amino acids on transmural and transmucosal electrical potential differences. J. Gen. Physiol. *57:*639–663.
Sawada, M., and Asano, T. (1963): Effects of metabolic disturbances on potential difference across intestinal wall of rat. Am. J. Physiol. *204:*105–108.
Schultz, S. G. (1972): Electrical potential differences and electromotive forces in epithelial tissues. J. Gen. Physiol. *59:*794–798.
Schultz, S. G., and Curran, P. F. (1968): Intestinal absorption of sodium chloride and water. In: *Handbook of Physiology. Alimentary Canal.* Washington, D.C., Am. Physiol. Soc. Sect. 6, Vol. III, Chap. 66, pp. 1245–1275.
Schultz, S. G., and Curran, P. F. (1970): Coupled transport of sodium and organic solutes. Physiol. Rev. *50:*637–718.
Schultz, S. G., Curran, P. F., Chez, R. A., and Fuisz, R. E. (1967): Alanine and sodium fluxes across mucosal border of rabbit ileum. J. Gen. Physiol. *50:*1241–1260.
Schultz, S. G., Fuisz, R. E., and Curran, P. F. (1967): Amino acid and sugar transport in rabbit ileum. J. Gen. Physiol. *49:*849–866.
Schultz, S. G., and Zalusky, R. (1963): Transmural potential difference, short circuit current and sodium transport in isolated rabbit ileum. Nature *198:*894–895.
Schultz, S. G., and Zalusky, R. (1964): Ion transport in isolated rabbit ileum. I. Short circuit current and Na^+ fluxes. J. Gen. Physiol. *47:*567–584.
Schultz, S. G., and Zalusky, R. (1964a): Ion transport in isolated rabbit ileum. II. The interaction between active sodium and active sugar transport. J. Gen. Physiol. *48:*1043–1059.
Schultz, S. G., and Zalusky, R. (1965): Interactions between active sodium transport and active amino acid transport in isolated rabbit ileum. Nature *205:*292–294.
Smith, M. W. (1964): Electrical properties and glucose transfer in the goldfish intestine. Experientia *20:*613–614.
Smyth, D. H., and Wright, E. M. (1966): Streaming potentials in the rat small intestine. J. Physiol. *182:*591–602.
Taylor, A. E., Wright, E. M., Schultz, S. G., and Curran, P. F. (1968). Effects of sugars on ion fluxes in intestine. Am. J. Physiol. *214:*836–842.
Tucker, A. M., and Kimmich, G. A. (1973): Characteristics of amino acid accumulation by isolated intestinal epithelial cells. J. Membrane Biol. *12:*1–22.
Ussing, H. H., and Windhager, E. E. (1964): Nature of shunt path and active transport path through frog skin epithelium. Acta Physiol. Scand. *61:*484–504.
White, J. F., and Armstrong, W. McD. (1970): Membrane potentials in bullfrog small intestine. Biophys. Soc. Abstr. p. 36a.
White, J. F., and Armstrong, W. McD. (1971): Effect of transported solutes on membrane potentials in bullfrog small intestine. Am. J. Physiol. *221:*194–201.
Whittembury, G. (1964): Electrical potential profile of the toad skin epithelium. J. Gen. Physiol. *47:*795–808.
Windhager, E. E., Boulpaep, E. L., and Giebisch, G. (1966): Electrophysiological studies on single nephrons. Proceedings of the 3rd International Congress on Nephrology, Washington, D.C. *1:*35.
Wright, E. M. (1966): The origin of the glucose-dependent increase in the potential difference across the tortoise small intestine. J. Physiol *185:*486–500.

DISCUSSION

WADDELL asked whether sugars and sodium ions pass through the membrane in a dehydrated form, then pick up water on the other side, and could this account for the decrease in the activity of the solvent water. ARMSTRONG replied that it is entirely reasonable to assume that sodium and sugar can pass through the membrane without any water of hydration and that water goes through another pathway. As an example he quoted the case of the ionophores, which are nice models for membrane carriers, and which transport ions stripped of their layer of hydration as an anhydrous complex. At present no clear-cut evidence exists connecting sugars with this kind of dry transport but it would not be surprising should such evidence be found. CURRAN made a comment about the puzzling observation that it is difficult to detect an increase in intracellular sodium concentration in the presence of actively transported nonelectrolytes. It is known that the cells swell under these conditions. Measurements of potassium concentration and activity clearly indicate this. ARMSTRONG replied that a number of studies indicate a swelling of the cells when exposed to actively transported sugars or amino acids. He agrees with Csáky's interpretation that the reason one cannot see an increase in intracellular sodium concentration is that water goes in with the sugar or amino acid and "dilutes" the extra sodium which enters at the same time. Water entry is also the reason for the rather drastic drop in potassium concentration and activity under these conditions.

KESTON made the point that quite a few studies indicate to him that the sodium-gradient hypothesis should be completely dismissed. ARMSTRONG replied that his data are not really antagonistic to the sodium-gradient hypothesis although he is aware of several studies which claim to disprove this theory. He does not want to take sides on this issue mainly because, in the absence of information concerning the thermodynamic efficiency of the coupling between the transport of sodium and that of sugars and amino acids, his work does not permit any categorical conclusions on the role of the sodium gradient in nonelectrolyte transport. CURRAN will review this topic later in the volume.

Intestinal Transport of Monosaccharides

V. Capraro, G. Esposito, and A. Faelli

Istituto di Fisiologia Generale, Università di Milano, Milan, Italy

I. INTRODUCTION

Since the well-known experiments of Riklis and Quastel (1958) on the transmural transfer of sugars in the guinea pig small intestine incubated *in vitro* in a Ringer bicarbonate solution, it has been confirmed that the accumulation of sugars and amino acids in the enterocyte, as well as its active transport across the intestinal wall, are dependent on the presence of sodium in the intestinal lumen.

The sodium dependence was interpreted by Crane (1965) as being caused by the existence of a sodium-sugar coupled process across the brush border, in which a ternary complex of the carrier with the transported substance and sodium is reversibly formed. The affinity of the carrier for the transported substance is sodium dependent, and the energy for cell accumulation derives from the downhill entry of sodium into the cell (the sodium gradient hypothesis). As emphasized by Csáky (1963) and later by Esposito (1972), the sodium effect on the brush border seems to be nonspecific.

The exit of the transported substance at the serosal pole of the enterocyte was initially supposed to be a simple diffusion process. Recently, Curran (1973) put forward another hypothesis, i.e., the extrusion (of amino acids) across the basolateral membrane should be a chemically facilitated sodium-independent process.

This chapter argues in favor of the presence of an efficient sugar pump located in the basolateral membrane of the enterocyte.

II. METHODS

Albino male rats weighing 200 to 300 g (Charles River Co., Italy) and hamsters (*Mesocricetus auratus*) were used. Under urethane narcosis, the abdomen was opened, and the first part of the jejunum (10 cm) was cannulated at both ends taking care not to occlude observable vessels. A continuous perfusion (6 ml/hr) was carried out by a peristaltic pump (Buchler, Fort Lee, New Jersey). The tested solution, gassed with 95% O_2 and 5% CO_2 entering the cranial end of the intestine, was previously warmed at 37°C in a water bath. The perfusate was then collected via the caudal cannula in a graduated cylinder. The intestinal loop was warmed and moistened throughout the experiment; care was taken in order to maintain normal blood circulation.

The lumen perfusing solution was a Krebs-Henseleit bicarbonate solution with 2 mg % of phenol red (basic solution) added; phenol red is a suitable nonabsorbable compound used to detect dilution in perfusion studies. According to the set of experiments, the basic solution was added with D-glucose 5.5 mM or 3-O-methyl-D-glucose 5.15 mM with trace amounts of 3-O-^{14}CH$_3$-D-glucose.

In order to determine the serosal extracellular space *in vivo* (ECS) (Esposito, Faelli, and Capraro, 1972), trace amounts of ^{14}C-polyethylene glycol (^{14}C-PEG, New England Nuclear Corporation) was continuously infused into the jugular vein (infusion/withdrawal pump, Model 904, Harward Apparatus Co. Inc., Dover, Mass.). In 3-O-methyl glucose experiments, instead of ^{14}C-PEG trace amounts of ^{3}H-inulin (Radiochemical Center, Amersham, England) were continuously infused.

Together with 3-O-methyl glucose perfusion a concentrated solution of 3-O-methyl glucose was continuously infused into the jugular vein. The specific activity of the perfusing and infusing sugar solutions was always the same. In a group of experiments, trace amounts of ^{14}C-PEG and a concentrated glucose solution were continuously infused into the jugular vein in order to raise and maintain a high blood-sugar concentration. In a last set of experiments 3-O-methyl glucose (cold and labeled) or xylose (cold and labeled) was only infused into the jugular vein in order to reach and maintain throughout the experiment a serum sugar concentration of 4 to 5 mM. Experiments were performed for 30, 60, and 120 min in order to investigate whether both sugars could reach an equilibration between blood and cell compartments. After 30 min (or otherwise in the last set of experiments), the intestine was removed, cut along the mesenteric edge, blotted on filter paper, and the mucosal layer was scraped off at 0°C and weighed; cells were broken by osmotic shock, frozen, and thawed. After centrifuging the supernatant, the perfusing fluid and the blood serum were analyzed for sugars, electrolytes, and radioactivity. The perfusing fluid was also analyzed to determine the phenol red concentration. The scraped mucosal layer and the remaining part of the intestine were dried overnight to constant weight and then weighed.

Fluid, sugars, and sodium absorbed from the lumen were expressed in milliliters, micromoles, and microequivalents per gram of dry tissue weight of the intestine per hour. Intracellular concentrations of sugars and electrolytes are given in millimoles per liter of enterocyte water and are calculated assuming a complete equilibration of these substances between blood serum and serosal ECS. The *in vivo* mucosal ECS is very low, only 3 to 4% of the total tissue water (*unpublished data from this laboratory*). For further details concerning the above methods see Esposito et al. (1973).

The technique we have employed for in vitro experiments was the everted and cannulated jejunal tract of the intestine (Esposito and Csáky, 1974).

III. RESULTS AND DISCUSSION

As reported in the introductory remarks, the commonly accepted mechanism of net sugar transepithelial transport implies a cellular accumulation depending on a favorable sodium gradient and a subsequent, presumably chemically facilitated, diffusion at the basolateral enterocyte membrane. As to the latter point, our present investigations performed in *in vivo* conditions

TABLE 1. *Rat jejunum in vivo*

Lumen perfusing solution	Net sugar transepithelial transport (micromoles $g^{-1} hr^{-1}$)	Net sodium transepithelial transport (microequiv. $g^{-1} hr^{-1}$)
Krebs-Henseleit bicarbonate + glucose 4.1 mM (11)	122 ± 15	1,536 ± 172
Krebs-Henseleit bicarbonate + 3-O-methyl glucose 4.9 mM (6)	70 ± 5	1,358 ± 106

Sugar and sodium transepithelial transport in the rat jejunum perfused *in vivo*. Time of perfusion, 30 min. Sugar lumen concentration is the average between the concentration of sugar entering the lumen and the concentration of sugar collected in the graduated cylinder at the end of the experiment. Transport values are referred to 1 g of dry tissue weight. Values ± SEM. Number of experiments are reported in parentheses.

seem to allow the conclusion that there exists an active extrusion mechanism from the cell to the blood, so that the transepithelial sugar transport should be reinterpreted in a different way.

In the rat jejunum *in vivo*, notwithstanding a highly favorable sodium gradient (intraluminal sodium concentration 143 mM, enterocyte sodium concentration 21 mM) and a high transepithelial net transport (Table 1), there is no cell accumulation of sugars (Fig. 1), and an uphill movement of sugars toward the blood should take place. The apparent sugar concentration in the absorbed fluid is 11 mM for D-glucose and 7 mM for 3-O-methyl glucose. In the hamster jejunum *in vivo*, in addition to a highly favorable gradient (intraluminal sodium concentration 143 mM, enterocyte sodium concentration 24 mM) as in the rat, there is a cellular D-glucose accumulation (Fig. 2); the net transepithelial movement is lower than in the rat and should take place against a cell to blood sugar gradient (Table 2, Fig. 2).

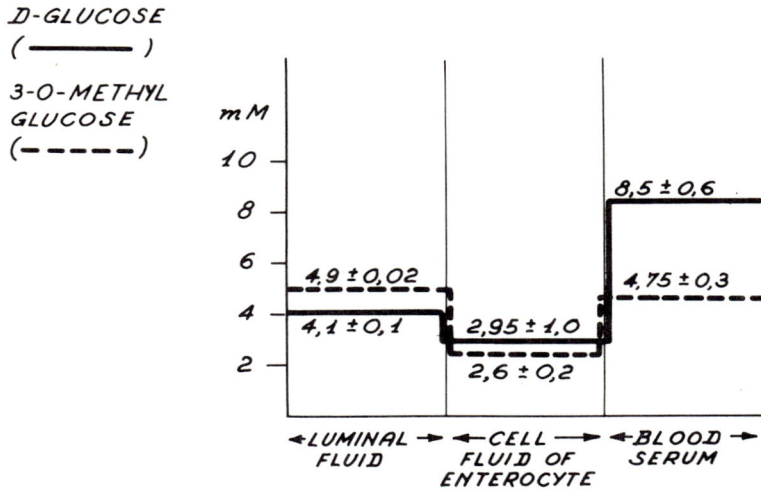

FIG. 1. Concentration profile of sugars (glucose or 3-O-methyl glucose) in lumen, enterocyte, and blood serum compartments of rat after 30 min of *in vivo* jejunal perfusion with a Krebs-Henseleit bicarbonate solution with sugar added.

These results suggest the conclusion that besides a sodium-sugar coupled mechanism across the brush border, which can sometimes produce a cell sugar accumulation (hamster), there is a pumping mechanism located at the basolateral membrane. The different behavior between the two species (rat and hamster) could be explained by a higher serum sugar concentration in the hamster, which hinders the extrusion from the cell into the blood; furthermore, there could be a lower efficiency of the basolateral sugar pump in the hamster jejunum in comparison with the rat jejunum. The lower efficiency results from the comparison of the *in vitro* behavior of the intestine of the two species (Table 3). In these conditions, notwithstanding the higher cell glucose concentration in the hamster intestine and the nearly equal glucose concentration in the serosal space in both species, the net glucose transepithelial transport is lower than in the rat intestine.

The hypothesis that the particular behavior of the hamster intestine is due to an underfunctioning of the sugar basolateral pump is further supported by the observation that by depressing the sugar pump in the rat a sugar enterocyte accumulation together with a lower sugar transport develops also in this species (Fig. 3, Table 4). The inhibition has been produced by increasing the blood sugar concentration. Some objections can now be raised against our data. One objection is that the calculated extracellular space is lower than the real one so that the sugar cell concentration could sometimes be overestimated. However, such an error seems to be negligible; a 20% increase of the extracellular space over our estimation should result in the worst condition in a calculated decrease of sugar cell concentration of only 5%. Another objection could arise from the histofunctional point of view

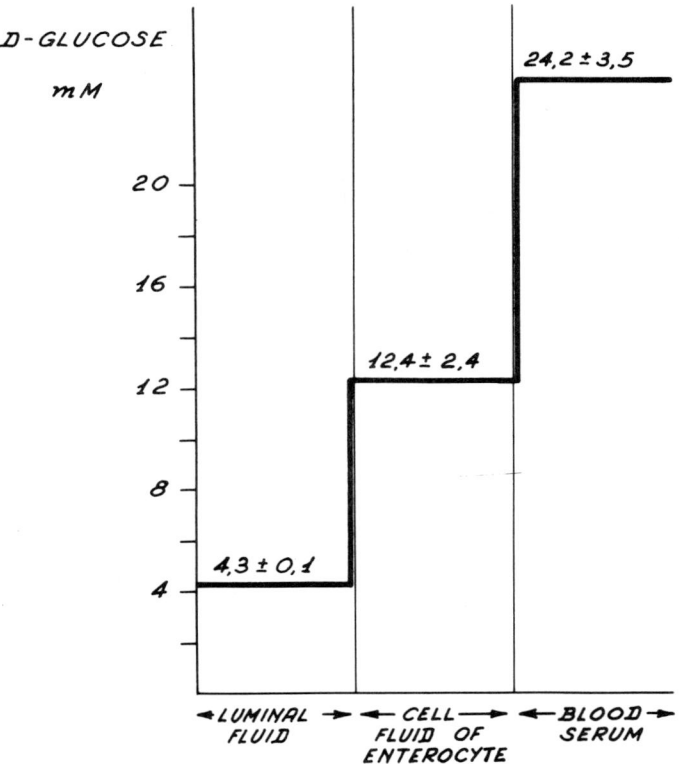

FIG. 2. Concentration profile of glucose in lumen, enterocyte, and blood serum compartments of hamster after 30 min of *in vivo* jejunal perfusion with a Krebs-Henseleit bicarbonate solution with glucose added.

TABLE 2. *Rat and hamster jejunum in vivo*

Lumen perfusing solution	Species	Glucose disappeared from the lumen (micromoles g^{-1} h^{-1})	Net sodium transepithelial transport (microequiv. g^{-1} hr^{-1})
Krebs-Henseleit bicarbonate + glucose 4.1 mM (11)	rat	180 ± 15	1,536 ± 172
Krebs-Henseleit bicarbonate + glucose 4.3 mM (6)	hamster	110 ± 10	405 ± 73

Sugar disappearing from the lumen and sodium transepithelial transport in the rat and hamster jejunum perfused *in vivo*. Time of perfusion 30 min. Sugar lumen concentration is the average between the concentration of sugar entering the lumen and the concentration of sugar collected in the graduated cylinder at the end of the experiment. Transport values are referred to 1 g of dry tissue weight. Values ± SEM. Number of experiments are reported in parentheses.

TABLE 3. *Rat and hamster jejunum in vitro* (28° C)

Lumen perfusing solution	Species	Cell glucose conc. (mM)	Serosal fluid glucose conc. (mM)	Net glucose transepithelial transp. (micromoles g^{-1} hr^{-1})	Net sodium transepithelial transp. (microequiv. g^{-1} hr^{-1})
Krebs-Henseleit bicarbonate + glucose 5.5 mM (5)	rat	7.24 ± 0.93	8.75 ± 0.62	144 ± 25	588 ± 54
Krebs-Henseleit bicarbonate + glucose 5.5 mM (6)	hamster	16.85 ± 1.17	7.92 ± 0.59	65 ± 14	337 ± 60

Cell and fluid sugar concentrations, sugar and sodium transepithelial transports in the rat and hamster jejunum incubated *in vitro*. Time of incubation 1 hr and temperature of incubation 28° C. Transport values are referred to 1 g of dry tissue weight and concentrations are referred to 1 liter water. Values ± SEM. Number of experiments are reported in parentheses.

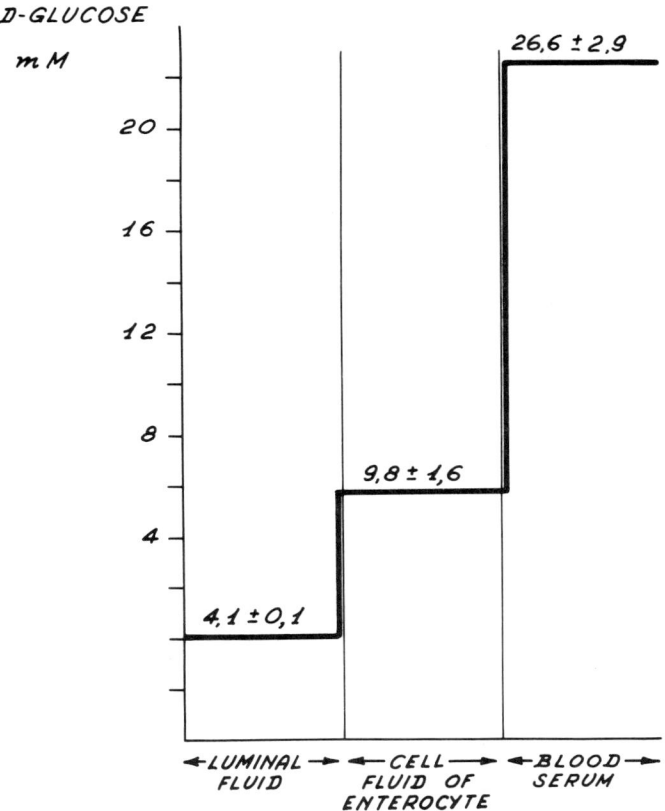

FIG 3. Concentration profile of glucose in lumen, enterocyte, and blood serum compartments of rat, after 30 min of in vivo jejunal perfusion with a Krebs-Henseleit bicarbonate solution with glucose added. In this case, a concentrated glucose solution was infused into the animal in order to increase the blood sugar concentration.

of the intestinal epithelium. Many cells of this epithelium are not absorbing cells; on the other hand, they are consuming glucose coming from the blood, and the glucose concentration in these cells may be very low. When we are perfusing the animal at a constant rate with 3-O-methyl glucose, which is not metabolized, a complete equilibration between serum and cell water should be expected in the absence of a sugar pump in the absorbing cells. This is not the case because a maximal sugar (cell)/sugar (serum) ratio of only 0.5 is reached after 1 hr of perfusion (Fig. 4). On the contrary, when the animal is perfused with xylose, which is characterized by a very low rate of intestinal absorption, a ratio close to one is found and a nearly complete equilibration is reached (Fig. 4). Also these results seem to suggest the hypothesis that the enterocyte is provided by a sugar pump located in the blood-facing membrane.

TABLE 4. *Rat jejunum in vivo*

Lumen perfusing solution	Blood sugar concentration	Glucose disappeared from the lumen (μmoles g^{-1} hr^{-1})	Net sodium transepithelial transp. (microequiv. g^{-1} hr^{-1})
Krebs-Henseleit bicarbonate + glucose 4.1 mM (11)	normal	180 ± 15	1,536 ± 172
Krebs-Henseleit bicarbonate + glucose 4.1 mM (5)	high	113 ± 14	966 ± 46

Sugar disappearing from the lumen and sodium transepithelial transport in jejunum perfused *in vivo* of rat at normal and high blood-sugar concentration. Time of perfusion, 30 min. Sugar lumen concentration is the average between the concentration of sugar entering the lumen and the concentration of sugar collected in the graduated cylinder at the end of the experiment. Transport values are referred to 1 g of dry tissue weight. Values ± SEM. Number of experiments are reported in parentheses.

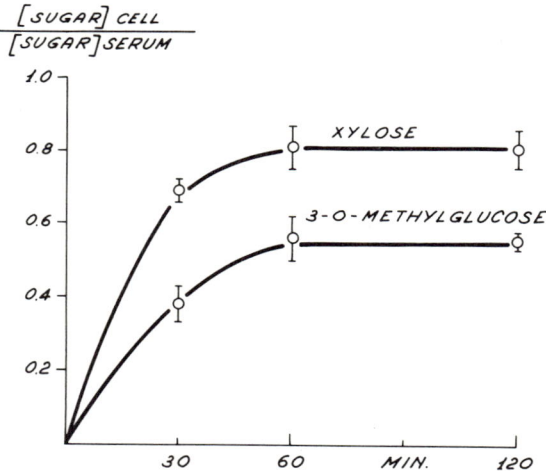

FIG. 4. Behavior of cell sugar concentration/serum sugar concentration ratio throughout 2 hr of infusion in the rat with a 3-O-methyl glucose or xylose solution at a concentration sufficient to maintain a serum concentration of 4 to 5 mM.

IV. CONCLUSIONS

The mechanism that can be suggested for *in vivo* intestinal absorption of sugars implies two chemically dependent steps: a sodium-sugar coupled entry across the brush border, which allows an increased rate of absorption and is not necessarily followed by a sugar cell accumulation, and a second step of sugar pumping, which allows an uphill movement of sugars from the cell to the blood. An increased capacity of concentrating sugars in the blood is thus reached, which in theory is equal to the product of the two single capacities of the brush border and of the basolateral membrane of the enterocyte.

REFERENCES

Crane, R. K. (1965): Na^+-dependent transport in the intestine and other animal tissues. Fed. Proc. *24:*1000–1006.
Csáky, T. Z. (1963): A possible link between active transport of electrolytes and non-electrolytes. Fed. Proc. *22:*3–7.
Curran, P. F. (1973): Amino acid transport in intestine. *Transport Mechanism in Epithelia,* Munksgaard, Copenhagen.
Esposito, G. (1972): A sodium-dependent, noncarrier-mediated transport of passively diffusing substances through the intestinal wall. Hoppe-Seyler's Zeitschr. Physiol. Chemie *353:*3.
Esposito, G., Faelli, A., and Capraro, V. (1972): The extracellular space of rat intestine *in vivo*. Pfluegers Arch. *331:*70–76.
Esposito, G., Faelli, A., and Capraro, V. (1973): Sugar and electrolyte absorption in the rat intestine perfused *in vivo*. Pfluegers Arch. *340:*335–348.
Esposito, G., and Csáky, T. Z. (1974): Extracellular space in the epithelium of the rat's small intestine. Am. J. Physiol. *226:*50–55.
Riklis, E., and Quastel, J. H. (1958): Effects of cations on sugar absorption by isolated surviving guinea pig intestine. Comp. Biochem. Physiol. *36:*347–361.

DISCUSSION

FARMANFARMAIAN questioned the measurement of extracellular space *in vivo*. CAPRARO replied that they determined the serosal extracellular space but not the mucosal because in the rat the mucosal extracellular space *in vivo* is very little, only about 3 to 4% of the total extracellular space. This is different from the *in vitro* condition when the extracellular space on both sides of the epithelium is approximately equal.

Someone else commented that in the hamster under *in vivo* conditions the extracellular space measured by inulin on the mucosal side is about one-third of that on the serosal side. CAPRARO replied that they did all the experiments in the rat and the difference could be due to variations between different species.

KESTON commented that, in case of the intestinal sugar absorption, attention should be paid to the particular anomeric forms which are present in various compartments, quoting an experiment in which it was shown that, if the gut is exposed to 3-O-methyl glucose in one anomeric form, the mutarotated mixture will be found within the intestinal cell. CAPRARO replied that, although such a possibility cannot be excluded, they did not examine in particular the effect of possible mutarotation on the transport of glucose or 3-O-methyl glucose.

Intestinal Absorption and Malabsorption,
edited by T. Z. Csáky.
Raven Press, New York © 1975

Amino Acid Transport by the Small Intestine

Stanley G. Schultz and Raymond A. Frizzell

Department of Physiology, University of Pittsburgh, School of Medicine, Pittsburgh, Pennsylvania 15261

I. INTRODUCTION

The ability of *in vitro* preparations of the small intestine to actively transport many amino acids from the mucosal solution to the serosal solution and to actively accumulate amino acids within the absorptive epithelium has been recognized for many years (Wiseman, 1968). Further, it is now well established that both active transepithelial transport and intracellular accumulation of amino acids are abolished in the absence of Na (Schultz and Curran, 1970). However, it should be clear from Fig. 1 that the location, properties,

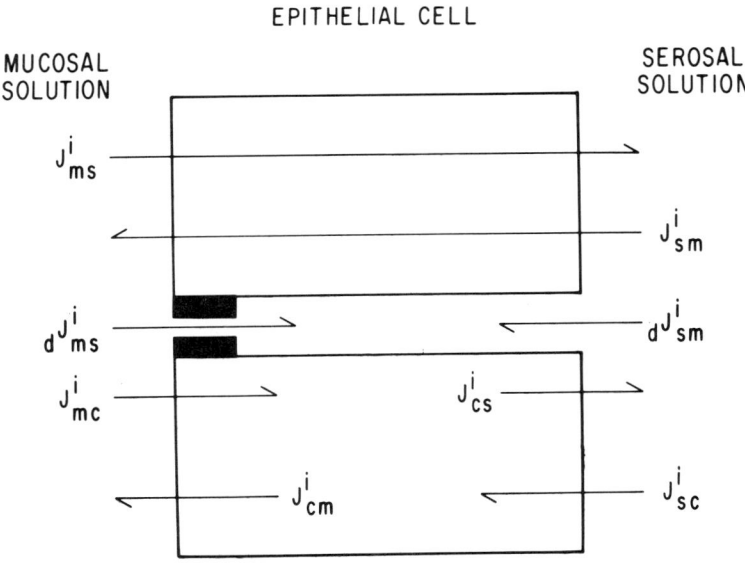

FIG. 1. Unidirectional movements of a solute, *i*, across the small intestinal epithelium, the mucosal and serosal membranes, and through the extracellular pathway. The subscripts *m*, *c*, and *s* designate the mucosal solution, intracellular compartment, and serosal solution, respectively. $J_{kj}{}^i$ designates the movement of species *i* (which in this paper will be represented by superscript A denoting amino acids) from compartment *k* to compartment *j*. The subscript *d* represents diffusional movements through the extracellular pathway.

and specificities of the mechanisms responsible for these phenomena cannot be deduced from studies of net transepithelial movements, bidirectional transepithelial fluxes, or intracellular accumulation alone, because the latter are the composite results of bidirectional movements across the mucosal (J_{mc}^A and J_{cm}^A) and serosal (J_{cs}^A and J_{sc}^A) limiting membranes; further transepithelial fluxes may be influenced by diffusional movements through extracellular shunt pathways. It follows that any attempt to elucidate the mechanisms responsible for the active transport of amino acids by the small intestine must be aimed at defining the individual characteristics of the transport of specific amino acids across the mucosal membrane, across the serosal membrane, and through the shunt pathway. The purpose of this communication is to summarize briefly the current status of our knowledge with respect to these three determinants of amino acid absorption by the small intestine.

II. AMINO ACID TRANSPORT ACROSS THE MUCOSAL MEMBRANES

Most of the information regarding the characteristics of the brush border transport mechanisms for amino acids has been derived from investigations on *in vitro* rabbit ileum. Studies of the unidirectional influxes of a number of amino acids from the mucosal solution across the mucosal membranes and into the epithelium (J_{mc}^A) have indicated that these processes conform reasonably well to a relatively simple kinetic model (Curran, Schultz, Chez, and Fuisz, 1967; Schultz and Curran, 1970). The central experimental observations underlying this model are (a) in the absence of Na, J_{mc}^A appears to be carrier-mediated inasmuch as it is a saturable function of the concentration of the amino acid in the mucosal solution, $[A]_m$, and subject to competitive inhibition; (b) increasing the Na concentration in the mucosal solution, $[Na]_m$, does not affect the maximal influx of this saturable process but progressively decreases the K_t, (the concentration of the amino acid necessary to elicit a half-maximal influx); (c) J_{mc}^A is not significantly affected by depletion of intracellular Na or by preloading the cells with the amino acid; (d) an increase in amino acid influx is associated with an increase in Na influx and the coupling coefficient ($\Delta J_{mc}^A/\Delta J_{mc}^{Na}$) is a function of $[Na]_m$; and (e) the influx process is reversible and can mediate the coupled efflux of alanine and Na (Curran, Hajjar, and Glynn, 1970; Hajjar, Lamont, and Curran, 1970).

The simplest kinetic model consistent with these experimental observations is one in which the amino acid (A) interacts with a membrane component or "carrier site" (X) to form a binary complex (XA). This complex may either translocate across the brush border and discharge the amino acid within the cell *or* it may combine with Na to form a ternary complex (XANa) which then translocates across the membrane and discharges both Na and A into the cell interior. The underlying assumptions and solution of this kinetic model have been discussed in detail (Curran et al., 1967) and will not be further elaborated upon. Two of the predictions of this model are that

$$J_{mc}^A = J_{mc}^{Amax} [A]_m/(K_t + [A]_m), \qquad (1)$$

and

$$K_t = (K_1 K_2)/(K_2 + [Na]_m), \qquad (2)$$

where $J_{mc}^A{}_{max}$ is the maximal influx; K_1 is the dissociation constant for the reaction $[A + X \rightleftharpoons XA]$ and K_2 is the dissociation constant for the reaction $[NA + XA \rightleftharpoons XANa]$. Thus, $1/K_1$ is the affinity for binding of the amino acid to the carrier site to form a binary complex and $1/K_2$ is the affinity for the binding of Na to the binary complex to form the ternary complex. Clearly, K_1 and K_2 can be calculated from kinetic studies of J_{mc}^A vs $[A]_m$ as a function of $[Na]_m$ employing Eqs. (1) and (2); these values, within the framework of this model, permit inferences regarding amino acid structure and charge that influence the binding of the amino acid to the transport site and the subsequent binding of Na to the binary complex.

A. Factors that Influence the Binding Affinity for the Amino Acid ($1/K_1$)

There are six factors that appear to influence the ability of a given amino acid to interact with *its* carrier site at the brush border:[1] (a) the α-carboxylate group; (b) the α-amino group; (c) the α-hydrogen atom; (d) the structure of the side chain; (e) the stereoisomeric form;[2] and (f) the net charge. The role of these factors will be discussed in sequence.

(a) Schultz, Yu-Tu, and Strecker (1972) found that the unidirectional influx of β-phenethylamine, which differs from L-phenyalanine only by the replacement of the α-carboxylate group with a H atom is a linear function of concentration and is not inhibited by a 20-fold greater concentration of L-phenylalanine. Further, 40-mM phenethylamine did not affect the unidirectional influx of phenylalanine at concentrations of 0.1 and 1 mM. These authors concluded that replacement of the α-carboxylate group with a H atom prevented binding of the amino acid to the carrier site responsible for phenylalanine influx and, more important, that phenethylamine is not trans-

---

[1] There is good reason to believe that there are separate transport mechanisms for neutral, basic, and acidic amino acids and imino acids in the small intestine that display overlapping specificities at least with respect to the ability of an amino acid from one group to inhibit the transport of amino acids from other groups. Furthermore, Schultz and Markscheid-Kaspi (1971) have presented evidence that there may be more than one influx mechanism for neutral amino acids across the brush border of the rabbit ileum. Thus, throughout this chapter we will refer to the movements of a given amino acid by *its transport mechanism or mechanisms* without inferring that the same mechanisms are involved in the movements of other amino acids.

[2] Throughout this chapter we will refer to the L-stereoisomeric form of the amino acid unless otherwise noted.

ported by the phenylalanine influx mechanism. In contrast, Hajjar and Curran (1970) reported that phenethylamine inhibits phenylalanine influx across the brush border and calculated that its affinity for the transport site is at least 12 times lower than that of phenylalanine; the K_1 for phenylalanine is approximately 18 mM, whereas the minimal K_1 for phenethylamine was estimated to be 229 mM. These authors did not investigate the influx of phenethylamine or the effect of phenylalanine on this movement.

Finally, Hajjar and Curran (1970) provided evidence that the negative charge of the α-carboxylate group may not be the essential characteristic for binding inasmuch as the phosphonic acid analogue of phenylalanine was a very poor inhibitor of phenylalanine influx, whereas phenylalanine-methyl-ester was a very strong inhibitor. Thus, the essential component of the carboxylate group may be the —C=O group; however, direct studies on the influx of phenylalanine-methyl-ester are necessary to determine whether this inhibitor is also transported by the mechanism responsible for phenylalanine influx.

(b) Schultz et al. (1972) found that the unidirectional influxes (J^A_{mc}) of hydrocinnamic acid (β-phenylpropionic acid, which differs from phenylalanine only by the absence of the α-amino group) and phenylacetic acid (an analogue of phenylglycine which differs from phenylalanine by the absence of the α-amino group and one methyl group in the side chain) are linear functions of concentration and are unaffected by the presence of phenylalanine at a 20-fold greater concentration. Furthermore neither of these compounds significantly affect phenylalanine influx. Again these results differ from those reported by Hajjar and Curran (1970) who found that phenylpropionic acid inhibited phenylalanine influx but that its affinity for the carrier site was 50 times lower than that of phenylalanine ($K_1 = 870$ mM).

Thus, there are some discrepancies regarding the effect of replacement of the α-carboxylate group or α-amino group with a H atom on phenylalanine influx across the brush border but these may be of secondary importance with respect to the principal question of the *requirements for amino acid transport*. Hajjar and Curran (1970) reported that phenethylamine and phenylpropionic acid competitively inhibit phenylalanine influx whereas no inhibition was observed by Schultz et al. (1972); the origin of this discrepancy is uncertain. But, perhaps more important, in the experiments reported by Schultz et al. (1972) the unidirectional influxes of phenethylamine, phenylpropionic acid, and phenylacetic acid were determined directly and where shown to be unaffected by high concentrations of phenylalanine; if these solutes were *transported* by the brush border carrier mechanism responsible for phenylalanine influx, a marked inhibition of influx should have been observed when the concentration of phenylalanine exceeded that of the analogue by a factor of 20.

In short, the available direct data strongly suggest that the influxes of phenethylamine, phenylpropionic acid, and phenylacetic acid are entirely the results of simple diffusion; whether or not they interact weakly with the phenylalanine carrier site is uncertain. Thus, it appears that replacement of *either* the α-carboxylate group or the α-amino group with a H atom prevents influx via the mechanism(s) responsible for phenylalanine influx so that the binding energies resulting from the interaction of these two α-groups with the phenylalanine carrier site are not additive but are cooperative; that is, there is an "all or none effect."

(c) The importance of the α-H atom in amino acid influx across the mucosal membranes has not been examined directly. Preston et al. (1974) reported that α-methyl methionine is a poor inhibitor of methionine influx and calculated that substitution of an α-methyl group for the α-H atom reduces the affinity of the analogue by a factor of 10. In view of the fact that the α-H atom is not likely to be very reactive this marked reduction in affinity is probably a consequence of steric factors. However, once again, studies on the influx of this analogue are necessary in order to determine whether it is transported by the methionine influx mechanism or whether it is simply a nontransported inhibitor. It is certainly feasible that a competitive inhibitor can result in an "abortive complex" which is incapable of translocation so that the demonstration of competitive inhibition (particularly in a complex system that is Na-dependent) does not necessarily imply that the inhibitor is also transported. For example, any substance that impairs the binding of Na would behave like a competitive inhibitor in spite of the fact that it may not interact with the amino acid binding site (see below and Schultz, 1969).

(d) The role of the amino acid side chain in influx across the mucosal membranes has been examined directly for glycine, alanine, valine, leucine, and phenylalanine, and the results strongly suggest that the affinity for binding ($1/K_1$) increases with increasing hydrophobicity of the side chain. This is illustrated in Fig. 2 where $1/K_1$ is plotted against the molecular weights of the neutral amino acids. The slope of the line is consistent with the notion that the addition of the equivalent of one methyl group increases the standard free energy of binding by 220 cal/mole, a value somewhat lower than that expected for strict hydrophobic bonding (Nemethy and Scheraga, 1962). However, from the values of K_1 (Table 1) it can be shown that the increase in standard free energy of binding resulting from the addition of one methyl group to glycine is 400 cal/mole, a value that is in excellent agreement with those reported for hydrophobic interactions. The increase in free energy of binding from valine to phenylalanine is less than that predicted for strict hydrophobic interactions. This may be attributed to the fact that partition coefficients of branched amino acids even into bulk lipids is lower than that of molecules with straight chains (England and Cohn, 1935) and that this reduction in hydrophobicity due to branching of the side chain is even more marked for the case of passive permeation of lipid soluble molecules across organized biological membranes (see discussion by Diamond and Wright, 1969). In addition, as discussed by Preston et al. (1974) steric factors may

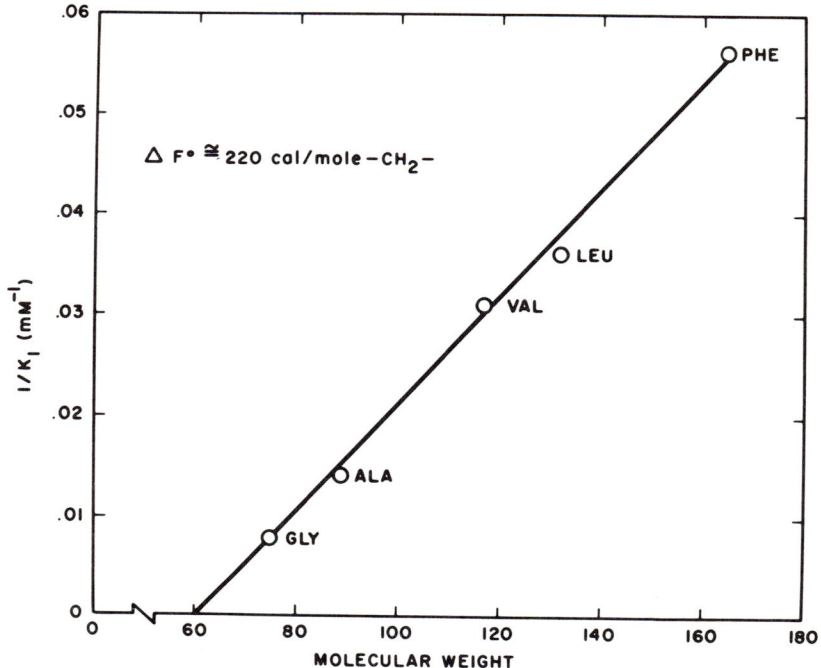

FIG. 2. Relation between $1/K_1$ and the molecular weights of five neutral amino acids (from Schultz and Curran, 1970).

restrict the ability of the hydrophobic region of the carrier site from fully accommodating branched or ring side chains.

Hajjar and Curran (1970) reported that the ability of analogues of phenylalanine with para-additions on the benzene ring to inhibit phenylalanine influx is increased if the added group possesses electron-withdrawing power (thereby rendering the ring more hydrophobic) but is decreased by electron-

TABLE 1. *Kinetic parameters for L-amino acid influxes*

Amino Acid	K_1 (mM)	K_2 (mM)
Glycine	125	25
Alanine	70	17
Valine	32	23
Leucine	29	24
Phenylalanine	18	25
Lysine	35	56
Glutamic acid	95	12
Aspartic acid	75	9

From Schultz, Yu-Tu, Alvarez, and Curran (1970); references to the sources of the original data are given in that paper.

releasing groups (which render the ring less hydrophobic); indeed, analogues containing electron-withdrawing groups such as -NO$_2$ and -Cl appear to have a greater affinity for the carrier site than phenylalanine itself and the reverse is the case for analogues containing electron-releasing groups such as -OH and -NH$_2$. Finally, Preston et al. (1974) have demonstrated that the ability of a number of amino acids to inhibit methionine influx is directly related to their octanol/water partition coefficients.

Thus, there appears to be little doubt that for the case of the neutral amino acids that have been investigated to date, the affinities for binding to their carrier sites and subsequent influx appear to be directly related to the hydrophobicity of the side chain.

TABLE 2. Kinetic parameters for L- and D- amino acid influxes

Amino Acid	L-Form		D-Form		
	J_{mc}^{Amax}	K_t	J_{mc}^{Amax}	K_t	K_1
Alanine	12	9	12	100	290
Valine	10	7	∞	∞	∞
Serine	12	12	12	20	38
Leucine	6	6	8	24	69
Phenylalanine	6	3.5	5	25	54
Tryptophan	8	6	8	32	62

J_{mc}^{Amax} is in μmoles/cm^2 hr; K_t and K_1 are in mM. Data from Schultz et al. (1972). Values of K_1 for L-amino acids are given in Table 1.

(e) Schultz et al. (1972) determined the influxes of the D-stereoisomers of alanine, valine, serine, leucine, phenylalanine, and tryptophan across the mucosal membranes of rabbit ileum. With the exception of D-valine, the influxes of these D-amino acids appear to be carrier-mediated, subject to classical competitive inhibition by their L-enantiomorphs, and Na-dependent. The influx of D-valine appears to be largely, if not entirely, attributable to simple diffusion, inasmuch as it is a linear function of concentration, is not significantly inhibited by L-valine, and is not significantly affected by removal of Na from the mucosal solution. The kinetic data for the L- and D-enantiomorphs obtained in this study are summarized in Table 2. It should be noted that in all instances, with the exception of D-valine, there is good agreement between the maximal influxes of the stereoisomers but that the K_t of the D-form significantly exceeds that of the L-form. Examination of the values for K_1 of the D-enantiomorphs indicates that stereospecificity is least marked for leucine, phenylalanine, and tryptophan, amino acids with bulky hydrocarbon side chains. Further, D-serine displays a much greater affinity than D-alanine, suggesting that the ability of the side chain to engage in hydrogen bonding is advantageous compared to the less reactive methyl group. Finally, the finding that D-valine has no detectable affinity for the carrier site suggests that β-branching of the side chain interferes with binding of this stereoisomer.

In view of the evidence that binding of both the α-carboxylate and α-amino groups is essential for amino acid influx, these findings suggest that when the D-enantiomorph binds to the carrier site the *mean* position of the β-carbon is displaced by 180° from the mean position assumed by the β-carbon of the more preferred L-enantiomorph, and that the affinity of the D-amino acid for the carrier site is determined by the ability of the displaced side chain to interact with neighboring groups. A similar model has been proposed for D-amino acid transport by Ehrlich ascites tumor cells (Oxender, 1965).

(f) The net charge of the amino acid appears to have a profound effect on its affinity for its carrier site. For example, both glutamic acid and aspartic acid form exceedingly weak interactions with their carrier site (the K_1 for glutamic acid is approximately 95 mM and that for aspartic acid is approximately 75 mM). In contrast, the positively charged amino acid lysine forms a relatively stable binary complex; its K_1 is 35 mM and thus compares favorably with valine and leucine (Table 1).

The possible implications of these findings will be discussed below.

B. Factors that Influence the Affinity of Na for the Binary Complex

1. *The Role of Anionic Groups*

A mechanistic interpretation of the kinetic model described by Curran et al. (1967) for amino acid influx across the brush border of the rabbit ileum is that the amino acid must bind to its carrier site first to form a binary complex and that this, in turn, permits the subsequent binding of Na thereby forming a ternary complex; that is to say, the binding of the amino acid somehow "creates" a configuration that has an affinity for Na (Schultz, 1969). Frizzell and Schultz (1970) demonstrated that in the presence of Na, alanine influx is inhibited by H, K, and Li, and kinetic analyses indicate that H and K behave as strict competitive inhibitors thus mimicking the effect of reducing $[Na]_m$. In the absence of Na, Li has a slight stimulatory effect on alanine influx but H and K are ineffective. Further, the data are consistent with the notion that the effect of H is a consequence of protonation of an anionic group with a pK_a of approximately 3.5; both carboxylate groups and phosphoryl residues would satisfy these findings.

Two models have been proposed to account for these findings (Frizzell and Schultz, 1970). The simplest and more attractive "single site model" is illustrated in Fig. 3. According to this model, *prior* to the binding of the amino acid the sequence of cation affinities for binding to the anionic group(s) is H > K > Rb > Li >> Na, Cs. This sequence corresponds closely to Eisenman's sequence IV (Eisenman, 1961) and describes an anionic field strength of intermediate intensity. However, if the amino acid binds to the carrier site (X) first, a conformational change occurs which alters the cation selectivity of the anionic group(s) so that the sequence of affinities is Na $\gg$ Li $\gg$ other cations. The latter sequence is consistent with Eisenman's sequence X (Eisenman, 1961) which corresponds to an anionic field strength of high intensity. This model is consistent with the kinetic data obtained by Frizzell and Schultz (1970) and may be considered in terms of the "induced fit" model suggested by Koshland (1964) in that the Na binding site may be viewed as existing in two possible states or conformations, a H-preferring state and a Na-preferring state. The transition from the former to the latter is brought about by the binding of the amino acid. Finally, the finding that low concentrations of La^{+++} and UO_2^{++}, agents that react strongly with carboxylate and phosphate groups, inhibit alanine influx in the presence of Na but not in its absence support the involvement of

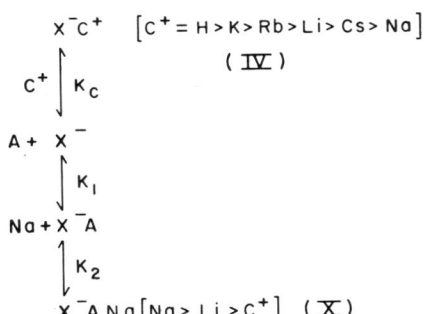

FIG. 3. Model for cation interactions with the alanine influx mechanism at the brush border of the rabbit ileum. A, X, and C designate alanine, the alanine carrier site, and other cations, respectively. K_c is the dissociation constant for the interaction between C and X. The sequences given in brackets represent the affinities of X and XA for the monovalent cations studied. The Roman numerals in parentheses indicate the corresponding cation sequences defined by Eisenman (1961). For further discussion of this model see Frizzell and Schultz (1970).

one or both of these groups in creating the anionic field and site responsible for Na binding to the binary complex (Frizzell and Schultz, 1970).

Schaeffer, Preston, and Curran (1973) reported that p-chloromercuriphenyl sulfonate (PCMBS) markedly inhibits phenylalanine, methionine, and alanine influxes across the brush border of the rabbit ileum. This effect is rapidly and completely reversed by ditriothreitol suggesting that the primary effect of PCMBS is on membrane sulfhydryl groups. Of particular interest is that, in the presence of PCMBS, phenylalanine influx is a saturable function of the amino acid concentration in the mucosal solution, that the K_t of the influx process is increased whereas the maximal influx is unaffected, and that although PCMBS somewhat reduces the affinity of the amino acid for its binding site its major effect is to substantially decrease the affinity of the transport site for Na (i.e., K_2 is markedly increased). Frizzell and Schultz (1970) also found that 10^{-3} M Hg^{++} or Ag^+ which reacts with sulfhydryl groups has a significantly greater inhibitory effect on alanine influx in the presence of Na than in its absence. Although the interpretation of these findings must remain speculative until more is known concerning the molecular nature of the carrier site, the data are consistent with (a) a direct involvement of sulfhydryl groups in the Na-binding site, and/or (b) the prevention of the conformational change necessary for forming the Na-binding site by these sulfhydryl binding agents. Finally, the observations of Schaeffer et al. (1973) verify the point that a competitive inhibitor of amino acid influx need not exert its effect by interacting with the amino acid binding site. Instead, as discussed by Schultz (1969), any agent that impairs the ability of the binary complex to bind Na would display the characteristics of a competitive inhibitor.

2. *The Nature of the Translocation Process*

Studies on amino acid uptake by Ehrlich ascites tumor cells have indicated that the uptake of amino acids coupled to the uptake of Na is accompanied by an extrusion of cellular K (Schultz and Curran, 1970). This observation suggested that the overall process of net amino acid influx may involve an obligatory exchange of Na for K mediated by the amino acid transport mechanism. Recent studies have demonstrated that the addition of actively transported amino acids to the mucosal solution results in a prompt depolarization of the electrical potential difference across the mucosal membrane (i.e., the cell interior becomes electrically more positive) (Rose and Schultz, 1971; White and Armstrong, 1971). These findings strongly suggest that the coupled Na-amino acid entry is rheogenic and does not involve an obligatory one-for-one exchange of Na for K (and/or another cation, e.g., H). These observations suggest the following:

(a) The extrusion of K by ascites cells in the presence of actively accumulated amino acids may be entirely nonspecific and may be simply the result of a decrease in intracellular negativity leading to an increased driving force for K diffusion out of the cell.

(b) Any Na-solute–coupled influx process that is rheogenic will be influenced by the electrical-potential difference across the membrane. Vidaver (1964) provided evidence that the electrical-potential difference across the membrane of pigeon erythrocytes influences Na-coupled glycine accumulation. Subsequently, Gibb and Eddy (1972) demonstrated that amino acid uptake by ascites tumor cells is markedly enhanced by treatment of the cells with valinomycin which renders the membrane readily permeable to K and presumably increases intracellular negativity; similar findings have been reported by Murer and Hopfer (1974) with respect to glucose uptake by brush border vesicles prepared from the rat small intestine.

Although a discussion of the ion-gradient hypothesis with respect to the active accumulation and absorption of amino acids by the small intestine is beyond the scope of this communication, one point is worthy of mention. If, in general, coupled–Na-amino acid influx mechanisms are rheogenic, *all* ion gradients and rheogenic transport processes that contribute to the transmembrane electrical-potential difference (PD) will influence influx, efflux, and accumulation. For example, the K-gradient need not affect amino acid transport through a direct interaction with the transport mechanism but could indirectly affect transport by influencing the transmembrane PD (the same would be true for all ion gradients that contribute to this PD). Further, if the energy-dependent active Na-K pump is rheogenic, as appears to be the case for the rabbit ileum (Rose and Schultz, 1971; Frizzell and Schultz, 1972; Schultz, 1973), it will directly contribute to the transmembrane PD and add to the contribution due to ionic gradients. Under these circumstances the use of poisoned cells and artificially established ion gradients may not be appropriate for testing the ion-gradient hypothesis. These considerations, together with the increasing evidence that overall intracellular Na concentrations overestimate the cytoplasmic Na activity due to possible binding as well as compartmentalization within nuclei (Terry and Vidaver, 1973), preclude a definitive conclusion regarding the adequacy of the ion-gradient hypothesis for active amino acid transport by epithelial as well as nonepithelial cells pending further investigation.

(c) Numerous studies have demonstrated that nonmetabolized, actively transported sugars inhibit active amino acid transport and *vice versa;* however, the underlying mechanism remains a subject of debate (Robinson and Alvarado, 1971). A possible explanation for this phenomenon is that any coupled Na-solute (amino acid or sugar) influx process that is rheogenic and causes depolarization of the PD across the mucosal membrane will, in turn, inhibit the unidirectional influx and/or accelerate the unidirectional efflux of any other rheogenic Na-coupled transport process across that membrane. A quantitative test of this hypothesis depends upon assumptions regarding the translocation mechanism and presents formidable experimental obstacles.

(d) It seems likely that the model suggested by Curran et al. (1967) must be modified to accommodate the possibility that the translocation constants (P) for the free "carrier" (X), the binary complex (XA), and the ternary complex ($XANa$) are not equal, in view of the fact that Na-coupled alanine influx is rheogenic whereas carrier-mediated alanine influx in the absence of Na is not (Rose and Schultz, 1971). It follows that the translocation constants for the bidirectional movements of X and XA, for the case of neutral amino acids, will not equal that for the ternary complex ($XANa$) when there is a significant PD across the mucosal membranes. Once again, any attempt to incorporate the effects of the PD across the mucosal membranes into kinetic models would require assumptions regarding the mechanism of translocation, the electrical-potential profile or potential-energy barriers across the membrane, etc. The fact that much of the data on the amino acid influx conforms reasonably well with the model suggested by Curran et al. (1967), within the limits of experimental error, suggests that inequalities in the translocation constants due to the transmembrane PD may be of secondary importance. However, further investigation is needed to resolve this issue.

C. The Effect of Amino Acid Charge on the Binding Affinity for Na

As discussed above, the binding affinities of neutral amino acids for their carrier sites is significantly influenced by the hydrophobicity of the side chain. At the same time, the complex between the cationic amino acid lysine and its carrier site has a relatively high stability, whereas the complexes between the anionic amino acids glutamic and aspartic acids and their carrier site(s) have very low stabilities.

The affinities for Na ($1/K_2$) of the binary complexes formed between several neutral, basic, and acidic amino acids with their carrier sites are given in Table 1. It is clear that in spite of the fact that K_1 for neutral amino acids ranges between 18 and 125 mM, the K_2's for these amino acids do not differ significantly and are approximately 20 to 25 mM. On the other hand, K_2 for lysine is approximately twice that of the neutral amino acids, whereas the K_2's for the anionic amino acids do not differ markedly and are approximately one-half that of the neutral amino acids. Thus, the binding of lysine to its carrier site forms a relatively stable binary complex that has a

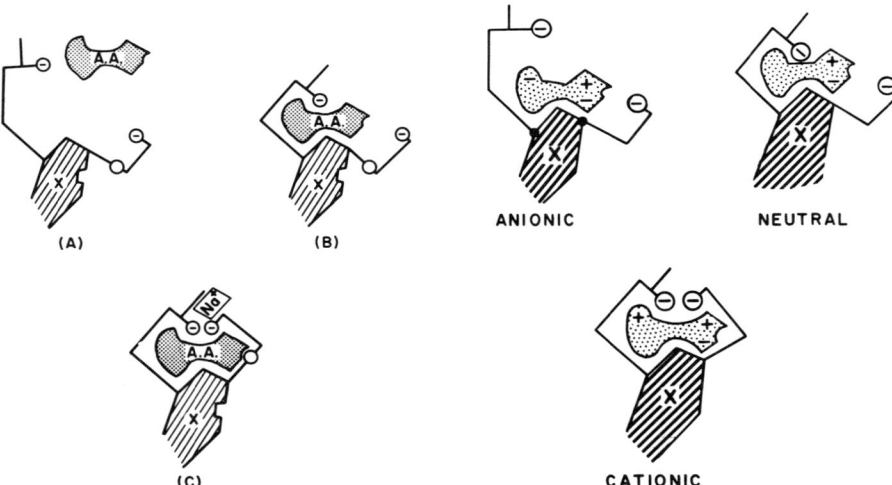

FIG. 4. Schematic illustration of the interaction between an amino acid and its binding site and the subsequent binding of Na. (Left) Sequences (A–C) depict the binding of the amino acid that results in a conformational change of mobile fixed anionic groups and the subsequent binding of Na. (Right) The effect of amino acid charge on the conformational changes involving fixed anionic groups which influence both K_1 and K_2. For further discussion of this mechanistic model see Schultz (1969) and Schultz et al. (1970). (Reproduced by permission of the Rockefeller University Press.)

relatively low affinity for Na, whereas the binding of anionic amino acids results in unstable complexes that have high affinities for the subsequent binding of Na.

Although these observations may be attributable to structural differences between the carrier sites for neutral, cationic, and anionic amino acids, a simpler explanation may be entertained. In view of the evidence that membrane-bound anionic groups are involved in the binding of Na to the binary complex and that the negative electrostatic field strength determines the affinity for Na binding, the following hypotheses seem reasonable:

The binding of a cationic amino acid could, through interaction with these anionic groups, mimic the action of Na, stabilize the binary complex, and, in turn, by reducing the anionic field strength, reduce the affinity for the subsequent binding of Na. Stated otherwise, the cationic amino acid may in part satisfy the need for the binding of Na in order to stabilize the carrier–amino acid complex.

In contrast, in the absence of Na the binding of an anionic amino acid would result in a highly unstable complex but the affinity for the subsequent binding of Na would be increased as a result of the increase in the total anionic field strength.

These admittedly speculative notions are illustrated in Fig. 4(a) and (b).

III. AMINO ACID TRANSPORT ACROSS THE SEROSAL MEMBRANES

It has long appeared reasonable to infer that amino acid transport across the basolateral membranes is carrier mediated inasmuch as it seems unlikely that relatively large, water soluble amino acids could readily exit from the cell by means of simple diffusion alone. Nonetheless, although the properties of the mucosal membranes with respect to amino acid entry into the absorptive cells have been fairly well characterized using direct methods for measurement of unidirectional influx, there is little direct information regarding the mechanisms of amino acid exit from the cell across the serosal membranes. This is principally due to the relative inaccessibility of the basolateral membranes, which precludes direct studies comparable to those that have been performed on the mucosal membranes.

Munck and Schultz (1969) presented evidence that J_{cs} (see Fig. 1) for lysine is a saturable function of intracellular lysine concentration and that the bidirectional fluxes of lysine across the basolateral membranes may be attributable to facilitated diffusion. Hajjar, Khuri, and Curran (1972) demonstrated that alanine transport across the serosal border of the turtle small intestine is the result of a Na-independent carrier-mediated process that has symmetrical properties (i.e., facilitated diffusion). The autoradiographic studies by Kinter and Wilson (1965) suggest that amino acid transport across the serosal membranes of the hamster small intestine is carrier-mediated and capable of active transport of valine from the serosal solution into the villus absorptive cells. Further, the active accumulation of valine was not inhibited by methionine.

These observations, although scanty, stress the importance of obtaining more detailed information regarding the kinetic characteristics and specificities of the mechanisms responsible for amino acid transport across the serosal membranes. If the net entry into the cell from the mucosal solution is more rapid than the exit into the serosal solution, the steady state would be characterized by a high intracellular amino acid concentration and a low rate of transepithelial transport; conversely, if entry is slow compared to exit, there would be a relatively rapid rate of transepithelial transport associated with a relatively low level of amino acid accumulation within the absorptive cells. Further, if the specificities of the transport mechanism(s) at the serosal membranes differ from those of the mucosal membranes, amino acid absorption and the effect of transported competitive inhibitors on transepithelial transport would reflect neither the properties of the transport mechanisms located at the mucosal membranes nor the properties of the mechanisms responsible for transport across the serosal membranes.

IV. THE SHUNT PATHWAY AND AMINO ACID TRANSPORT

In recent years it has become abundantly clear that the mammalian small intestine is characterized by a relatively high conductance extracellular pathway whose anatomic counterpart appears to be the junctional complexes and the lateral intercellular spaces. This route appears to have relatively large dimensions compared to passive permeation pathways through cell membranes, is water-filled, and permits rapid transepithelial diffusion of a number of ions presumably in their hydrated forms (Frizzell and Schultz, 1972; Munck and Schultz, 1974; also see Moreno and Diamond, 1974, for a detailed review of this issue). This extracellular (or paracellular) pathway across the rabbit ileum and the rat jejunum is impermeable to lysine and tetraethylammonium ions (Munck and Schultz, 1969; Munck and Schultz, 1974, and *unpublished observations*) suggesting that the dimensions of this route are such that they restrict the diffusion of solutes whose effective radii are greater than 5 to 6 Å. Estimates of equivalent pore radii or slit widths for the junctional complexes in the renal proximal tubule (Bentzel, Parsa, and Hare, 1969) and the rabbit gallbladder (Moreno and Diamond, 1974) also suggest that the limiting diameter or width of the paracellular pathway is approximately 10 to 15 Å. Assuming that these estimates are reasonable, it is quite possible that transepithelial movements of glycine and to a lesser extent those of alanine and valine are influenced by diffusion through the extracellular pathway; it is unlikely that this pathway contributes significantly to the transepithelial movements of larger amino acids. On the other hand, as pointed out by Moreno and Diamond (1974), molecules whose dimensions are smaller than the limiting dimensions of the extracellular pathway may be restricted from permeation through that pathway due to unfavorable Coulombic as well as non-Coulombic interactions with the ligands that line the pathway and determine its permselectivity. Furthermore, solutes whose dimensions in free solution appear to exceed the limiting dimensions of the extracellular pathway, may traverse this route because interactions with the ligands that line this pathway may reduce their dimensions as a result of proton withdrawal or other conformational changes that are not observed in free aqueous solution. Thus, a definitive conclusion regarding the contribution of the extracellular route to the transepithelial movements of amino acids awaits further study.

ACKNOWLEDGMENTS

Investigations carried out in the authors' laboratories were supported by research grants from the U.S. Public Health Service, National Institute of Arthritis, Metabolism, and Digestive Diseases and the American Heart Association.

REFERENCES

Bentzel, C. J., Para, B., and Hare, D. K. (1969): Osmotic flow across proximal tubule of Necturus. Correlation of physiologic and anatomic studies. Am. J. Physiol. *217:*570–580.
Curran, P. F., Hajjar, J. J., and Glynn, I. M. (1970): The sodium-alanine interaction in rabbit ileum: Effect of alanine on sodium fluxes. J. Gen. Physiol. *55:*297–308.
Curran, P. F., Schultz, S. G., Chez, R. A., and Fuisz, R. E. (1967): Kinetic relations of the Na-amino acid interaction at the mucosal border of intestine. J. Gen. Physiol. *50:*1261–1286.
Diamond, J. M., and Wright, E. M. (1969): Molecular forces governing non-electrolyte permeation through cell membranes Proc. Roy. Soc. B (London) *1972:*273–316.
Eisenman, G. (1961): On the elementary atomic origin of equilibrium ionic specificity. In: *Membrane transport and metabolism,* edited by A. Kleinzeller and A. Kotyk, Academic Press, New York, pp. 163–179.
England, A., Jr., and Cohn, E. J. (1935): Studies of the physical chemistry of amino acids, peptides and related substances. IV. The distribution coefficients of amino acids between water and butyl alcohol. J. Am. Chem. Soc. *57:*634–637.
Frizzell, R. A., and Schultz, S. G. (1970): Effects of monovalent cations on the sodium-alanine interaction in rabbit ileum: Implication of anionic groups in sodium binding. J. Gen. Physiol. *56:*462–490.
Frizzell, R. A., and Schultz, S. G. (1972): Ionic conductances of extracellular shunt pathway in rabbit ileum: Influence of shunt on transmural sodium transport and electrical potential differences. J. Gen. Physiol. *59:*318–346.
Gibb, L. E., and Eddy, A. A. (1972): An electrogenic sodium pump as a possible factor leading to concentration of amino acids by mouse ascites tumour cells with reversed sodium ion concentration gradients. Biochem. J. *129:*979–981.
Hajjar, J. J., and Curran, P. F. (1970): Characteristics of the amino acid transport system in the brush border of rabbit ileum. J. Gen. Physiol. *56:*673–691.
Hajjar, J. J., Khuri, R. N., and Curran, P. F. (1972): Alanine efflux across the serosal border of turtle intestine. J. Gen. Physiol. *60:*720–734.

Hajjar, J. J., Lamont, A. S., and Curran, P. F. (1970): The sodium-alanine interaction in rabbit ileum: Effect of sodium on alanine fluxes. J. Gen. Physiol. 55:277–296.
Kinter, W. B., and Wilson, T. H. (1965): Autoradiographic study of sugar and amino acid absorption by everted sacs of hamster intestine. J. Cell Biol. 25:19–39.
Koshland, D. E., Jr. (1964): Conformation changes at the active site during enzyme action. Fed. Proc. 23:719.
Moreno, J. H., and Diamond, J. M. (1974): Cation permeation mechanisms and cation selectivity in "tight junctions" of gall-bladder epithelium. In: *Membranes—A series of advances,* edited by G. Eisenman, Marcel Dekker, New York.
Munck, B. G., and Schultz, S. G. (1969): Lysine transport across isolated rabbit ileum. J. Gen. Physiol. 53:157–182.
Munck, B. G., and Schultz, S. G. (1974): Properties of the passive conductance pathway across in vitro rat jejunum. J. Membrane Biol. 16:163–174.
Murer, H., and Hopfer, U. (1974): Demonstration of an electrogenic Na-dependent D-glucose transport in intestinal brush border membranes. Proc. Nat. Acad. Sci. 71:484–488.
Nemethy, G., and Scheraga, H. A. (1962): The structure of water and hydrophobic bonding in proteins. III. The thermodynamic properties of hydrophobic bonds in proteins. J. Phys. Chem. 66:1773–1789.
Oxender, D. L. (1965): Stereospecificity of amino acid transport for Ehrlich tumor cells. J. Biol. Chem. 240:2976–2982.
Peterson, S. C., Goldner, A. M., and Curran, P. F. (1970): Glycine transport in rabbit ileum. Am. J. Physiol. 219:1027–1032.
Preston, R. L., Schaeffer, J. F., and Curran, P. F. (1974): Structure-affinity relationships of substrates for the neutral amino acid transport system in rabbit ileum. J. Gen. Physiol. 64:443–467.
Robinson, J. W. L., and Alvarado, F. (1971): Interaction between the sugar and amino-acid transport systems at the small intestinal brush border: A comparative study. Pflügers Arch. 326:48–75.
Rose, R. C., and Schultz, S. G. (1971): Studies on the electrical potential profile across rabbit ileum: Effects of sugars and amino acids on transmural and transmucosal electrical potential differences. J. Gen. Physiol. 57:639–663.
Schaeffer, J. F., Preston, R. L., and Curran, P. F. (1973): Inhibition of amino acid transport in rabbit intestine by p-chloromercuriphenyl sulfonic acid. J. Gen. Physiol. 62:131–146.
Schultz, S. G. (1969): The interaction between sodium and amino acid transport across the brush border of rabbit ileum: A plausible molecular model. In: *The molecular basis of membrane function,* edited D. C. Tosteson, Prentice Hall, New Jersey, pp. 401–420.
Schultz, S. G. (1973): Shunt pathway, sodium transport and the electrical potential profile across rabbit ileum. In: *Transport Mechanisms in Epithelia,* edited by H. H. Ussing and N. A. Thorn, Munksgaard, Copenhagen, pp. 147–160.
Schultz, S. G., and Curran, P. F. (1970): Coupled transport of sodium and organic solutes. Physiol. Rev. 50:637–718.
Schultz, S. G., and Markscheid-Kaspi, L. (1971): Competitive interactions between L-alanine and L-phenylalanine in rabbit ileum. Biochim. Biophys. Acta 241:857–860.
Schultz, S. G., Yu-Tu, L., Alverez, O. O., and Curran, P. F. (1970): Anionic amino acid influx across brush border of rabbit ileum: effects of amino acid charge on the Na-amino acid interaction. J. Gen. Physiol. 56:621–639.
Schultz, S. G., Yu-Tu, L., and Strecker, C. K. (1972): Influx of neutral amino acids across the brush border of rabbit ileum: Stereospecificity and the roles of the α-amino and α-carboxylate groups. Biochim. Biophys. Acta 288:367–379.
Terry, P. M., and Vidaver, G. A. (1973): The effect of gramacidin on sodium-dependent accumulation of glycine by pigeon red cells: A test of the cation gradient hypothesis. Biochim. Biophys. Acta 323:441–455.
Vidaver, G. A. (1964): Some tests of the hypothesis that the sodium ion gradient furnishes the energy for glycine active transport by pigeon red cells. Biochemistry 3:803–808.

White, J. F., and Armstrong, W. McD. (1971): Effect of transported solutes on membrane potentials in bullfrog small intestine. Amer. J. Physiol. 221:194–201.

Wiseman, G. (1968): Absorption of amino acids. In: *Handbook of physiology,* Section 6: Alimentary Canal, Vol. III, Intestinal Absorption, edited by C. F. Code, Am. Physiol. Soc., Washington, D.C., pp. 1277–1307.

DISCUSSION

CSÁKY quoted experiments indicating a competition between sugar and amino acid uptake by intestinal cells and asked for Frizzell's thoughts about this. FRIZZELL replied that such studies should be interpreted with caution inasmuch as all driving forces influencing Na-coupled nonelectrolyte uptake may not have been taken into account. One of these is likely to be the electrical potential difference across the mucosal membrane. Recent studies by Hopfer and Murer (*Proc. Natl. Acad. Sci.* 71:484, 1974) suggest that agents which are likely to increase the electrical potential difference (PD) across brush border vesicles (e.g., valinomycin in K-loaded vesicles) accelerate sugar uptake. Thus, the PD across the brush border may be one driving force for Na-coupled nonelectrolyte uptake that is often overlooked. Indeed, the studies of Rose and Schultz (*J. Gen. Physiol.* 57:639, 1971) and White and Armstrong (*Am. J. Physiol.* 221:194, 1971) have indicated that the coupled entry of Na with either sugars or amino acids in small intestine of rabbit and bullfrog is a rheogenic (current generating) process which must, in turn, be influenced by the PD across the brush border. Thus, the mutual inhibition between the uptake of sugars and amino acids observed in a variety of intestinal preparations need not reflect interactions of these solutes with a common (polyfunctional) carrier mechanism but may reflect the effects of these solutes on the transmucosal PD. More specifically, a depolarization of the transmucosal potential difference due to Na-coupled amino acid uptake across the brush border may reduce the driving force for concomitant Na-coupled sugar uptake and vice versa. Clearly, more direct experimental evaluation of this possibility is required to assess the quantitative importance of the transmucosal potential difference as a driving force for Na-coupled nonelectrolyte uptake by intestinal cells.

Intestinal Absorption and Malabsorption,
edited by T. Z. Csáky.
Raven Press, New York © 1975

Intestinal Transport of Peptides

D. M. Matthews

Department of Experimental Chemical Pathology, Vincent Square Laboratories of Westminster Hospital, 124 Vauxhall Bridge Road, London SW1V 2RH, England

I. INTRODUCTION

There is little doubt that mucosal uptake of small peptides, followed by hydrolysis and entry into the blood in the form of amino acids, plays an important part in protein absorption. Nevertheless, the idea that peptides may be transported into the absorptive cells by a specific, active transport mechanism is still somewhat unfamiliar and tends to evoke a skeptical reaction. It might be easier to accept if it were more widely known that it has long been established that transport of intact peptides to the cell interior plays an important part in the nutrition of microorganisms (Payne, 1972) and that examples of active transport of di- and tripeptides in the mammalian body have already been described in kidney, erythrocytes, and brain (see Matthews and Payne, *in press*). The aim of this account is to set out the evidence for intestinal peptide transport and to describe the phenomena associated with this process. Accounts of the history of protein absorption and of the development of the classical hypothesis of protein absorption, according to which proteins were completely hydrolyzed to amino acids within the intestinal lumen and taken up in this form, have been given elsewhere (Matthews, 1971, 1974, *in press*) and will not be repeated here. Suffice it to say that until the work of Newey and Smyth (1959, 1960, 1962) it was generally believed, and had been believed for many years, that the intestinal mucosa took up only free amino acids. Newey and Smyth, as the result of their investigations of dipeptide absorption *in vivo* and *in vitro,* put forward the hypothesis that there was a second mode of protein absorption, apart from the uptake of free amino acids—mucosal uptake of peptides with intracellular hydrolysis. Since 1968, a number of striking observations have given increasing support to this hypothesis, and it is now apparent that intralumen or brush border hydrolysis of peptides followed by uptake of amino acids from free solution is a totally inadequate explanation of protein absorption. The observations referred to include more rapid absorption of amino acids from peptides than from the equivalent free amino acids, avoidance of competition for intestinal transport between amino acids when they are presented to the intestinal mucosa as peptides, findings indicating the independence of mucosal uptake of peptides and amino acids, and the ability of patients with hereditary defects of amino acid absorption to absorb "affected" amino acids from peptides. Very recently, the use of peptides that have structural features that make them resistant to hydrolysis but do not interfere with their transport has made it possible to put forward direct evidence for active transport of di- and tripeptides by the intestinal mucosa.

The amount of information accumulated in the last few years on intestinal handling of peptides is quite extensive and cannot be dealt with in detail in a short account such as this. Full-length reviews are available elsewhere (Matthews, 1974, in press), and the first of these summarizes findings on peptide absorption in intestinal disease.

Standard three-letter abbreviations for free and peptide-bound amino acids will be used throughout. Amino acids should be taken to be the L-forms unless otherwise indicated.

II. RELATIVE RATES OF ABSORPTION OF PEPTIDES AND AMINO ACIDS

The observation that amino acids can be absorbed from a peptide more rapidly than from the equivalent free amino acid or amino acid mixture (i.e., the amino acid or amino acid mixture produced by hydrolysis of the peptide) was first made in man by means of tolerance tests using Gly, Gly-Gly, and Gly-Gly-Gly (Craft, Geddes, Hyde, Wise, and Matthews, 1968) and jejunal perfusion using Gly-Gly and Gly-Leu (Adibi and Phillips, 1968). Similar observations were made in the rat *in vivo* using di- and tripeptides of Gly and Met (Matthews, Craft, Geddes, Wise, and Hyde, 1968; Matthews, Lis, Cheng, and Crampton, 1969). Not only was total absorption of amino acids greater from the peptides than from the equivalent amino acids, but competition for absorption between amino acids was partly or completely avoided during absorption of mixed peptides. These findings showed that peptide absorption could not be the result of intralumen or brush border hydrolysis of peptides with uptake of amino acids from free solution. The early observations have now been confirmed and extended by a large number of investigations in man and several species of laboratory animal, using methods *in vivo* and *in vitro* and a wide variety of di- and tripeptides consisting of various combinations of neutral, basic, and acidic amino acids (e.g., Adibi, 1971; Cheng, Navab, Lis, Miller, and Matthews, 1971; Lis, Crampton, and Matthews, 1971; Burston, Addison, and Matthews, 1972; Cook, 1972; Hellier, Holdsworth, McColl, and Perrett, 1972; Silk, Perrett, and Clark, 1973b—for further references see Matthews 1972, 1974, *in press*). More rapid absorption of one or more amino acids from peptides than from the equivalent amino acid mixtures has been shown with most, although not all, of the di- and tripeptides so far studied. In the limited number of cases in which absorption, or uptake *in vitro*, of peptides and the equivalent amino acids has been measured at more than one concentration, it has been found that with some peptides, including Met-Met and Gly-Gly, transport is more rapid from the peptides than the amino acids at high concentrations but not at lower ones; with others (Lys-Lys, α-Glu-Glu, β-Ala-His), it is more rapid from the peptides than the amino acids at low concentrations but not at higher ones (Matthews et al., 1968; Cheng et al., 1971; Burston et al., 1972; Matthews, Addison, and Burston, 1974). Such findings might be expected if peptides and the equivalent amino acids are taken up by separate mechanisms with different kinetic characteristics. The uptake of two amino acids A and B from a dipeptide is often unequal, uptake of A being greater than that of B, whether the peptide is AB or BA. This would not be expected if a single mechanism, peptide uptake followed by intracellular hydrolysis, were entirely responsible for peptide absorption (unless the rates of exit of amino acids from the absorptive cells were unequal). It has usually been found that the amino acid more extensively taken up from a peptide is the one that is more extensively taken up from the equivalent amino acid mixture. The evidence so far available suggests that in many cases the inequality in uptake is due to the fact that in addition to peptide uptake followed by hydrolysis, intralumen or brush border hydrolysis with uptake of amino acids from free solution also plays some part in peptide absorption. A survey of the uptake of amino acids from 22 dipeptides of neutral, basic, and acidic amino acids by hamster jejunum *in vitro* (Burston, Addison, and Matthews, 1972) and a comparison of the characteristics of absorption of a partial hydrolysate of casein and the equivalent amino acid mixture in man (Silk, Marrs, Burston, Addison, Clark, and Matthews, 1973) have suggested that an important feature of peptide absorption is that amino acids which are particularly slowly absorbed from free solution may be very much more rapidly absorbed from peptides. For example, Glu, which was relatively slowly taken up on its own and taken up still more slowly in the presence of Met, was taken up nearly 10 times as rapidly from Met-Glu as from the equivalent mixture of Met and Glu (Burston et al., 1972).

III. KINETICS OF INTESTINAL PEPTIDE TRANSPORT

Few investigations of the kinetics of peptide transport by the intestine have yet been made. The early work with peptides of Gly and Met suggested that peptide absorption was the result of a saturable process. Cheng et al. (1971) showed that uptake of Met from Met-Met by rat small intestine *in vitro* apparently conformed to Michaelis-Menten kinetics at low concentrations. At low concentrations, uptake of Met from Met-Met took place at about the same rate as uptake of the equivalent free Met. At higher concentrations (above 10 μmoles/ml Met or 5 μmoles/ml Met-Met) the uptake curves diverged, and uptake of Met from the peptide continued to increase with increasing concentration over a concentration range in which uptake of free Met was saturated. Rubino, Field, and Shwachman (1971) studied 1-min uptake of ^{14}C-Gly from Gly-Pro by rabbit ileal mucosa *in vitro*. This appeared to be the result of two saturable processes, one with a high apparent affinity and a low maximal velocity and the other with a low apparent affinity and a high maximal velocity. An investigation of influx of β-Ala-His (carnosine, Car), a peptide which undergoes very little hydrolysis, into hamster jejunum *in vitro* (Matthews et al., 1974) showed that this apparently conformed to Michaelis-Menten kinetics. There was no evidence of uptake by more than one mechanism. Adibi and Soleimanpour (1974) have shown by jejunal perfusion in man that Gly-Gly and Gly-Leu have substantially higher maximal transport velocities than either of the constituent amino acids.

IV. INDEPENDENCE OF AMINO ACID AND PEPTIDE TRANSPORT

It has recently become clear that mucosal uptake of peptides is independent of that of free amino acids The evidence for this is of several kinds. In the amino acid transport defects of Hartnup disease and cystinuria, it has been shown that amino acids are relatively well absorbed from peptides even when these peptides are composed entirely of an "affected" amino acid. The findings in these diseases are discussed more fully later. Experiments with the small intestine *in vitro* (Rubino et al., 1971; Addison, Burston, and Matthews, 1972; 1973; Caspary, 1973; Addison, Matthews, and Burston, 1974a) have indicated that amino acids and peptides do not compete for transport. It is true that there is usually some inhibition of amino acid uptake by peptides and some inhibition of amino acid uptake from peptides by amino acids, but these effects appear to be the result of partial hydrolysis of peptides in the brush border with release of amino acids in free solution. Evidence supporting the concept of the independence of amino acid and peptide transport has been supplied by observations showing that the sites of maximal absorption of peptides and amino acids along the length of the small intestine are not the same, that for peptides being more proximal than that for amino acids (Lis, Matthews, and Crampton, 1972a; Crampton, Lis, and Matthews, 1973) and that the effects of dietary alterations on absorption of amino acids and absorption of peptides are different (Lis, Crampton, and Matthews, 1972b; Lis et al., 1972a).

V. COMPETITION FOR INTESTINAL TRANSPORT BETWEEN DI- AND TRIPEPTIDES

Rubino et al. (1971) showed that a number of dipeptides of neutral amino acids inhibited uptake of Gly from Gly-Pro by rabbit ileal mucosa *in vitro,* and in the case of Leu-Leu the kinetics of the inhibition were shown to be competitive. Caspary (1973) reported that several dipeptides of neutral amino acids inhibited uptake of Gly from Gly-Gly by the rat small intestine. Adibi and Soleimanpour (1974) have recently shown that absorption of

Gly-Gly in man is competitively inhibited by Gly-Leu but not significantly affected by Gly or Leu or a mixture of these amino acids. Very clear-cut results have been obtained with peptides which are well transported but unusually slowly hydrolyzed, appear intact in the intestinal tissue on incubation *in vitro,* and probably undergo almost no hydrolysis in the brush border. Uptake of these, which include glycylsarcosine (Gly-Sar), Car, and glycylsarcosylsarcosine (Gly-Sar-Sar), is not at all inhibited by free amino acids. Uptake of Gly-Sar by hamster jejunum was inhibited by Met-Met but not by Met (Addison et al., 1972) and uptake of Car was inhibited by a number of dipeptides of neutral amino acids but not by the equivalent free amino acids (Addison et al., 1973, 1974a). In the case of Gly-Pro, inhibition was shown to be competitive. Recent work from the author's laboratory using Gly-Sar-Sar indicates that in hamster jejunum transport of tripeptides, like that of dipeptides, is independent of free amino acids and suggests that di- and tripeptides share a common transport system (Addison, Burston, Matthews, Payne, and Wilkinson, 1974b). The tetrapeptide Gly-Sar-Sar-Sar did not inhibit uptake of Gly-Sar-Sar. Combined with the observation that uptake of the tetrapeptide is extremely poor, this suggests that tetrapeptides are unsuitable for carrier-mediated transport by the small intestine.

It is not yet clear whether the intestine possesses only one or more than one peptide uptake system. Rubino et al. (1971) observed that uptake of Gly from Gly-Pro was not inhibited by a high concentration of Pro-Gly. Addison et al. (1974a) found that uptake of Car was unaffected by equimolar Lys-Lys or Glu-Glu, and that Lys-Lys and Glu-Glu had no significant effect on uptake of each other. Although these observations suggest the possibility of more than one system, they are preliminary only, and much more investigation will be required before the point can be settled.

VI. ACTIVE TRANSPORT OF PEPTIDES BY THE SMALL INTESTINE

Most small peptides are hydrolyzed so rapidly by the small intestine that they are not detectable in the intestinal wall and do not appear in the serosal fluid of everted sacs of the small intestine *in vitro.* Until very recently this prevented any conventional demonstration of active transport of peptides by the intestine, since there appeared to be no chance of showing concentration of a peptide against a gradient. Work on transport of peptides by microorganisms (see Payne, 1972) suggested that this difficulty might be overcome by the use of peptides whose structure is such that they fulfill the structural requirements for transport but are exceptionally resistant to hydrolysis. The first such peptide to be tried was Gly-Sar, in which a methyl group is attached to the N of the peptide bond. It was shown that Gly-Sar was accumulated in hamster jejunum *in vitro* against an electrochemical gradient by a Na^+-dependent and energy-dependent process (Addison et al., 1972). Similar findings were obtained with the tripeptide Gly-Sar-Sar (Addison et al.,

1974b). A second dipeptide, Car, was also actively accumulated by an Na⁺-dependent process (Addison et al., 1973; Matthews et al., 1974). Somewhat unusual findings were obtained with the tripeptide β-Ala-Gly-Gly (Addison, Burston, and Matthews, 1974c; Burston, Addison, Matthews, Payne, and Wilkinson, 1974). This appeared intact in hamster jejunum *in vitro* but was not concentrated in the ICF of the whole intestinal wall, and its uptake was linearly related to concentration over a wide range of concentrations. However, uptake of β-Ala-Gly-Gly was inhibited by anoxia, 2:4 dinitrophenol and Na⁺ replacement, and by other di- and tripeptides including Gly-Sar and Gly-Sar-Sar but not by the equivalent amino acids, so that it is probable that this peptide is also actively transported, although its transport is relatively poor.

Since uptake of Gly-Sar, Gly-Sar-Sar, Car, and β-Ala-Gly-Gly, which all seem to share the same uptake system, is inhibited by other di- and tripeptides which do not appear intact in the small intestine *in vitro* (Addison et al., 1972, 1974b, 1974c; Burston et al., 1974), it seems likely that these also share the uptake system and are also actively transported into the mucosal cells. In the case of the tripeptides, however, the possibility that the inhibition is due to dipeptides liberated extracellularly has not been excluded.

The likelihood that most of the di- and tripeptides produced in the course of protein digestion are extremely rapidly hydrolyzed suggests that they enter the absorptive cells down a steep concentration gradient. This would tend to assist active transport in accelerating their entry.

VII. THE INFLUENCE OF MOLECULAR STRUCTURE ON PEPTIDE TRANSPORT AND HYDROLYSIS

The structural requirements for peptide transport by the intestine have not yet been systematically studied. The following is a brief summary of the observations that have been made so far with the rat, hamster, or rabbit small intestine. It appears that substitution of the *N-terminal amino group* of a dipeptide abolishes or substantially reduces affinity for transport. Methylation of this group, in Sar-Gly, resulted in poor uptake and slow hydrolysis (Burston et al., 1972). Acetylation, in N-acetyl-Gly-Gly, resulted in failure to inhibit uptake of Gly from Gly-Pro (Rubino et al., 1971) and Pro-Hyp did not appear to be actively transported (Hueckel and Rogers, 1972). However, Pro-Hyp was a weak inhibitor of Car uptake (Addison et al., 1974a). Attachment of the N-terminal amino group to a β-carbon atom, in Car, was compatible with active uptake but led to slow hydrolysis (Matthews et al., 1974). Amidation of the *C-terminal carboxyl group,* in Gly-Gly amide, resulted in failure to inhibit uptake of Car and Gly-Sar-Sar (Addison et al., 1974a, 1974b). The influence of the *amino acid side-chains* and their charge on peptide transport is uncertain (Addison et al., 1974a). Methylation of the nitrogen of peptide bonds, in Gly-Sar and Gly-Sar-Sar, was compatible with active transport but led to slow hydrolysis (Addison et al., 1972; 1974b). A γ-linkage, in γ-Glu-Glu, caused poor uptake and slow hydrolysis (Burston et al., 1972) while γ-Glu-Cys-Gly (glutathione), which is also slowly hydrolyzed, was also poorly transported, probably by diffusion (Evered and Wass, 1970). The behavior of Gly-Sar-Sar-Sar (Addison et al., 1974b) suggests that active transport of α-linked peptides is limited to those of two and three amino acid residues. Like the transport mechanisms for free amino acids, the mechanism for peptide transport shows stereochemical specificity, peptides containing D-amino acids being very poorly taken up (as well as very slowly hydrolyzed) (Burston et al., 1972; Asatoor, Chadha, Milne, and Prosser, 1973). There is, however, some interaction between peptides of L-amino acids and those containing D-amino acids, since Cheeseman and Smyth (1973) showed that uptake of D-Leu-Gly was inhibited by Leu-Ala.

VIII. PEPTIDE ABSORPTION IN HARTNUP DISEASE AND CYSTINURIA

Investigations of peptide absorption in the hereditary renal and intestinal transport defects of Hartnup disease and cystinuria have provided results of great interest, showing the independence of intestinal amino acid and peptide transport in man and suggesting that mucosal peptide uptake is of considerable quantitative importance in protein absorption. For some years after the demonstration that these diseases involved severe defects of absorption of certain amino acids, including essential ones (Milne, 1964), there was no satisfactory explanation of why the patients showed no evidence of protein malnutrition and had no disturbance after protein meals. In 1970 it was shown that two patients with Hartnup disease could absorb "affected" amino acids relatively well when these were given in the form of dipeptides. In the first case (Asatoor, Cheng, Edwards, Lant, Matthews, Milne, Navab, and Richards, 1970; Navab and Asatoor, 1970) it was shown that absorption of free His and free Trp was defective, but that absorption of these amino acids from Car and Gly-Trp, respectively, was relatively normal. Since these peptides might have entered the mucosal cells through the intact entry sites for β-Ala and Gly, whose absorption was normal, a peptide composed entirely of an "affected" amino acid, Phe-Phe, was given. Although absorption of free Phe was very poor, absorption of Phe from Phe-Phe was almost normal. This indicated the independence of mucosal uptake of amino acids and peptides in the human subject. In the second case (Tarlow, Seakins, Lloyd, Matthews, Cheng, and Thomas, 1970, 1972) it was shown that absorption of free Tyr was defective, but that Tyr was well absorbed from Gly-Tyr. Uptake of His from Gly-His by a jejunal biopsy was more than three times as great as that of free His, which was subnormal. Very recently, a third case has been studied (Leonard, Marrs, Addison, Burston, Clegg, Lloyd, Seakins, and Matthews, 1974). Tolerance tests were carried out following administration of an amino acid mixture simulating casein, and an enzymic hydrolysate of casein containing about 60% oligopeptides. The results suggested that absorption of free His, Leu, Tyr, Phe, Ser, Met, Gly, and Glu was defective, but that all these amino acids were comparatively well absorbed from the enzymic hydrolysate (the apparent impairment of absorption of Gly and Glu was unexpected).

Analogous findings to those in Hartnup disease have been obtained in cystinuria, in which it has been shown that Lys and Arg are very much better absorbed from peptides than in the free form (Hellier, Perrett, and Holdsworth, 1970; Asatoor, Crouchman, Harrison, Light, Loughridge, Milne, and Richards, 1971; Asatoor, Harrison, Milne, and Prosser, 1972; Hellier, Holdsworth, Perrett, and Thirumalai, 1972). The finding that absorption of Lys from Lys-Lys is within normal limits in cystinuria whereas absorption of free Lys is very poor (Hellier et al., 1970, 1972) provides additional evidence for the independence of mucosal uptake of peptides and amino acids.

There can be no doubt that retention of the ability to take up peptides is a major factor in maintaining protein nutrition in patients with the amino acid transport defects of Hartnup disease and cystinuria. Unless mucosal uptake of peptides is abnormally effective in these patients, the results suggest that peptide uptake must play an important part in protein absorption in normal man. It may be noted that the ability of patients with these diseases to absorb amino acids from peptides adds to evidence that the defects involved are defects of transport of amino acids into the mucosal cells, not defects of the mechanisms responsible for exit of amino acids from them.

IX. EFFECTS OF DIETARY ALTERATIONS AND PYRIDOXINE DEFICIENCY ON ABSORPTION OF PEPTIDES AND AMINO ACIDS

Although there have been many investigations of the effects of dietary alterations on the absorption of amino acids by laboratory animals (see Lis et al., 1972b), the effects of such alterations on the absorption of peptides and the absorption of peptide–amino acid mixtures have hardly begun to be explored. The two investigations so far made, in the rat *in vivo* (Lis et al., 1972a, b), have shown that the effects of dietary alterations on absorption of amino acids and the absorption of peptides are not the same. For example, absorption of Met was increased by short-term restriction of dietary intake, a high Met diet and a high protein diet, but these alterations had no effect on the absorption of Met-Met (Lis et al., 1972b); prolonged feeding on an almost protein-free diet decreased absorption of an amino acid mixture simulating casein but had no significant effect on absorption of a tryptic hydrolysate of casein consisting mainly of oligopeptides (Lis et al., 1972a). In general, absorption of amino acids appeared to be much more readily influenced by dietary alterations than that of peptides. The results so far available indicate that the effects of altering the diet on absorption of amino acids cannot be taken to represent the effects on absorption of the normal products of intralumen digestion of proteins, oligopeptides and amino acids, and that much work in this area will have to be done again. The fact that the effects of dietary alterations on amino acid and peptide absorption are different has interesting theoretical implications. It suggests that these effects are on entry rather than exit mechanisms and is consistent with the hypothesis of the independence of mucosal uptake of peptides and amino acids.

Asatoor, Chadha, Dawson, Milne, and Prosser (1972) studied the effects of pyridoxine deficiency (which is known to depress amino acid absorption) on absorption of amino acids and peptides in the rat *in vivo*. They found that both peptide and amino acid absorption were reduced and, in view of the strong evidence for independence of the entry of amino acids and peptides into mucosal cells, concluded that pyridoxine deficiency probably impaired exit of amino acids from the mucosal cells.

X. QUANTITATIVE IMPORTANCE OF MUCOSAL PEPTIDE UPTAKE IN PROTEIN ABSORPTION

Apart from the evidence from Hartnup disease and cystinuria, enough work has been done in animals to suggest that mucosal uptake of peptides must play an important part in protein absorption, although no estimate of the relative importance of peptide uptake and uptake of free amino acids can yet be arrived at. It seems quite possible that peptide uptake is more important in the absorption of some amino acids, for example, Glu, Asp, Lys, Gly, Pro, and Hyp, than in the absorption of others.

Crampton, Gangolli, Simson, and Matthews (1971) studied absorption by the rat small intestine *in vivo* of amino acid mixtures simulating several proteins and tryptic hydrolysates of the proteins that contained about two-thirds oligopeptides of mean chain length two to six amino acid residues and one-third free amino acids. In all cases, absorption of the tryptic hydrolysates was substantially more rapid than that of the corresponding amino acid mixtures. In the case of lactalbumin and serum albumin, 10-min absorption of the tryptic hydrolysates was approximately double that of the amino acid mixtures. In an extension of the work to human volunteers (Silk et al., 1973a) absorption of an amino acid mixture simulating casein and of a tryptic hydrolysate of casein were studied by jejunal perfusion. Total absorption of α-amino nitrogen was greater from the tryptic hydrolysate than from the amino acid mixture, as in the rat. Moreover, there was a striking difference in the pattern of absorption of individual amino acids from the mixture and from the tryptic hydrolysate. The extent of absorption of individual amino acids from the mixture of free amino acids varied widely, from 73% (Met) to only 26% (Asp). When the tryptic hydrolysate was perfused, several amino acids which were relatively slowly absorbed from the amino acid mixture were absorbed considerably more rapidly. The difference was significant for Phe, Ala, His, Lys, Glu, and Asp. As a result, the range of percentage absorption of individual amino acids was substantially reduced, becoming 73% (Phe) to 47% (Gly).

These results provide additional evidence indicating that mucosal peptide uptake plays a significant part in the absorption of protein digestion products and confirm previous evidence suggesting that the characteristics of absorption of amino acid mixtures do not represent those of the normal products of intralumen digestion of protein, oligopeptides and amino acids. Nasset (1965) pointed out that during protein absorption, the molar ratios between individual amino acids in the intestinal lumen did not alter with time and distance from the pylorus as might be expected if some amino acids were preferentially absorbed as they are from an amino acid mixture, although this could not be accounted for at the time. Nixon and Mawer (1970a,b) in a careful study of protein absorption in man also emphasized that the rates of absorption of amino acids from mixtures did not appear to correspond to their rates of absorption from protein meals. They found that some amino acids, such as Glu and Asp, were absorbed from protein very much more rapidly than expected from the results of work on absorption of amino acid mixtures. They also showed that some amino acids were released so slowly by intralumen digestion that it did not seem possible that they could be absorbed entirely in the free form and suggested that these must either be liberated in the region of the brush border, or taken up by the mucosa as peptides. These slowly liberated amino acids included Gly, Thr, Ser, Pro, Hyp, Glu, Asp, Ala, Ileu, and His, and the work suggested that intralumen hydrolysis followed by uptake of free amino acids could account for the absorption of only a minority of the amino acids present in proteins. Coulson and Hernandez (1970), investigating absorption in the cayman, also obtained results indicating that intralumen hydrolysis followed by amino acid uptake could not account for protein absorption. It seems to me that any attempt to categorize amino acids into those which are absorbed in the free form and those which are taken up as peptides (Gray and Cooper, 1971) is premature and that it is likely that most if not all amino acids leave the intestinal lumen both in the free form and as peptides, the proportion of each leaving as amino acid or as peptide varying from one amino acid to another.

The possible nutritional significance of the differences in the patterns of absorption of amino acids from proteins and from amino acid mixtures simulating these proteins is discussed elsewhere (Payne and Matthews, 1975).

XI. CONTENTS OF THE INTESTINAL LUMEN AFTER PROTEIN MEALS, AND FORMS IN WHICH PROTEIN DIGESTION PRODUCTS ENTER THE PORTAL BLOOD

These topics have been dealt with in detail elsewhere (Matthews, 1974, *in press*) and will only be touched on here. Comparatively little is known about the composition of the contents of the intestinal lumen after protein meals, and much more information is needed on the concentrations of amino acids and peptides likely to be presented to the intestinal mucosa for absorption. As early as 1912, it was reported that during protein digestion the intestinal lumen contained a mixture of free amino acids and short-chain peptides probably of two to three amino acid residues (see Van Slyke, 1917). More recent investigations have confirmed that after protein meals the lumen contains a mixture of amino acids and peptides, and estimates of the chain length of the peptide fraction suggest that it is largely made up of small peptides of a few (three to six) amino acid residues (Chen, Rogers, and Harper, 1962; Adibi and Mercer, 1973). It is probable that digestion to peptides of two to three amino acid residues and free amino acids takes place mainly in the brush border (Ugolev, 1968; Peters, 1970; Peters, Donlon, and Fottrell, 1972).

There is no reasonable doubt that protein digestion products enter the portal blood almost entirely as free amino acids, but it is also well established that a few small peptides, which are unusually slowly hydrolyzed, may enter the blood intact, at least when given in large doses. These include Gly-Gly (Newey and Smyth, 1959; Adibi, 1971), peptides of Hyp (Prockop, Keiser, and Sjoerdsma, 1962; Bronstein, Haeffner, and Kowlessar, 1966), Car and Ans (β-Ala-MeHis) (Perry, Hansen, Tischler, Bunting, and Berry, 1967), β-aspartyl di- and tripeptides (Dorer, Haley, and Buchanan, 1966) and peptides containing D-amino acids (Asatoor et al., 1973). Boullin, Crampton, Heading, and Pelling (1974) have shown that during the absorption of high concentrations (100 μmoles/ml) of Gly-Gly, Gly-Phe, Gly-Pro, Pro-Gly, Gly-D-Phe, and Car in the rat, low concentrations of intact peptides appear in the portal blood, the extent of entry into the blood being inversely related to the rate of hydrolysis by the intestinal mucosa.

XII. POSSIBLE SCHEMES OF PEPTIDE ABSORPTION

There can be little doubt that more than one process is involved in the absorption of small peptides. Intralumen and/or brush border hydrolysis with release of amino acids in free solution, followed by amino acid uptake by the usual amino acid uptake mechanisms probably plays some part in the absorption of all peptides. With some peptides, such as Gly-Gly and Gly-Leu, this mode of absorption may be negligible (Fogel and Adibi, 1973); with others, it may be quantitatively important. For example, during the absorption of Met-Met in the rat, much free Met appears in the intestinal lumen, especially in the ileum, and it appears to be liberated largely by intralumen hydrolysis (Crampton et al., 1973); during absorption of Gly-Ala and Ala-Gly in man, there is evidence suggesting both intralumen hydrolysis and some hydrolysis at the brush border (Silk et al., 1973b). Several features of peptide absorption, however, cannot possibly be explained by extracellular hydrolysis followed by uptake of amino acids from free solution. These include more rapid absorption of amino acids from peptides than from the equivalent free amino acids, avoidance of competition for transport between amino acids when peptides are absorbed, the independence of amino acid and peptide uptake with competition for absorption between peptides but not between peptides and amino acids, and retention of the ability to absorb amino acids from peptides in Hartnup disease and cystinuria. At least two schemes may be proposed to explain these phenomena: (1) Peptides undergo hydrolysis on or in the outer layers of the plasma membrane of the absorptive cells with uptake of amino acids by sites closely associated with the hydrolase, available only to amino acids released by the hydrolase, and involving different carriers from those responsible for uptake of amino acids from free solution (Matthews, 1972; Ugolev, 1972). (2) Peptides are taken up by the mucosal cells by one or more specific transport mechanisms, independent of those for free amino acids, and hydrolyzed deep to the transport mechanism, probably within the cells deep to the plasma membrane (Matthews, 1972). The first scheme has some attractions, in particular its similarity to a scheme put forward to explain disaccharide absorption (Crane, Malathi, Caspary, and Ramaswamy, 1970) and the fact that it conforms to the concept of "membrane digestion" and the "digestive-absorptive surface." On the other hand, there is no positive evidence in its favor. Observations suggesting that peptide hydrolysis precedes the transport step (Ugolev, Iesuitova, Timofeeva, and Fediushina, 1964; Kushak and Ugolev, 1966; Ugolev and Kooshuck, 1966; Ugolev, Iesuitova, Timofeeva, and Kushak, 1967; Fern, Hider, and London 1969; Kooshuck, 1971; Ugolev, 1972; Caspary, 1973) appear to be related to the extracellular hydrolysis that admittedly plays some part in peptide absorption. The second scheme is strongly supported by the demonstration that di- and tripeptides that are poorly hydrolyzed accumulate in the intestinal wall as the result of active transport. It is also favored by the results of investigations of the subcellular distribution of peptidase activity (Das and Radhakrishnan, 1972; Kim, Birtwhistle, and Kim, 1972; Peters, Donlon, and Fottrell, 1972). It seems to this writer that all observations so far made on peptide absorption can be accounted for by the hypothesis that this is due to a combination of two processes—mucosal peptide uptake followed by hydrolysis and extracellular hydrolysis followed by uptake of amino acids from free solution. The evidence presently available does not justify the invocation of any additional mode of peptide absorption.

XIII. SUMMARY

It is evident that mucosal uptake of small peptides, followed by hydrolysis, plays an important part in protein absorption. It is likely that intralumen and brush border digestion produce a mixture of small peptides and amino acids. Dipeptides and probably tripeptides are taken up in addition to free amino acids, subsequently undergoing intracellular hydrolysis. Uptake of peptides is the result of Na-dependent active transport and is independent of that of free amino acids. Di- and tripeptides compete for uptake, but there is no competition for uptake between amino acids and peptides. In the amino acid transport defects of Hartnup disease and cystinuria the ability to absorb amino acids from peptides is retained and is largely responsible for maintaining protein nutrition in patients with these disorders. When peptides are taken up, the competition for transport occurring between free amino acids is avoided. In many instances peptide uptake has been shown to be more rapid than that of the constituent amino acids. Amino acids that are particularly slowly absorbed from free solution may be very much more rapidly absorbed from peptides. The relatively rapid uptake of peptides, combined with the independence of peptide and amino acid uptake and avoidance of competition for uptake between amino acids when peptides are taken up, helps to account for the rapidity of protein absorption, and the absorptive capacity of the intestine for the normal products of protein digestion, small peptides and amino acids, is much greater than its absorptive capacity for amino acid mixtures. The patterns of absorption of amino acids from proteins and mixtures of free amino acids simulating proteins are different, and the differences are due at least in part to the occurrence of mucosal uptake of peptides.

ACKNOWLEDGMENTS

Work on peptide absorption in the author's laboratory is currently supported by a grant from the Medical Research Council. This and previous support from the British Nutrition Foundation, the Governors' Discretionary Fund of the Westminster Hospital, and the Variety Club of Great Britain are gratefully acknowledged.

REFERENCES

Addison, J. M., Burston, D., and Matthews, D. M. (1972): Evidence for active transport of the dipeptide glycylsarcosine by hamster jejunum *in vitro*. Clin. Sci. *43*:907–911.

Addison, J. M., Burston, D., and Matthews, D. M. (1973): Carnosine transport by hamster jejunum *in vitro* and its inhibition by other di- and tripeptides. Clin. Sci. Molec. Med. *45*:3–4P.

Addison, J. M., Matthews, D. M., and Burston, D. (1974a): Competition between carnosine and other peptides for transport by hamster jejunum *in vitro*. Clin. Sci. Molec. Med. *46*:707–714.

Addison, J. M., Burston, D., Matthews, D. M., Payne, J. W., and Wilkinson, S. (1974b): Evidence for active transport of the tripeptide glycylsarcosylsarcosine by hamster jejunum *in vitro*. Clin. Sci. Molec. Med. *46*:30P.

Addison, J. M., Burston, D., and Matthews, D. M. (1974c): Transport of the tripeptide β-alanyl-glycyl-glycine by hamster jejunum *in vitro*. Clin. Sci. Molec. Med. *46*:5–6P.

Adibi, S. A. (1971): Intestinal transport of dipeptides in man: Relative importance of hydrolysis and intact absorption. J. Clin. Invest., *50*:2266–2275.

Adibi, S. A., and Phillips, E. (1968): Evidence for greater absorption of amino acid from peptides than from free form by human intestine. Clin. Res. *16*:446.

Adibi, S. A., and Mercer, D. W. (1973): Protein digestion in human intestine as reflected in luminal, mucosal and plasma amino acid concentrations after meals. J. Clin. Invest. 52:1586–1594.
Adibi, S. A., and Soleimanpour, M. R. (1974): Functional characterization of dipeptide transport system in human jejunum. J. Clin. Invest., 53:1368–1374.
Asatoor, A. M., Cheng, B., Edwards, K. D. G., Lant, A. F., Matthews, D. M., Milne, M. D., Navab, F., and Richards, A. J. (1970): Intestinal absorption of two dipeptides in Hartnup disease. Gut 11:380–389.
Asatoor, A. M., Crouchman, M. R., Harrison, A. R., Light, F. W., Loughridge, L. W., Milne, M. D., and Richards, A. J. (1971): Intestinal absorption of oligopeptides in cystinuria. Clin. Sci. 41:23–33.
Asatoor, A. M., Harrison, B. D. W., Milne, M. D., and Prosser, D. I. (1972): Intestinal absorption of an arginine-containing peptide in cystinuria. Gut 13:95–98.
Asatoor, A. M., Chadha, A. K., Dawson, I. M. P., Milne, M. D., and Prosser, D. I. (1972): The effect of pyridoxine deficiency on intestinal absorption of amino acids and peptides in the rat. Brit. J. Nutr. 28:417–423.
Asatoor, A. M., Chadha, A., Milne, M. D., and Prosser, D. I. (1973): Intestinal absorption of stereoisomers of dipeptides in the rat. Clin. Sci. Molec. Med. 45:199–212.
Boullin, D. J., Crampton, R. F., Heading, C. E., and Pelling, D. (1973): Intestinal absorption of dipeptides containing glycine, phenylalanine, proline, β-alanine or histidine in the rat. Clin. Sci. Molec. Med. 45:849–858.
Bronstein, H. D., Haeffner, L. J., and Kowlessar, O. D. (1966): The significance of gelatin tolerance in malabsorptive states. Gastroenterology 50:621–630.
Burston, D., Addison, J. M., and Matthews, D. M. (1972): Uptake of dipeptides containing basic and acidic amino acids by rat small intestine in vitro. Clin. Sci. 43:823–837.
Burston, D., Addison, J. M., Matthews, D. M., Payne, J. W., and Wilkinson, S. (1974): Intestinal transport of two tripeptides. In preparation.
Caspary, W. F. (1973): Interaction of dipeptide absorption and transport of free amino acids. In: *Biochemical and clinical aspects of peptide and amino acid absorption,* edited by K. Rommel and H. Goebell, F. K. Schattauer Verlag, Stuttgart and New York, pp. 29–40.
Cheeseman, C. I., and Smyth, D. H. (1973): Specific transfer process for intestinal absorption of peptides. J. Physiol. 229:45–46P.
Chen, M. L., Rogers, Q. R., and Harper, A. E. (1962): Observations on protein digestion in vivo. IV. Further observations on the gastrointestinal contents of rats fed different dietary proteins. J. Nutr. 76:235–241.
Cheng, B., Navab, F., Lis, M. T., Miller, T. N., and Matthews, D. M. (1971): Mechanisms of dipeptide uptake by rat small intestine in vitro. Clin. Sci. 40:247–259.
Cook, G. C. (1972): Comparison of intestinal absorption rates of glycine and glycylglycine in man and the effect of glucose in the perfusing fluid. Clin. Sci. 43:443–453.
Coulson, R. A., and Hernandez, T. (1970): Protein digestion and amino acid absorption in the cayman. J. Nutr. 100:810–826.
Craft, I. L., Geddes, D., Hyde, C. W., Wise, I. J., and Matthews, D. M. (1968): Absorption and malabsorption of glycine and glycine peptides in man. Gut 9:425–427.
Crampton, R. F., Gangolli, S. D., Simson, P., and Matthews, D. M. (1971): Rates of absorption by rat intestine of pancreatic hydrolysates of proteins and their corresponding amino acid mixtures. Clin. Sci. 41:409–417.
Crampton, R. F., Lis, M. T., and Matthews, D. M. (1973): Sites of maximal absorption and hydrolysis of two dipeptides by rat small intestine in vivo. Clin. Sci. 44:583–594.
Crane, R. K., Malathi, P., Caspary, W. F., and Ramaswamy, K. (1970): Evidence for a second glucose transport system in hamster small intestine specific for glucose released by brush border digestive enzymes. Fed. Proc. 29:595.
Das, M., and Radhakrishnan, A. N. (1972): Substrate specificity of a highly active dipeptidase purified from monkey small intestine. Biochem. J. 128:463–465.
Dorer, F. E., Haley, E. E., Buchanan, D. L. (1966): Quantitative studies of urinary β-aspartyl oligopeptides. Biochemistry 5:3236–3240.

Evered, D. F., and Wass, M. (1970): Transport of glutathione across the small intestine of the rat *in vitro*. J. Physiol. *209:*4–5P.
Fern, E. B., Hider, R. C., and London, D. R. (1969): The sites of hydrolysis of dipeptides containing leucine and glycine by rat jejunum *in vitro*. Biochem. J., *114:*855–861.
Fogel, M. R., and Adibi, S. A. (1973): Assessment of physiological function of brush border peptide hydrolases in human jejunum. Clin. Res. *21:*826.
Gray, G. M., and Cooper, H. L. (1971): Protein digestion and absorption. Gastroenterology *61:*535–544.
Hellier, M. D., Perrett, D., and Holdsworth, C. D. (1970): Dipeptide absorption in cystinuria. Brit. Med. J. *IV:*782–783.
Hellier, M. D., Holdsworth, C. D., McColl, I., and Perrett, D. (1972): Dipeptide absorption in man. Gut *13:*965–969.
Hellier, M. D., Holdsworth, C. D., Perrett, D., and Thirumalai, C. (1972): Intestinal dipeptide transport in normal and cystinuric subjects. Clin. Sci. *43:*659–668.
Hueckel, H. J., and Rogers, Q. R. (1972): Prolylhydroxyproline absorption in hamsters. Canad. J. Biochem. *50:*782–790.
Kim, Y. S., Birtwhistle, W., and Kim, Y. W. (1972): Peptide hydrolysis in the brush border and soluble fractions of small intestinal mucosa of rat and man. J. Clin. Invest. *51:*1419–1430.
Kooshuck, R. J. (1971): Site of the peptidase action in the cells of the small intestine epithelium of mammals, birds, and fishes of different age. Sechenov Physiol. J. USSR. *57:*1053–1057.
Kushak, R. I., and Ugolev, A. M. (1966): On the localisation of peptidase activity in the cells of the small intestine of white rats. Dokl. Biol. Sci. *168:*411–413.
Leonard, J. V., Marrs, T. C., Addison, J. M., Burston, D., Clegg, K. M., Lloyd, J., Seakins, J. M., and Matthews, D. M. (1974): Absorption of amino acids and peptides in Hartnup disease. Clin. Sci. Molec. Med. *46:*15P.
Lis, M. T., Crampton, R. F., and Matthews, D. M. (1971): Rates of absorption of a dipeptide and the equivalent free amino acid in various mammalian species. Biochim. Biophys. Acta *233:*453–455.
Lis, M. T., Matthews, D. M., and Crampton, R. F. (1972a): Effects of dietary restriction and protein deprivation on intestinal absorption of protein digestion products in the rat. Brit. J. Nutr. *28:*443–446.
Lis, M. T., Crampton, R. F., and Matthews, D. M. (1972b): Effect of dietary changes on intestinal absorption of L-methionine and L-methionyl-L-methionine in the rat. Brit. J. Nutr. *27:*159–167.
Matthews, D. M. (1971): Protein absorption. J. Clin. Path. *24*, Suppl. (Roy. Coll. Path.) *5:*29–40.
Matthews, D. M. (1972): Rates of peptide uptake by small intestine. In: *Peptide transport in bacteria and mammalian gut.* A Ciba Foundation Symposium, edited by K. Elliott and M. O'Connor, Associated Scientific Publishers, Amsterdam, pp. 71–88.
Matthews, D. M. (1974): Absorption of peptides by mammalian intestine. In: *Peptide transport in protein nutrition,* edited by D. M. Matthews and J. W. Payne. Associated Scientific Publishers, Amsterdam, *in press.*
Matthews, D. M. (*in press*): Peptide absorption. *Physiol. Rev.*
Matthews, D. M., Craft, I. L., Geddes, D. M., Wise, I. J., and Hyde, C. W. (1968): Absorption of glycine and glycine peptides from the small intestine of the rat. Clin. Sci. *35:*415–424.
Matthews, D. M., Lis, M. T., Cheng, B., and Crampton, R. F. (1969): Observations on the intestinal absorption of some oligopeptides of methionine and glycine in the rat. Clin. Sci. *37:*751–764.
Matthews, D. M., Addison, J. M., and Burston, D. (1974): Evidence for active transport of the dipeptide carnosine (β-alanyl-L-histidine) by hamster jejunum *in vitro*. Clin. Sci. Molec. Med. *46:*693–705.
Matthews, D. M., and Payne, J. W. (*in press*): Occurrence and biological activities of

peptides. In: *Peptide transport in protein nutrition,* edited by D. M. Matthews and J. W. Payne, Associated Scientific Publishers, Amsterdam.

Milne, M. D. (1964): Disorders of amino acid transport. Brit. Med. J. *1:*327–336.

Nasset, E. M. (1965): Role of the digestive system in protein metabolism. Fed. Proc. *24:*953–958.

Navab, F., and Asatoor, A. M. (1970): Studies on intestinal absorption of amino acids and a dipeptide in a case of Hartnup disease. Gut *11:*373–379.

Newey, H., and Smyth, D. H. (1959): The intestinal absorption of some dipeptides. J. Physiol. *145:*48–56.

Newey, H., and Smyth, D. H. (1960): Intracellular hydrolysis of dipeptides during intestinal absorption. J. Physiol. *152:*367–380.

Newey, H., and Smyth, D. H. (1962): Cellular mechanisms in intestinal transport of amino acids. J. Physiol. *164:*527–551.

Nixon, S. E., and Mawer, G. E. (1970a): The digestion and absorption of protein in man. 1. The site of absorption. Brit. J. Nutr. *24:*227–240.

Nixon, S. E., and Mawer, G. E. (1970b): The digestion and absorption of protein in man. 2. The form in which digested protein is absorbed. Brit. J. Nutr. *24:*241–258.

Payne, J. W. (1972): Mechanisms of bacterial peptide transport. In: *Peptide transport in bacteria and mammalian gut.* A Ciba Foundation Symposium, edited by K. Elliott and M. O'Connor, Associated Scientific Publishers, Amsterdam, pp. 15–32.

Payne, J. W., and Matthews, D. M. (*in press*): Peptides in the nutrition of microorganisms and peptides in relation to animal nutrition. In: *Peptide transport in protein nutrition,* edited by D. M. Matthews and J. W. Payne, Associated Scientific Publishers, Amsterdam.

Perry, T. L., Hansen, S., Tischler, B., Bunting, R., and Berry, K. (1967): Carnosinaemia: A new metabolic disorder associated with neurologic disease and mental defect. New Engl. J. Med. *277:*1219–1227.

Peters, T. J. (1970): Intestinal peptidases. Gut *11:*720–725.

Peters, T. J., Donlon, J., and Fottrell, P. F. (1972): The subcellular localization and specificity of intestinal peptide hydrolases. In: *Transport across the intestine,* edited by W. L. Burland and P. D. Samuel, Churchill Livingston, Edinburgh and London, pp. 153–167.

Prockop, D. J., Keiser, H. R., and Sjoerdsma, A. (1962): Gastrointestinal absorption and renal excretion of hydroxyproline peptides. Lancet *2:*527–528.

Rubino, A., Field, M., and Shwachman, H. (1971): Intestinal transport of amino acid residues of dipeptides. 1. Influx of the glycine residue of glycyl-L-proline across mucosal border. J. Biol. Chem. *246:*3542–3548.

Silk, D. B. A., Marrs, T. C., Addison, J. M., Burston, D., Clark, M. L., and Matthews, D. M. (1973a): Absorption of amino acids from an amino acid mixture simulating casein and a tryptic hydrolysate of casein in man. Clin. Sci. Molec. Med. *45:*715–719.

Silk, D. B. A., Perrett, D., and Clark, M. L. (1973b): Intestinal transport of two dipeptides containing the same two neutral amino acids in man. Clin. Sci. Molec. Med. *45:*291–299.

Tarlow, M. J., Seakins, J. W. T., Lloyd, J. K., Matthews, D. M., Cheng, B., and Thomas, A. J. (1970): Intestinal absorption and biopsy transport of peptides and amino acids in Hartnup disease. Clin. Sci. *39:*18P.

Tarlow, M. J., Seakins, J. W. T., Lloyd, J. K., Matthews, D. M., Cheng, B., and Thomas, A. J. (1972): Absorption of amino acids and peptides in a child with a variant of Hartnup disease and coexistent coeliac disease. Arch. Dis. Childhood, *47:*798–803.

Ugolev, A. M. (1968): *Physiology and pathology of membrane digestion,* Plenum Press, New York.

Ugolev, A. M. (1972): Membrane digestion and peptide transport. In: *Peptide transport in bacteria and mammalian gut.* A Ciba Foundation Symposium, edited by K. Elliott and M. O'Connor, Associated Scientific Publishers, Amsterdam, pp. 123–137.

Ugolev, A. M., Iesuitova, N. N., Timofeeva, N. M., and Fediushina, I. N. (1964): Location of hydrolysis of certain disaccharides and peptides in the small intestine. Nature *202:*807–809.

Ugolev, A. M., and Kooshuck, R. I. (1966): Hydrolysis of dipeptides in cells of the small intestine. Nature *212:*859–860.
Ugolev, A. M., Iesuitova, N. N., Timofeeva, N. M., and Kushak, R. I. (1967): On the microtopography of the distribution in the intra- and extracellular fluids of hexoses and amino acids formed by hydrolysis of disaccharides and dipeptides. Nahrung *11:*595–606.
Van Slyke, D. D. (1917): The present significance of the amino acids in physiology and pathology. Arch. Int. Med. *19:*56–78.

DISCUSSION

ARMSTRONG asked if the peptides pass unchanged through the cell and appear in the blood as such. MATTHEWS answered that a few peptides, which are slowly hydrolyzed, do; in experiments *in vitro* it is difficult to quantitate the appearance of peptides in the serosal fluid because the latter contains surprisingly high peptidase activity so that some splitting of the peptides always occurs.

ESPOSITO asked if monosaccharides or disaccharides interfere with the uptake of peptides. MATTHEWS answered that this question was not yet investigated.

Intestinal Absorption and Malabsorption,
edited by T. Z. Csáky.
Raven Press, New York © 1975

Cation Effects on Intestinal Transport of Nonelectrolytes

Peter F. Curran*

Department of Physiology, Yale University School of Medicine, New Haven, Connecticut 06510

Other chapters in this volume discuss several aspects of the transport of hexoses and amino acids by the intestinal epithelium and mention the effects of cations on these processes. My assignment is to discuss these cation effects in more detail and to attempt to provide some idea of our current understanding of their nature. The discussion will be mainly in the nature of a summary, because detailed reviews of the cation dependence of nonelectrolyte transport have appeared in recent years (Schultz and Curran, 1970; Heinz, 1972; Kimmich, 1973) and another one seems unnecessary at present.

The most striking cation effect on transport of nonelectrolytes by the small intestine clearly involves the Na ion. Complete removal of Na from solutions bathing *in vitro* preparations of intestine essentially abolishes active transport of hexoses and amino acids. As shown by the data in Table 1 taken from studies in my laboratory, this effect is observed in studies of tissue accumulation of hexoses or amino acids and in studies of transmural transport of the nonelectrolytes. In the presence of normal (140 mM) Na the epithelial cells of the intestine accumulate sugars and amino acids to concentrations several times higher than those in the external solutions and can bring about net transport of these substances across the tissue from the mucosal to the serosal side in the absence of a concentration difference between the bathing solutions. In the complete absence of Na both of these manifestations of active transport disappear. However, these simple observations provide no information about the nature of the Na effect; it could be due to an effect on transport process at the brush border membrane, the serosal membrane, or both, or to a disturbance of the supply of energy required for the active transport phenomena. Whatever the nature of the Na effect on nonelectrolyte transport, the relationship is a reciprocal one. The addition of actively transported sugars or amino acids to the solution bathing the mucosal surface of *in vitro* intestinal preparations causes an increase in the rate of net active transport of Na across the tissue (Schultz and Zalusky, 1964). A similar stimulation of Na absorption by sugars and amino acids is observed *in vivo* (see, for example, Adibi, 1970).

In an effort to obtain some insight into the nature of the Na effect in the rabbit ileum, Schultz, Curran, Chez, and Fuisz (1967) studied the influx

---

* Deceased October 16, 1974.

TABLE 1. *Effect of Na on hexose and amino acid transport in the rabbit ileum*

Solute	C_i/C_e		J_{net} (μmoles/hr cm^2)	
	Na	Choline	Na	Choline
3-O-methyl glucose	2.8	0.5	0.6	0.0
Alanine	8.5	1.0	1.2	0.0
Glycine	4.6	0.8	0.6	0.0

C_i/C_e is the ratio of intracellular to extracellular concentration in strips of mucosa incubated for 30 min. J_{net} is the net transmural flux from mucosa to serosa observed with identical nonelectrolyte concentrations in mucosal and serosal solutions. Data are from Schultz et al. (1966), Field et al. (1967), and Goldner et al. (1969).

of alanine across the brush border membrane from the mucosal solution to the cells using the technique described by Schultz and Frizzell (*this volume*). The method measures the initial rate of amino acid uptake across the brush border and avoids any possible complications due to uptake into the cells across the serosal membrane because this side of the tissue is not exposed to the amino acid. In addition, in our hands, the technique does not appear to be seriously compromised by the presence of unstirred fluid layers (Preston, Schaeffer, and Curran, 1974). The results shown in Table 2 indicate that removal of Na from the bathing solution causes a 75% reduction in alanine influx across the brush border at the concentration tested (5 mM). Similar results were obtained by Goldner, Schultz, and Curran (1969) for the actively transported hexose 3-O-methyl glucose. Thus the brush border membrane is clearly one locus for the cation effect on nonelectrolyte transport. Table 2 also indicates that the requirement of Na for the normal influx of nonelectrolyte is mainly a requirement for external Na. If the tissue is preincubated in a Na-free solution to deplete cell Na and the influx is then measured by brief exposure to a solution containing 140-mM Na plus alanine, a normal influx is observed. In other words, the influx is little altered by a marked reduction in cell Na.

TABLE 2. *Effect of Na on alanine influx across the brush border of the rabbit ileum*

Preincubation	Test	Influx (μmoles/hr cm^2)
Na	Na	2.2 ± 0.1
Choline	Choline	0.6 ± 0.1
Choline	Na	2.1 ± 0.2

Alanine concentration was 5 mM. Preincubation was for 30–45 min. Influx was measured over a 1-min period using the test solution indicated. Data from Schultz et al. (1967).

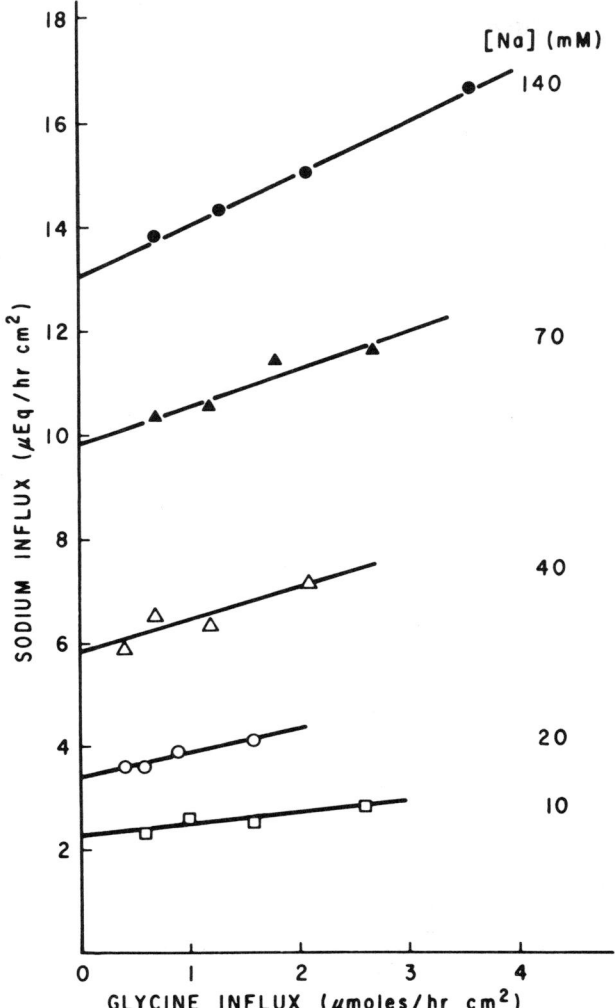

FIG. 1. Relationship between influxes of Na and glycine across the brush border of the rabbit ileum. Reproduced from Peterson et al. (1970) with permission of Rockefeller University Press.

As shown in Fig. 1, reciprocal effects between Na and nonelectrolyte transfer are also observed at the level of the brush border. There is a linear relationship between the Na influx and the simultaneously measured influx of glycine, indicating a close relationship between the transfer of these two solutes across the membrane. Qualitatively similar results were obtained for actively transported hexoses (Goldner et al., 1969). This stimulation of Na entry into the cells by nonelectrolytes is presumably the initial step involved in the overall increase in active Na transport across the epithelial cell layer caused by the presence of these solutes in the mucosal solution. Studies of this type led us to specific kinetic models to explain the interaction of Na and nonelectrolyte transport in the brush border membrane (see Schultz and Curran, 1970, for a general discussion). These models involve transport systems that can combine with both Na and nonelectrolyte and mediate the transfer of both solutes across the membrane via a process that has become known as cotransport. Schultz and Frizzell have already discussed the specific model developed for amino acid transport and indicated that it can be characterized in part in terms of dissociation constants for the reaction between amino acid and transport site and between Na and transport site (*this volume*). The details of this model need not concern us here.

A fuller explanation of the effects of cations on nonelectrolytes requires study of the behavior of ions other than Na. Can any other ions substitute for Na? Do they compete with Na? The most detailed study of these questions is probably that of Frizzell and Schultz (1970) on alanine influx across the brush border of the rabbit ileum. Some of their results are shown in Fig. 2. In experiments carried out in the presence of 20-mM Na, 115-mM K, Rb,

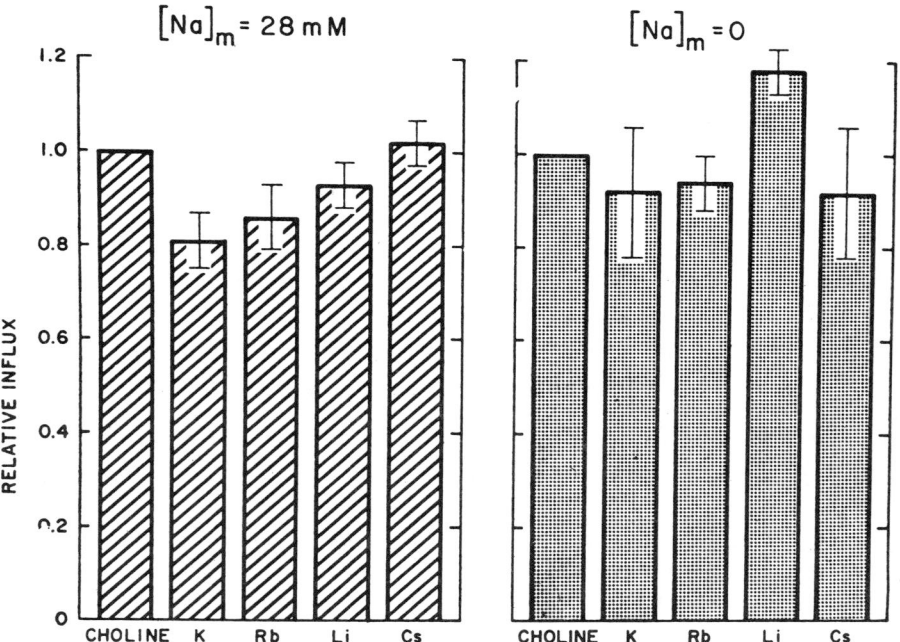

FIG. 2. Effect of various Na substitutes on alanine influx across the brush border of the rabbit ileum. Fluxes are expressed relative to those observed in the presence of choline. Reproduced from Frizzell and Schultz (1970) with permission of Rockefeller University Press.

and Li, all inhibited alanine influx compared to the influx observed in the presence of 115-mM choline and 25-mM Na; Cs was essentially equivalent to choline. Similar results were obtained by Goldner et al. (1969) in identical studies of 3-O-methyl glucose influx in the rabbit ileum. In this case, Li, K, and guanidinium ions were found to reduce the influx below that observed when choline or Tris was substituted for all but 28-mM Na. Frizzell and Schultz (1970) showed that the effect of K on alanine influx had the kinetics of competitive inhibition, a point to which we shall return later. The nature of the other cation effects has not been explored in comparable detail.

However, when Frizzell and Schultz examined the effect of various cations on alanine influx in the complete absence of Na, they obtained different results shown on the right side of Fig. 2. Under these conditions, K, Rb, and Cs were equivalent to choline, but Li caused a significant increase in the influx compared to the other cations, suggesting that it would function poorly as a substitute for Na. Some results of Hayashi, Siato, and Hoshi (1971) suggest that this may also be true for the sugar transport system in the toad intestine. Addition of glucose to the mucosal solution in the presence of Na causes a substantial increase in the electrical potential difference (PD) across the intestine. A similar but smaller glucose-induced increase in PD was observed in experiments in which all of the Na was replaced by Li, again indicating that Li may substitute for Na in the process. Actually Li appears to have a dual effect on nonelectrolyte transfer at the brush border since the results of Frizzell and Schultz showed that it inhibits alanine influx in the presence of Na but stimulates it in the complete absence of Na.

In addition to these results, Frizzell and Schultz (1970) also showed that the hydrogen ion inhibited alanine influx in the presence of Na but had only a small effect on the mediated influx of alanine in the complete absence of Na. The effect of the hydrogen ion was also shown to have the kinetic characteristics of competitive inhibition. The interpretation of these effects of cations other than Na in terms of kinetic models is complex. They could involve a site on the transport system other than the specific site occupied by Na or, perhaps in part, the Na site itself. A final model of the cation sensitivity of these systems will require more information than is now available.

We have little information about the nature of the Na site in the transport system. As indicated by Schultz and Frizzell, this site may be "created" by a confirmational change caused by the binding of an amino acid to the transport site. This suggestion is based on the finding for the rabbit ileum that the binding of an amino acid appears to precede the binding of Na. Observations on the effects of the hydrogen ion on the system suggest that the Na site could involve a carboxyl group with a pK of approximately 4. Some additional information comes from recent studies by Schaeffer, Preston, and Curran (1973) on the effect of a sulfhydryl reagent, p-chloromercuribenzenesulfonic acid (PCMBS), on phenylalanine influx in the rabbit ileum. As shown in Fig. 3, this reagent rapidly inhibits amino acid influx by 80% but

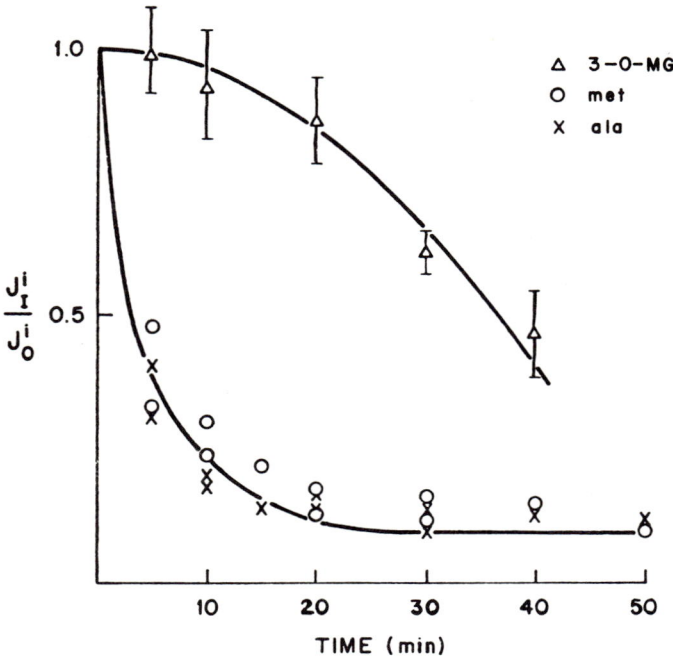

FIG. 3. Effect of time of exposure to 5 mM PCMBS on nonelectrolyte influx across the brush border of the rabbit ileum. Fluxes are expressed relative to control values. The lower solid line shows the time course for inhibition of phenylalanine influx. Reproduced from Schaeffer et al. (1973) with permission of Rockefeller University Press.

has a much lesser effect on 3-O-methyl glucose influx at least at short times. However, kinetic studies of influx as a function of phenylalanine concentration indicate that the transport system is not inactivated by treatment with PCMBS. Instead there is a marked decrease in the Na sensitivity of the influx process. This conclusion is indicated by the finding that treatment of the tissue with PCMBS does not alter the maximum influx of phenylalanine but causes a marked increase in the apparent Michaelis constant for the process. When these studies are interpreted in terms of the model for amino acid transport discussed by Schultz and Frizzell, they indicate approximately a fivefold decrease in the apparent affinity of the transport system for Na with only a small decrease in the apparent affinity for phenylalanine itself. These and other results obtained in this study suggest that PCMBS may react with the transport system in such a way as to prevent or seriously impede the confirmational change that creates the Na site without causing a major change in the ability of the system to bind the amino acid. The possibility of such a mode of action of inhibitors was suggested several years ago by Schultz (1969).

Regardless of the nature of the Na site or the molecular details of the action of cations on nonelectrolyte transport, it is important to note that the cation dependence of these processes led to the proposal of the Na-gradient hypothesis for intestinal transport of nonelectrolytes (Crane, 1962, 1965). This concept has of course been discussed extensively in terms of a variety of cells and tissues but I will restrict my remarks about it mainly to studies on the intestine. According to this hypothesis, the energy required for the active accumulation of sugars and amino acids in intestinal cells is supplied by the Na-concentration gradient across the brush border membrane, high in the mucosal solution, low in the cytoplasm. The cotransport systems in the brush border membrane are driven by this Na gradient in the direction to cause cellular accumulation of nonelectrolyte to concentrations above those in the mucosal solution, so that there is no need to postulate direct input of metabolic energy. In thermodynamic terms the apparent active transport of nonelectrolyte is driven by coupling to Na flow (via the cotransport system), not by direct coupling to the metabolism. It is important to note that cell Na is maintained low by extrusion of Na from the cell at the lateral serosal membrane by an active, energy-requiring process. A variety of evidence for and against this hypothesis has been presented based on studies of several different cell types, and much of this information has been reviewed recently (Schultz and Curran, 1970; Heinz, 1972; Christensen, de Cespedes, Handlogten, and Ronquist, 1973; Kimmich, 1973. It is not my intent to review this evidence further. Rather I would like to pose four specific questions relating to the status of the Na-gradient hypothesis for the intestine and to see what conclusions we might draw from the answers. The questions are each related to the fundamental question of whether or not the Na-gradient hypothesis can be ruled out for the intestine. Similar questions can be posed for other cell types as well, but we will consider mainly the intestinal cell.

QUESTION 1. *Can ion concentration differences between the external solution and the cytoplasm cause net movements of nonelectrolyte against their concentration difference?* If the answer to this question is no, the ion-gradient hypothesis is untenable. However, I believe the answer to the question is yes. Crane (1964) has demonstrated that in isolated villi from the hamster an "active" extrusion of hexose from the cells caused by arranging conditions so that cellular-Na concentration was higher than that in the external solution. Hajjar, Lamont, and Curran (1970) obtained similar results for alanine movement in strips of mucosa from the rabbit ileum, and Curran, Hajjar, and Glynn (1970) showed that net Na movements could be caused in ouabain-poisoned tissue by concentration differences of alanine between inside and outside of the cells. Finally, in studies on the turtle intestine, Hajjar, Khuri, and Curran (1972) demonstrated that alanine extrusion from cells caused by an outwardly directed Na-concentration difference was a property of the brush border membrane, not the basolateral membrane.

QUESTION 2. *Is there enough energy available from the Na gradient to account for the uphill accumulation of nonelectrolytes by intestinal cells?* The question is essentially a thermodynamic one. The minimum free energy required for accumulation of nonelectrolyte, *s*, is given by the steady-state difference in chemical potential, $\Delta\mu_s$ across the membrane:

$$\Delta\mu_s = RT \ln \frac{C_{s(\text{cell})}}{C_{s(\text{out})}}$$

The maximum free energy available from the Na gradient is given by the chemical potential difference for Na, $\Delta\mu_{\text{Na}}$:

$$\Delta\mu_{\text{Na}} = RT \ln \frac{a_{\text{Na(out)}}}{a_{\text{Na(cell)}}},$$

in which *a* is activity. If the electrical potential difference is included, the maximum free energy available will be given by the electrochemical potential difference for Na, $\Delta\bar{\mu}_{\text{Na}}$:

$$\Delta\bar{\mu}_{\text{Na}} = \Delta\mu_{\text{Na}} + F(\Psi_{\text{out}} - \Psi_{\text{cell}}),$$

in which *F* is the Faraday and Ψ is the electrical potential.

To the best of my knowledge, there is only one study that really approaches this question for the intestine. It was carried out by Armstrong, Byrd, and Hamang (1973) and has already been mentioned by Armstrong (*this volume*). The study involved measurements of Na activities (not concentrations), electrical potentials, and galactose accumulation under identical experimental conditions in the bullfrog intestine. The results of this study are presented on *P*. They indicate that $\Delta\mu_{\text{Na}} < \Delta\mu_{\text{gal}}$ but that $\Delta\bar{\mu}_{\text{Na}} > \Delta\mu_{\text{gal}}$. In other words the maximum free energy available in the difference in activity between mucosal solution and cytoplasm is not sufficient to account for galactose accumulation but the energy available in the electrochemical potential difference for Na is sufficient. These considerations neglect a possible role of K, which is a competitive inhibitor of the Na effect in the rabbit ileum. Thus, the high cellular-K concentration could have the effect of reducing the effective cellular activity of Na with respect to the process of nonelectrolyte transport. This effect cannot be quantitatively evaluated at present but, if it occurs, it would tend to increase the maximum energy available from the ion gradients. These points lead in a natural way to my third question.

QUESTION 3. *Should the effects of the electrical potential difference (PD) be included in evaluations of the ion gradient hypothesis?* The above discussion indicates clearly that this question is important for thermodynamic arguments. It is equally important for kinetic arguments regarding these systems and to any interpretation or experimental results. I am prepared to argue, on the basis of the results of White and Armstrong (1971) and Rose and Schultz (1971), that the PD must be considered as a driving force for these systems. The studies cited demonstrated clearly that the addition of actively transported hexoses or amino acids to the mucosal bathing solution caused an immediate depolarization of the PD across the brush border membrane. This result strongly suggests that cotransport of nonelectrolyte and Na into the cell involves movement of a charged species. Such behavior would clearly be expected on the basis of models of the cotransport system since combination of the transport site with a cation means that the loaded and unloaded site must differ in charge and a single cycle of the system would lead to the transfer of positive charge into the cell. If operation of the transport system involves movement of charge, the PD must clearly be included as contributing to the total driving force for the system.

These results and this conclusion are consistent with the recent observation of Murer and Hopfer (1974) on sugar transport by isolated membrane vesicles prepared from the brush border of the rat intestine. They found that experimental maneuvers that should make the interior of the vesicle electrically negative increased sugar accumulation by the vesicles. The concept that the PD plays a role in the cotransport process has several important implications. First, it implies that the PD must be included in the thermodynamic considerations outlined under Question 2. Thus, on the basis of the very limited information now available on the intestine, I do not think that the Na-gradient hypothesis can be rejected on thermodynamic or energetic grounds. [A similar conclusion was recently reached by Heniz and Geck (1974) for amino acid transport by Erlich ascites cells.] Second, if the PD plays a role, it must be considered in interpretation of experiments in which the relationship between nonelectrolyte transport and ion gradients are examined. To state the case simply, observation of cellular accumulation of a nonelectrolyte in the absence of or against a Na-concentration difference does not *necessarily* rule out the Na-gradient hypothesis. In order to interpret such a study fully, knowledge of the PD and of ion activities (not concentrations) is required.

On the basis of my considerations of the first three questions posed, I am led to conclude that ion gradients can provide energy for apparent active transport of nonelectrolytes and in the one case for which enough information is available to make the calculation, it is *thermodynamically* possible that all the energy for galactose accumulation could be provided by the electrochemical potential gradient for Na. I am thus led naturally to a fourth question.

QUESTION 4. *Are sources of energy other than ion and electrical gradients involved in the active transport of nonelectrolytes by the intestine?* For example, is direct utilization of ATP involved? I regret to say that I cannot answer this question on the basis of the information now available, nor can anyone else in my opinion. Clearly, there are observations available that are not consistent with the Na-gradient hypothesis in its simple form (see for example Kimmich, 1970), but I am not convinced that we know enough about the systems involved to rule out entirely the gradient hypothesis. On the other hand, I am not convinced that these observations can be explained entirely by an extended form of the hypothesis; they may indeed indicate that other sources of energy are used, at least under certain conditions, for active nonelectrolyte transport by the intestine. In this regard, it is of interest to note that Ried and Eddy (1971) have found that amino acid transport by ascites cells under given conditions is altered by the cellular-ATP level; they suggested that the effect might not involve ATP splitting but rather an effect of the cellular-ATP level on characteristics of the cotransport system. Perhaps the truth lies somewhere in between the concept of transport systems driven only by ion and electrical gradients and ones driven only by direct input of metabolic energy.

I would like to comment briefly on one final point. Virtually all of the discussion so far has involved the brush border membrane, because the movement of nonelectrolytes across that membrane has been shown very clearly to depend on cations, particularly Na. It is, however, appropriate to ask whether transfer of sugars and amino acids across the basolateral membrane is cation dependent and whether that membrane could be involved in any of the effects we have been discussing. We have minimal information on the properties of this membrane because it is much less accessible to direct experimental measurement than is the brush border membrane. The information we have available indicates that hexoses and amino acids probably cross the basolateral membrane by a process of facilitated transfer. The transfer appears to be in the direction of the concentration difference of the solute and to be entirely independent of Na. Results consistent with these conclusions have been obtained in the turtle intestine for alanine (Hajjar et al., 1972), in the rabbit ileum for galactose (Naftalin and Curran, 1974), and in the hamster small intestine for hexoses (Bihler and Cybulsky, 1973). Each study involved quite different techniques but in no case could a significant Na effect be detected at the basolateral membrane. Thus it seems safe to conclude that the cation effects that we have been discussing are localized entirely to the brush border membrane, and it is perhaps attractive to speculate that the membranes at the two sides of the intestinal cell contain rather similar "carrier" systems for nonelectrolytes but that the brush border systems have developed or maintained a Na sensitivity whereas the basolateral ones have failed to develop or lost this cation sensitivity. Thus the asymmetry of the membranes at the two sides of the cell that is required for active transepithelial nonelectrolyte may reside almost entirely in the cation sensitivity of the transfer systems in these membranes.

REFERENCES

Adibi, S. A. (1970): Leucine absorption rate and net movements of sodium and water in human Jejunum. J. Appl. Physiol. 28:753–757.

Armstrong, W. M., Byrd, B. J., and Hamang, P. M. (1973): The Na^+ gradient and D-galactose accumulation in epithelial cells of bullfrog small intestine. Biochim. Biophys. Acta 330:237–241.

Bihler, I., and Cybulsky, R. (1973): Sugar transport of the basal and lateral aspects of the small intestinal cell. Biochim. Biophys. Acta *298:*429.
Christensen, H. N., de Cespedes, C., Handlogten, M. E. and Ronquist, G. (1973). Energization of amino acid transport, studied for the Erlich ascites tumor cell. Biochim. Biophys. Acta. *300:*487–522.
Crane, R. K. (1962): Hypothesis for mechanism of intestinal active transport of sugars. Fed. Proc. *21:*891–895.
Crane, R. K. (1964): Uphill outflow of sugar from intestinal cells induced by reversal of the Na^+ gradient: its significance for the mechanism of Na^+-dependent active transport. Biochem. Biophys. Res. Commun. *17:*481–485.
Crane, R. K. (1965): Na^+-dependent transport in the intestine and other animal tissues. Fed. Proc. *24:*1000–1005.
Curran, P. F., Hajjar, J. J., and Glynn, I. M. (1970): The sodium-alanine interaction in rabbit ileum: effect of alanine on Na fluxes. J. Gen. Physiol. *55:*297–308.
Field, M., Schultz, S. G., and Curran, P. F. (1967): Alanine transport across isolated rabbit ileum. Biochim. Biophys. Acta *135:*236–243.
Frizzel, R. A., and Schultz, S. G. (1970): Effects of monovalent cations on the sodium-alanine interaction in rabbit ileum. Implication of anionic groups in sodium binding. J. Gen. Physiol. *56:*462–490.
Goldner, A. M., Schultz, S. G. and Curran, P. F. (1969): Sodium and sugar fluxes across the mucosal border of rabbit ileum. J. Gen. Physiol. *53:*362–383.
Hajjar, J. J., Khuri, R. N., and Curran, P. F. (1972): Alanine efflux across the serosal border of turtle intestine. J. Gen. Physiol. *60:*720–734.
Hajjar, J. J., Lamont, A. S., and Curran, P. F. (1970): The sodium-alanine interaction in rabbit ileum: effect of Na on alanine fluxes. J. Gen. Physiol. *55:*277–296.
Hayashi, H., Saito, Y., and Hoshi, T. (1971): Sugar-dependent increment of the transmural potential of isolated small intestine in Li^+-medium. Tohoku J. Exp. Med. *103:*119–128.
Heinz, E. (Ed.) (1972): *Na^+-linked transport of organic solutes,* Springer, Berlin.
Heinz, E., and Geck, P. (1974): The efficiency of energetic coupling between Na^+ flow and amino acid transport in Erlich cells—A revised assessment. Biochim. Biophys. Acta *339:*426–431.
Kimmich, G. A. (1970): Active sugar accumulation by isolated intestinal epithelial cells. A new model for sodium dependent metabolite transport. Biochemistry *9:*3669–3677.
Kimmich, G. A. (1973): Coupling between sodium and sugar transport in small intestine. Biochim. Biophys. Acta *300:*31–78.
Murer, H., and Hopfer, U. (1974): Demonstration of electrogenic Na^+-dependent D-glucose transport in intestinal brush border membranes. Proc. Nat. Acad. Sci. *71:*484–488.
Naftalin, R., and Curran, P. F. (1974): Galactose transport in rabbit ileum. J. Memb. Biol. *16:*257–278.
Peterson, S. C., Goldner, A. M. and Curran, P. F. (1970): Glycine transport in rabbit ileum. Am. J. Physiol. *219:*1027–1032.
Preston, R. L., Schaeffer, J. F., and Curran, P. F. (1974): Structure-affinity relationships of substrates for the neutral amino acid transport system in rabbit ileum. J. Gen. Physiol., in press.
Reid, M., and Eddy, A. A. (1971): Apparent metabolic regulation of the coupling between the potassium ion gradient and methionine transport in mouse ascites tumor cells. Biochem. J. *124:*951–952.
Rose, R. C., and Schultz, S. G. (1971): Studies on the electrical potential profile across rabbit ileum. Effect of sugars and amino acids on transmural and transmucosal electrical potential differences. J. Gen. Physiol. *57:*639.
Schaeffer, J. F., Preston, R. L., and Curran, P. F. (1973): Inhibition of amino acid transport in rabbit intestine by *p*-chloromercuriphenylsulfonic acid. J. Gen. Physiol. *62:*131–146.
Schultz, S. G. (1969): The interaction between sodium and amino acid transport across the brush border of rabbit ileum: A plausible molecular model. In: *The molecular*

basis of membrane function, edited by D. C. Tosteson, Prentice-Hall, Englewood Cliffs, N.J., p. 401.

Schultz, S. G., and Curran, P. F. (1970): Coupled transport of sodium and organic solutes. Physiol. Rev. *80:*637–718.

Schultz, S. G., Curran, P. F., Chez, R. A., and Fuisz, R. E. (1967): Alanine and sodium fluxes across the mucosal border of rabbit ileum. J. Gen. Physiol. *50:*1241–1260.

Schultz, S. G., Fuisz, R. E., and Curran, P. F. (1966): Amino acid and sugar transport in rabbit ileum. J. Gen. Physiol. *49:*849–866.

Schultz, S. G. and Zalusky, R. (1964): Ion transport in isolated rabbit ileum. II. The interaction between active sodium and active sugar transport. J. Gen. Physiol. *47:*1043–1059.

White, J. F., and Armstrong, W. M. (1971): Effect of transported solutes on membrane potentials in bullfrog small intestine. Am. J. Physiol. *221:*194–201.

DISCUSSION

HANKE asked how it is possible that PCMBS affects the transport of amino acids but has very little effect on the transport of 3-O-methyl glucose. CURRAN replied that in his views there are two entirely different transport systems for sugars and for amino acids. One cannot even state that the nature of the sodium effect is exactly the same on the sugar transport as it is on the amino acid system; in fact some kinetic evidence in rabbit ileum suggests that these are two entirely different effects so that even the nature of the sodium binding site may be quite different. Alternatively, the difference in PCMBS effects could be due to different accessibility of important -SH groups; at longer times of exposure PCMBS also has a significant effect on sugar influx.

Concerning the nature of the sodium-sugar interaction, ARMSTRONG commented that, in the experiments carried out in his laboratory on the bullfrog's intestine, both actively transported sugars and amino acids cause an increase of the potential difference. Phlorizin instantly abolished the increment in potential difference due to sugars but had no effect on that of amino acids; from this they have concluded that the two effects must be different.

USSING remarked that one of the basic questions is: if the potential difference has to be taken into account as a possible driving force in the coupled transport of sugars and amino acids, how can one explain the splitting of the complex when it arrives on the interior surface of the membrane. In the ionic gradient theory the dissociation of the sugar-carrier-sodium complex was achieved due to the fact that the intracellular concentration of sodium was low; therefore, the whole complex splits. If this occurs with a solution which has the same sodium concentration on the inside and the outside, why does the complex split at all? It seems to him that the electrical potential would need to affect the complex in order to cause dissociation if one wants to invoke the latter as a driving force. CURRAN answered that this may not necessarily be true if one assumes that the major electrical effect may be on the translocation of the charged complex across the membrane. The kinetic properties of models are such that net solute flux depends in a complex manner on the rate coefficients for translocation, but he indicated that he didn't have a chance to calculate this out so that he could not answer the question in detail.

FRIZZELL asked if the anionic groups influence the nature of the interaction between the amino acids and the carrier sites and the subsequent binding of sodium; and whether PCMBS changes in the same way the influx of cationic and anionic amino acids in the absence of sodium. CURRAN replied that they did not do any experiments in this area.

INDEPENDENT COMMENTS MADE WITHOUT DISCUSSION

Farmanfarmaian commented on experiments (conducted by Lipp and Farmanfarmaian at Rutgers University) that were designed to evaluate the cation gradient hypothesis under *in vivo* conditions in the hamster jejunum. In separate experiments Tris, Mannitol, and K^+ were substituted for Na^+ in Krebs-Henseleit incubation solutions in order to reverse the lumen-to-cell gradient of Na^+ and eliminate the cell-to-lumen gradient of K^+. Quabain was used in preincubation solutions to raise the intracellular Na^+ concentration of the mucosal epithelium. ^{3}H- and ^{14}C-inulin were added to lumen and blood, respectively, to determine correction factors for the steady-state contribution of extracellular fluid from those compartments to the tissue. Na^+ and K^+ were determined by flame photometry; D-glucose was assayed with purified glucose oxidase. Experimental conditions and results are summarized in the following Table 1. The terminal distribution ratios of Na^+, K^+, and glucose show that, under all cation gradient conditions tested, accumulation transport of glucose

TABLE 1. Terminal distribution of Na^+, K^+, and glucose in the jejunum of the hamster, in vivo

Preincubation	Incubation	Mean intracellular concentration mean terminal lumen concentration		
		Na^+	K^+	GLU
KH	KH	0.18	28.68	1.86
None	KHTS	N.D.	33.80	2.42
Ouabain	KH	0.13	31.30	2.39
Ouabain	KHTS	6.20	28.82	1.83
Ouabain	KHMS	4.83	32.66	2.22
Ouabain	KHKCl	5.30	1.62	1.72
Ouabain	KHKCl-PLZ	4.10	1.74	0.29

KH (Krebs-Henseleit saline); KHTS (Krebs-Henseleit saline with Tris-Cl substituted for NaCl and NaHCO$_3$); N.D. (nondetectable); ouabain (1 mM ouabain in Krebs-Henseleit saline); KHMS (Krebs-Henseleit saline with mannitol substituted for NaCl and Tris-Cl for NaHCO$_3$); KHKCl (Krebs-Henseleit saline with K^+ substituted for all Na^+); PLZ (5×10^{-4} M phloridzin in Krebs-Henseleit saline with K^+ substituted for all Na^+). Preincubation 20 min; incubation 1 min; all incubation solutions contained 4 mM D-glucose as substrate is approximately the same as in normal controls (KH, KH). Glucose transport therefore appears to be independent of the energy available in the chemical gradients of Na^+ and K^+. By contrast, the inclusion of phloridzin nearly abolishes glucose transport. In the K^+ substitution experiments, electrical potential across the brush border and the cell was probably close to zero or even negative with respect to the mucosal surface (see Lyon and Crane, 1967. *BBA* 135:61; Schultz and Zalusky, 1964. *J. Gen. Physiol.* 47:1043). This reduces the possibility of Na^+ back fluxes across the cell or through the paracellular shunt which may be attributed to electrical potential differences under normal or KHTS and KHMS conditions. Therefore the energy required for the observed accumulation of glucose cannot be due to electric potentials.

Although the electrochemical energy of the normal Na^+ and K^+ gradients may be substantial (Armstrong et al., 1973. *BBA* 330:237) and may serve other energy transducing processes in the cell, our results do not support a direct energetic coupling of these gradients to the accumulative transport of organic solutes in normally functioning intestine, *in vivo*. The results, however, do not eliminate the possibility that Na^+ or K^+ ions are "cofactors" which are efficiently coupled to "carrier" proteins (Heinz and Geck, 1974. *BBA* 339:426) or act as agents essential to membrane integrity.

Intestinal Absorption and Malabsorption,
edited by T. Z. Csáky.
Raven Press, New York © 1975

15 Years of Struggle with the Brush Border

Robert K. Crane

Department of Physiology, College of Medicine and Dentistry of New Jersey, Rutgers Medical School, Piscataway, New Jersey 08854

For the brush border 1960 was a big year. It was identified as the locale of sugar-active transport (McDougal, Little, and Crane, 1960). It was isolated as an intact, subcellular organelle and was found to possess the enzymes responsible for the terminal phases of carbohydrate digestion (Miller and Crane, 1960). It was claimed to absorb pancreatic amylase and thereby to contribute a major role in the digestion of starch (Ugolev, 1960). It was proposed (in August of that year) that the brush border carrier for sugar also cotransported Na^+, thereby coupling the energy used in Na^+ pumping to accumulation of sugar. In 1960 the brush border had finally "arrived" as a digestive-absorptive surface and was so depicted (Fig. 1).

In 1974 the figure one would draw would not be so strikingly different. The brush border as the locale of active transport, as the site of specificity and phlorizin inhibition has been amply and elegantly confirmed (Stirling 1967; Stirling and Kinter, 1967; Stirling, Schneider, Wong, and Kinter, 1972). The brush border enzymes are still where we said they were: namely, "at a locus external to a diffusion barrier sensitive to phlorizin and external to the active transport process for sugars" (Miller and Crane, 1961a, p. 292), which is now known to be clearly associated with the plasma-membrane fraction (Eichholz and Crane, 1965; Overton, Eichholz, and Crane, 1965), but they have increased some three- to fourfold in number (Table 1). The sodium pump has been moved out of the brush border membrane and into the lateral cell surface most particularly in response to the findings of Csáky and Hara (1965) relative to the sidedness of ouabain inhibition but also in keeping with the ideas of Schultz and Zalusky (1964) and Schultz and Curran (1968) among others. Also, early findings of Taylor (1962), Berg and Chapman (1965), and Rosenberg and Rosenberg (1968) apparently confirming our postulate of an ATP-utilizing cation pump in the brush border seem to be losing out to more recent fractionations which suggest that most, if not all, pump ATPase is in the lateral membranes (Quigley and Gotterer, 1969; Fujita, Ohta, Kawai, Matsui, and Nakao, 1972).

Cotransport of Na^+ and sugar, however, remains a property of the brush border as confirmed by extensive *in vitro* studies that were designed to be particularly relevant to the question and extended to amino acids (Schultz

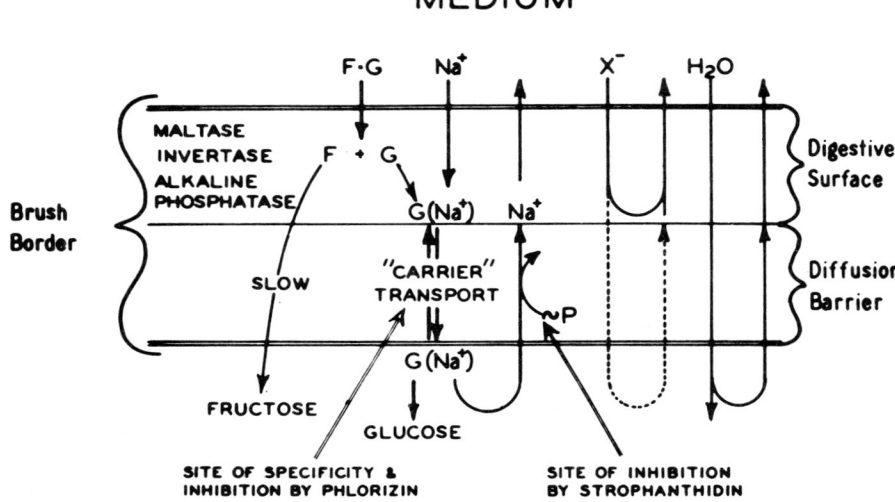

FIG. 1. Model of brush border digestive and absorptive functions (from Crane, Miller, and Bihler, 1961).

and Curran, 1970). Besides that, the "breakthrough" studies of Hopfer, Nelson, Perrotto, and Isselbacher (1973) show that vesicles prepared from brush border microvilli membranes exhibit this specific property. Cotransport appears to be a fact.

Early on (Crane, 1962) we modified Fig. 1 to better indicate the carrier basis of fructose transport across the brush border, although we did not change the fundamental concept of the independence of the glucose and fructose pathways (Crane, 1960). The single route we showed for glucose transport has now (Honegger and Semenza, 1973) become at least two, but we would not further change our indication (Crane, 1962) of a carrier-mediated but facilitated diffusion mechanism for fructose. Gracey, Burke, and Oshin (1972) have, indeed, reported an Na^+-dependent fructose uptake in the rat gut but application of this finding to other species or to normal functions of the digestive-absorptive process is disputed by the results of others (Schultz and Strecker, 1970; Guy and Deren, 1971; Honegger and Semenza, 1973). Not shown in Fig. 1 are (a) the many other transport activities known to be functions of the brush border and (b) the adsorbed pancreatic enzymes of Ugolev. I will omit discussion of the other transport activities because they have been well taken care of in other chapters. I will, however, discuss Ugolev's ideas.

In 1965 Ugolev brought together his thoughts on "membrane digestion" and indicated a location for adsorbed pancreatic enzymes which, by its description, would be substantially the same as indicated in Fig. 1 for maltase, invertase, and alkaline phosphatase: "adsorbed on the pillar base of lecithin of the intestinal membrane" (DeLaey, 1967). In a later version (Ugolev, 1972a) the adsorbed pancreatic enzymes were moved, for the most part, away from the surface and into the "fuzzy coat" as we had earlier argued was more reasonable (Crane, 1968). Also, I am gratified to find greatly increased emphasis placed on the intrinsic brush border enzymes. However, from the point of view of functional requirement it would look, today, as though the pancreatic enzymes should probably be eliminated. So far as can be found in the published literature, the observations of Ugolev and his colleagues on pancreatic enzymes appear not to have withstood the tests of time and experiments in other laboratories. Confirmation has generally not been forth-

TABLE 1. *Brush border enzyme activities*

oligopeptidase[a]
γ-glutamyl transpeptidase[b]
enterokinase[c]
glucoamylase (oligosaccharidase)[d]
maltase[e]
sucrase[e]
isomaltase (α-dextrinase)[f]
lactase[g]
trehalase[h]
phlorizin hydrolase (glycosylceramidase)[i]
alkaline phosphatase[j]

Significant, but not necessarily the earliest, indications of the brush border localization of the enzymes listed are to be found in the following references:

[a] Holt and Miller, 1962; Rhodes, Eichholz, and Crane, 1967; Peters, 1970.
[b] Cohen, Gartner, Blumenfeld, and Arias, 1969.
[c] Holmes and Lobley, 1970; Nordstrom and Dahlquist, 1971; Schmitz, Preiser, Maestracci, Crane, Troesch, and Hadorn, 1974.
[d] Alpers and Solin, 1970; Kelly and Alpers, 1973.
[e] Miller and Crane, 1961b; Lojda, 1965.
[f] Jos, Frezal, Rey, and Lamy, 1967; Gray, 1970.
[g] Doell, Rosen, and Kretchmer, 1965; Crane, 1962.
[h] Jos et al., 1967; Malathi and Crane, 1968.
[i] Malathi and Crane, 1969; Diedrich, 1968; Leese and Semenza, 1973.
[j] Deane and Dempsey, 1945; Holt and Miller, 1962.

coming (Alpers and Solin, 1970; Dahlquist, 1973), but more specifically a direct attempt (Hubel and Parsons, 1971) to find evidence of the enhancement of amylase activity by jejunal mucosa proposed by Jesuitova, Delaey, and Ugolev (1964) has failed to show any effect that could be a significant factor in the digestion of a meal containing starch. It is, of course, correct to say that some amounts of pancreatic enzymes, proteases (Goldberg, Campbell, and Roy, 1971), as well as amylase (Alpers and Solin, 1970), do bind to the mucosal surface of the gut, but there is as yet no evidence that this binding is to any degree an essential feature of the process of digestion. The pancreatic enzymes can be left out of the figure because they do not have a clear function to perform in it.

In Fig. 1, first exhibited in 1960, the brush border is shown to be both a "digestive surface" and a "diffusion barrier" with the hydrolytic enzymes clearly shown to be external to the carriers responsible for glucose active transport. There is no specific provision in this drawing for the superficial region that we felt obliged to postulate in order to account for our observations, which indicated "that hydrolysis occurs in a restricted portion of the cell to give a zone of relatively high concentration from which diffusion of the hydrolytic products occurs into the tissue as whole and into the medium" (Miller and Crane, 1961a). We had observed tissue accumulation of the passively transported sugar, fructose from sucrose, to high levels relative to the medium, and we had observed an apparent failure of phlorizin (10^{-3} M) to prevent tissue accumulation of glucose from maltose. These observations seemed to us to be out of keeping with the sense that the interface between hydrolysis (enzyme activity) and transport (carrier activity) was in immediate and complete contact with the bulk medium. Consequently, we used the term "intracellular" to describe the location of the hydrolase, with the explicit understanding in Fig. 1 and in our discussions (e.g., Crane, 1962) that morphologic identification of the location of the diffusion barrier would identify, as well, the location of the "digestive surface" and its hydrolases.

As Smyth (1972) has commented, "it is easy to get lost in the niceties of terminology," and I find myself in heartfelt agreement with him. For example, whatever the word "intracellular" may be taken to mean, our description of hydrolase location, in words and in diagrams, has been clear; clear enough certainly to obviate the possibility of such a gross distortion as represented by the figure that appears in a recent Ciba Foundation Symposium volume (Ugolev, 1972b, p. 142). The figure Ugolev used originated with one I drew in 1965 (Crane, 1966), wherein I represented the diffusion barrier for carrier transport, in accordance with current thought, as being the lipid leaflet of the trilaminar plasma membrane. I placed the digestive hydrolases in the relative location shown in Fig. 1, i.e., on the outside of the diffusion barrier. If one may assume that Ugolev, in reproducing my drawing, intended to mean the same thing by it, then it is clear that Ugolev (1972b) has misrepresented us; that is (Miller and Crane, 1963)[1] as having placed the hydrolases on the cytoplasm side of the diffusion barrier.

In 1960–61 we used the term "intracellular" and, as indicated above, we have suffered for it. However, the argument can be made that, at the time, there wasn't a very large choice in the matter. As already mentioned, we had observations on the accumulation of fructose from sucrose and on the effects of phlorizin which seemed anomalous. We also had clear indications from experiments with glucose oxidase that the brush border enzyme sucrase is in some way more intimately associated with transport than is the brush border enzyme alkaline phosphates (Crane and Miller, 1961a; G. G. Syme, *unpublished observations*). It was our opinion that these phenomena were not merely the result of local high concentrations of hydrolysis products in the interstices between the microvilli. The phenomena seemed not to be "extracellular" in the usual sense of that word. Hence, we said they were "intracellular." Alternatively, we might have used the term "periplasmic," except that Mitchell (1961) invented it a little later, too late for our use and, anyway, its special meaning for bacteria with their clearly defined cell wall outside of a plasma membrane is not replicated in the brush border pole of the mammalian gut cell. At the brush border, there is no morphologically identifiable compartment to credit as the underlying cause for our observations. Consequently, by 1962–1963 we had stopped thinking in terms of a compartment and favored a concept of close spatial organization that we called "kinetic advantage" (Crane, 1966).

Meanwhile, Ugolev, Jesuitova, and Delaey (1964) failed to confirm our findings with sucrose as a substrate but they did not measure the tissue concentrations of fructose, as we had, nor did they test for the effect of phlorizin. At about the same time, Rutloff, Friese, and Taüfel (1964) tried the glucose oxidase experiment and found, as expected, interference with the transport of glucose from sucrose. However, failing to note that it was the difference in the degree of interference between sucrose and the alkaline phosphatase substrate glucose 1-phosphate, which had so impressed us, they did not try the comparative experiment. Hence, their conclusion differed from ours and agreed with that of Ugolev et al. (1964). Hamilton and McMichael (1968) invoked differential rates of diffusion of glucose and disaccharide within the fuzzy coat lining the microvilli to explain our findings. None of the explanations offered seemed satisfactory, although we could recognize the merit in each.

---

[1] This reference contains no original data and has a 1963 date of publication because it is an inordinately long-delayed printing of a paper presented, as noted on its first page, at the 16th Annual Meeting of the National Vitamin Foundation, Inc., on March 7, 1961, a full two years earlier. This paper does not represent my 1963 views or, indeed, my 1961 views. The paper was written and given by Dr. Miller after he had left my laboratory.

There was one supportive line of work. Parsons and Prichard (1965) began a series of studies with a preparation of perfused amphibian gut (Parsons and Prichard, 1968) and achieved results that suggested a very close relationship, perhaps even an identity, between the brush border disaccharidases and the glucose transport system (Parsons and Prichard, 1971). The "kinetic advantage" for the transfer of hexose released by disaccharidase that we saw in the hamster gut was matched by a highly efficient capture of glucose units released by disaccharidase in the amphibian gut.

For several years my laboratory focused on other questions inasmuch as "kinetic advantage" seemed not to be yielding to experiment. However, about 5 years ago (as I reported at Evian: Crane, 1970a, and elsewhere during 1969), we (Crane, Malathi, Caspary, and Ramaswamy, 1970) finally began to see our way through the puzzle. We believe now that the correct explanation for the apparent "intracellular" location and for a good deal of "kinetic advantage" as well is to be found in a new variety of transport based upon the direct transfer of hexose through the diffusion barrier as the hexose is produced by hydrolysis. We have recently published full documentation for this direct transfer (Malathi, Ramaswamy, Caspary, and Crane, 1973; Ramaswamy, Malathi, Caspary, and Crane, 1974), and I am gratified to find that our work is already substantially confirmed (Hanke and Diedrich, 1974). Although I intend to develop the subject more fully, I should note at this point that the data base for direct transfer exhibits substantial and fundamental differences from the observations in amphibia by Parsons and Prichard (1971), although the concepts independently developed will be seen to have some resemblance.

Our "breakthrough" came when we observed that the theoretical maximal rate of glucose transport was exceeded when glucose was provided in the form of a disaccharide on top of a saturating concentration (30 mM) of free glucose (Fig. 2). We found that all disaccharides having a counterpart brush border enzyme gave a similar result; we found that the disaccharides added to one another as well as to glucose, and, consistent with our early results with glucose 1-phosphate relative to sucrose (Miller and Crane, 1961a), we now found that glucose 1-phosphate, the substrate for alkaline phosphatase, did not give this result.[2] It was clear that we had uncovered a membrane transport system for glucose, which was in addition to the well-known Na^+-dependent glucose transport system and which required the glucose to be presented to it in the form of a disaccharide. We (Ramaswamy et al., 1974) have subsequently found that this disaccharidase-related transport or, better, hydrolase-related transport (HRT) is independent of Na^+, that both moieties, fructose as well as glucose, are transferred, and that the sugars are transferred directly into and through the membrane barrier *without being mixed*

---

[2] More recent experiments indicate that there is a small component of direct transfer from glucose 1-phosphate that can be detected in the absence of Na^+.

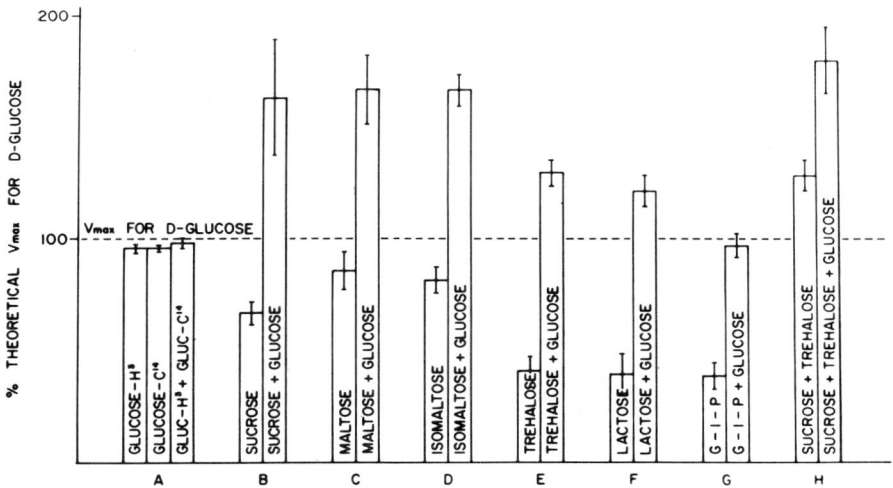

FIG. 2. Glucose uptake from mixtures of D-[U-¹⁴C]glucose and a disaccharide or D-[1-³H] glucose or glucose 1-phosphate (G-1-P). Intestinal rings were incubated in 50 ml of Krebs-phosphate buffer with single or mixed substrates in concentrations, as follows: ³H-glucose, ¹⁴C-glucose, sucrose, maltose, isomaltose, and glucose 1-phosphate, 30 mM; trehalose and lactose, 50 mM. Incubations were for 2 min. Results are expressed as percentage of the theoretical maximal rate derived for glucose assuming a K_m of 1.5 mM (Crane, 1960). The standard deviation of the mean of at least four experiments is indicated for each variation A to G. In H two experiments were done. For B to F, the difference between disaccharide plus glucose and the theoretical V_{max} (or the measured rate at 60-mM total glucose in A) has a p value by Student's t test of less than 0.0005. In G, glucose 1-phosphate plus glucose does not differ from A. From Malathi et al., 1973.

with a pool of free sugar added in high concentration to the incubation medium. Here, at last, is clear, unequivocal "intracellular" release of hexose. In the experiment shown in Table 2 the entry of free glucose into the tissue was largely prevented by the absence of Na⁺. We used sucrose labeled in the glucose moiety with carbon 14. The ¹⁴C-glucose was transferred and there was no dilution of the label by the added cold glucose.

TABLE 2. *Direct transfer of glucose from sucrose into the cell*

External compartment at 0 time	Internal compartment at 2 min
50 mM ¹⁴C-sucrose	6.0 μm/ml of glucose at sa = 3,520 cpm/μM
50 mM ¹⁴C-sucrose plus 30 mM "Cold"-glucose	6.3 μm/ml of glucose at sa = 3,660 cpm/μM

Everted segments of hamster jejunum prepared on polyethylene tubing to restrict sugar access to the mucosal side only were incubated for 2 min at 37° C in 10 ml of choline⁺ buffer. Data from Ramaswamy et al., 1974.

The functional basis of HRT is not yet clear. There seem to be three possibilities. First, the disaccharidases could be spatially integrated with specific glucose carriers, which are themselves oriented in such a way that they can accept glucose only from disaccharide and not from free solution. This was our first proposal (Fig. 3). Second, disaccharides could enter the cell across the diffusion barrier and be split intracellularly. This seems highly unlikely. Third, the disaccharidases could impart an inward vectorial component to some of the hexoses liberated from glycosidic linkage at the membrane interface and thus directly subserve a transport function. It is difficult experi-

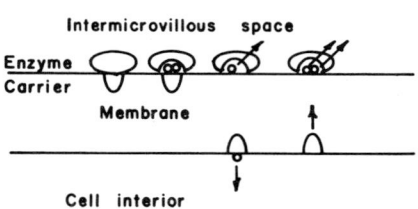

FIG. 3. Speculative organization between disaccharidases and the disaccharidase related carriers. The figure is intended to indicate (a) that these carriers are shielded from interaction with glucose free in the lumen, (b) that one moiety of the disaccharide is transferred to the carrier and one to the intermicrovillous space, and (c) that the disaccharidase hydrolyzes substrate faster than the carrier can transport it (from Crane, Malathi, Caspary, and Ramaswamy, 1970). See also Crane, 1970b.

mentally to choose from among these, but our later preference has been for the third, and recent findings would tend to confirm this preference. For one thing, in Semenza's laboratory it has been found (Storelli, Vogeli, and Semenza, 1972) that purified sucrase-isomaltase complex can be incorporated into black lipid membranes that are normally impermeable to sucrose, glucose, fructose, and mannitol. Membranes containing the complex are more permeable to glucose and fructose presented in the form of sucrose than they are to free glucose and fructose. For another, although phlorizin does not penetrate the brush border membrane (Crane, 1960; Alvarado, 1970; Stirling et al. 1972) it does contribute its glucose moiety in a direct transfer (Diedrich, Hanke, and Evans, *this volume*) like the one we have shown for disaccharides. There is, thus, reason to believe that the disaccharidases have a carrier function. However, one must not lose sight of the fact that, in all cases, hydrolysis outruns transport. Only a portion of the glucose and fructose released are transferred across the membrane. This is, likewise, as true in the model experiments of Semenza's laboratory as it is for our hamster gut data. What does it mean? Does it mean that HRT is a function of all of the disaccharidase molecules some of the time or does it mean that HRT is a function of some of the disaccharidase molecules all of the time? We do not know. In an effort to get an answer we studied HRT in developing hamsters between age 2 weeks and age 10 weeks. Over this period, sucrase increased nearly 10-fold, whereas HRT increased by only one-third. It is not a clear answer. However, a possible way in which HRT takes place is illustrated in Fig. 4.

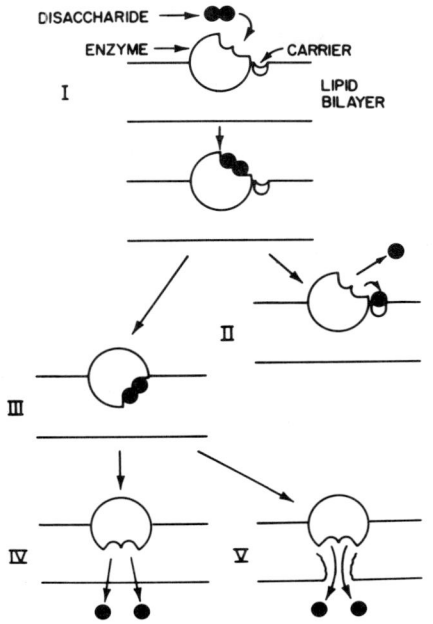

FIG. 4. Illustration of hydrolase-related transport. The assumption is made that the enzyme is continuously changing the orientation of its active site with respect to the lipoidal matrix of the membrane. When the active site is oriented toward the intermicrovillous space the enzyme can accept disaccharide (I). If this orientation is maintained during hydrolysis, the products are released (II) into the intermicrovillous space to be subsequently transported by their respective carriers. If the orientation changes (III) before hydrolysis can take place, the hexose product may be released within the matrix. The point of release may be halfway or more than halfway through the bilayer (IV) or may be next to an aqueous channel in contact with the cytoplasmic space (V). This sequence of diagrams would represent the condition that "all of the enzymes carry out HRT some of the time." The relationship between the enzymes and carriers is assumed to be as previously visualized (Crane, 1966, 1969).

A functional significance for HRT also escapes our understanding. On the one hand, I am gratified to have such complete, if belated, corroboration of our very early results (Miller and Crane, 1961a). On the other hand, I am finally disappointed that so much effort has been expended on elucidating a transport system that is not obviously related to a major physiological event. An efficient capture mechanism (ECM) is one thing and HRT, quite another, as may be seen by the contrast in Table 3 of the properties of HRT in the hamster with ECM in amphibia. Although it is true that some apparent properties of HRT change when Na^+ is present and there are indications that this may be due to an Na^+-induced closer proximity of HRT to the sodium-dependent glucose transport system, HRT is nonetheless a separate transport system on the clear grounds exhibited in Fig. 2, namely, the transport of disaccharide-glucose is additive to the transport of a saturating level of free glucose.

HRT exists but its activity for sugars cannot be detected *in vivo*. If it were to be detected, it should then be advantageous for the absorption of sugar to feed it as disaccharide. This is not a new idea. The idea that it may be advantageous to the absorption of hexose to provide it in the form of disaccharide has a history that goes back at least to 1960 and that I recently reviewed (Crane, 1973). Briefly, Chain, Mansford, and Pocchiari (1960) studied sugar absorption with the *in vitro* technique of Fisher and Parsons (1949). Their conclusions were that fructose is better absorbed when given

TABLE 3. *Comparison of hydrolase-related transport (HRT) in hamster gut[a] with the efficient capture mechanism (ECM) in amphibian gut[b] and their relationships to sodium-dependent glucose transport (SDGT)*

Measured Parameter	HRT[c]	ECM
Competition for hydrolysis between disaccharides	no	no
Competition for translocation between species of disaccharide-glucose	no	yes
Translocation inhibited by phlorizin	no	yes
Translocation requires Na^+	no	yes
Competition for translocation between free glucose and disaccharide glucose	no	yes
Both moieties of disaccharide are transported	yes	not tested[d]
The functional relationship with SDGT	independent	sequential

[a] See Malathi et al., 1973 and Ramaswamy et al., 1974.
[b] See Parsons and Prichard, 1971.
[c] Refers to the Na^+-free condition.
[d] Not tested. Amphibian gut contains no sucrose. The moieties of maltose and trehalose are indistinguishable.

as sucrose and that oligosaccharides are better than glucose. This has also been claimed to be the case *in vivo* in man (MacDonald and Turner, 1968). However, the most recent and, in my opinion, the best-controlled comparison of the absorption of sucrose and its monosaccharides (Cook, 1970) shows no difference between them. This last agrees with our assessment of the capability of HRT (Crane, 1973) based on what we have seen (Malathi et al., 1973) of inhibitory effects both of Na^+ and the local concentrations of glucose produced in excess of the gut capacity for transport (Gray and Ingelfinger, 1966).[3]

Let me now briefly take up one more point raised by Fig. 1. This point is, naturally, the coupling which is indicated between the cotransport of Na^+ with glucose and the ATP-utilizing Na^+ pump. As noted above, the pump has been moved to the lateral membranes in response to many findings. Cotransport itself, however, has been retained because it seems to be the only explanation for a large number of findings which are generally well-known (Schultz and Curran, 1970) and the phenomena predicted by it have apparently been seen in brush border membrane vesicles (Hopfer et al., 1973).

[3] Nonetheless, it should theoretically be possible for HRT to function as a bypass mechanism for the absorption of some amounts of hexose when carrier function is deleted as in glucose-galactose malabsorption. As a practical matter, it would not be expected to be effective, at least at normal dietary loads of di- and oligosaccharides, because diarrhea would still ensue from the large amounts of luminal hexose also produced. However, this line of reasoning raises the question of whether the ability of peptides to bypass amino acid carrier function may not be, at least in some cases, the result of an HRT contributed by brush border membrane oligopeptidase. Diarrhea does not seem to be an important symptom of amino acid carrier deletion disease and nutritionally valuable amounts of an essential amino acid could be obtained by the HRT route without an accompanying life-threatening loss of fluid.

I do not intend to try to deal with all the data. However, I would like to point out once again (see Crane, 1974) that the existence of a carrier for the cotransport of glucose and Na^+ in the brush border membrane establishes the capacity for energy to be coupled to glucose transport by means of an imposed gradient or flux of Na^+ across the membrane. Under these circumstances the relevant question is not whether gradient-coupling exists (Crane, 1967) but whether the energy in the gradient or flux of Na^+ is sufficient to drive sugar accumulation to the observed levels and whether that is the sole or principal means by which metabolic energy is so coupled.

Kimmich (1973) has recently, comprehensively and thoroughly, reviewed the question of coupling between Na^+ and sugar transport in the small intestine. Earlier, Kimmich (1970) visualized a mechanism in which, if I understand it correctly, the energized (phosphorylated?) intermediate of the Na^+–K^+ pump was alternatively utilized as the direct driving force for sugar and amino acid accumulation. There was no provision for cotransport in this original proposal. In a more recent version (Kimmich, 1973) cotransport was included. I am unable to foresee what Kimmich's next position may be. As noted earlier, the amount of Na^+-pump ATPase in the brush border membrane (which is where Kimmich's proposal absolutely requires it to be) gets smaller and smaller (Fujita et al., 1972). Also others are now testing the transport capabilities of isolated cells and in at least one very recent instance (Gall, Butler, Tepperman, and Hamilton, 1974) the authors conclude that their results are "consistent with the ion-gradient model" and "not compatible with the direct energy-coupling model" of Kimmich.

It has also been recorded that there is not enough energy in cation gradients to account for the observed solute gradients at least in Ehrlich ascites tumor cells (Schafer and Heinz, 1971). In comment, I would only bring to your attention two very recent reports from Heinz's laboratory (namely, Geck, Heinz, and Pfeiffer, 1974 and Heinz and Geck, 1974). The former of these two papers provides evidence (for the Ehrlich cell) against a direct coupling between amino acid transport and ATP hydrolysis. The second one put the Na^+-gradient back in business through a revised assessment of the energy demands which amino acid transport places on the ion gradient. Heinz and Geck (1974) conclude (a) that the energy in the electrochemical potential gradient of Na^+ has been "found to be approximately adequate to account for the highest accumulation ratios" reported for α-aminoisobutyrate and (b) that "the gradient hypothesis cannot be rejected on energetic grounds."

ACKNOWLEDGMENT

The research work of the author and his colleagues has been supported by grants from the National Institutes of Health and the National Science Foundation.

REFERENCES

Alpers, D. H., and Solin, M. (1970): The characterization of rat intestinal amylase. Gastroenterology 58:833–842.
Alvarado, F. (1970): Effect of phloretin and phlorizin on sugar and amino acid transport systems in small intestine. Fed. Eur. Biochem. Symp. 20:131.
Berg, G. G., and Chapman, B. (1965): The sodium and potassium activated ATPase of intestinal epitheliam. I. Location of enzymatic activity in the cell. J. Cell. Comp. Physiol. 65:361–372.
Chain, E. B., Mansford, K. R. L., and Pocchiari, F. (1960): The absorption of sucrose maltose and higher oligosaccharides from the isolated rat small intestine. J. Physiol. 154:39–51.
Cohen, M. I., Gartner, L. M., Blumenfeld, O. O., and Arias, I. M. (1969): Gamma glutamyl transpeptidase: Measurement and development in guinea pig small intestine. Pediat. Res. 3:5–10.
Cook, G. C. (1970): Comparison of the absorption and metabolic products of sucrose and its monosaccharides in man. Clin. Sci. 38:687–697.
Crane, R. K. (1960): Intestinal absorption of sugars. Physiol. Rev. 40:789–825.
Crane, R. K. (1962): Hypothesis of mechanism of intestinal active transport of sugars. Fed. Proc. 21:891–895.
Crane, R. K. (1966): Structural and functional organization of an epithelial cell brush border. In: *Symposia of the International Society for Cell Biology*, Vol. 5, edited by K. B. Warren, Academic Press, New York, pp. 71–102.
Crane, R. K. (1967): Gradient coupling and the membrane transport of water soluble compounds: A general biological mechanism? In: *Colloquia on the Protides of the Biological Fluids*, edited by H. Peeters, Elsevier, Amsterdam, pp. 227–235.
Crane, R. K. (1968): A concept of the digestive-absorptive surface of the small intestine. In: *Handbook of Physiology*, Sec. 6, Alimentary Canal, Vol. 5, Digestion, edited by C. F. Code, Amer. Physiol. Soc., Washington, D. C., pp. 2535–2542.
Crane, R. K. (1969): Functional organization contributing to carbohydrate economy. In: *Comprehensive Biochemistry*, Vol. 17, edited by M. Florkin and E. Stotz, Carbohydrate Metabolism, pp. 1–14.
Crane, R. K. (1970a): Functional organization at the brush border membrane. In: *7th International Congress Clinical Chemistry*, Geneva, Evian, Vol. 4, Digestion and Intestinal Absorption, Karger, Basel, pp. 23–30.
Crane, R. K. (1970b): Organisation der digestiv-absorptiven funktion an der membran des Bürstensaums. In: K. Rommel and P. H. Clodi *Biochemische and Klinische Aspekte der Zuckerabsorption*, F. K. Schattauer Verlag, Stuttgart, pp. 75–83.
Crane, R. K. (1973): Digestive-absorptive organization in the brush border membrane. In: *Intestinal enzyme deficiencies and their nutritional implications, Symposia of the Swedish Nutrition Foundation XI*, edited by B. Borgstrom, A. Dahlqvist, L. Hambraeus, Stockholm, pp. 15–19.
Crane, R. K. (1974): Intestinal absorption of glucose. In: *Intestinal Absorption*, edited by D. H. Smyth, Vol. L, Chap. 10, Plenum, New York.
Crane, R. K., Malathi, P., Caspary, W. F., and Ramaswamy, K. (1970): Evidence for a second glucose transport system in hamster small intestine specific for glucose release by brush border digestive enzymes. Fed. Proc. 29:1952.
Crane, R. K., Miller, D., and Bihler, I. (1961): The restrictions on the possible mechanisms of intestinal active transport of sugars. In: *Membrane transport and metabolism*, edited by A. Kleinzeller and A. Kotyk, Czechoslovak Academy of Science Press, Prague, pp. 439–450.
Csaky, T. Z., and Hara, Y. (1965): Inhibition of active intestinal sugar transport by digitalis. Am. J. Physiol. 209:467–472.
Dahlqvist, A. (1973): General survey on the digestion and absorption of carbohydrates. In: *Intestinal enzyme deficiencies and their nutritional implications, Symposia of the Swedish Nutrition Foundation*, edited by B. Borgstrom, Dahlqvist and Hambraeus, Stockholm, pp. 9–14.

Deane, H. W., and Dempsey, E. W. (1945): The localization of phosphatase in the Golgi region of intestinal and other epithelial cells. Anat. Rec. 93:401–417.
DeLaey, P. (1967): Die membramverdauung der Starke. 6. Mitt. Die Bindung der Amylase auf der Intestinal-mucosa. Die Nahrung 11:17–30.
Diedrich, D. F. (1968): Is phloretin the sugar transport inhibitor in intestine. Arch. Biochem. Biophys. 127:803–812.
Doell, R. G., Rosen, G., and Kretchmer, N. (1965): Immunochemical studies of intestinal disaccharidases during normal and precocious development. Proc. Nat. Acad. Sci. 54:1268–1273.
Eichholz, A., and Crane, R. K. (1965): Studies on organization of the brush border in intestinal epithelial cells. I. Tris-disruption of isolated hamster brush borders and density gradient separation of fractions. J. Cell Biol. 26:687–691.
Fisher, R. B., and Parsons, D. S. (1949): A preparation of surviving rat small intestine for the study of absorption. J. Physiol. 110:36–46.
Fujita, M., Ohta, H., Kawai, K., Matsui, H., and Nakao, M. (1972): Differential isolation of microvillous and basolateral plasma membranes from intestinal mucosa: Mutually exclusive distribution of digestive enzymes and ouabain-sensitive ATPase. Biochim. Biophys. Acta 274:336–347.
Gall, D. G., Butler, D. G., Tepperman, F., and Hamilton, J. R. (1974): Sodium ion transport in isolated intestinal epithelial cells: The effect of actively transported sugars on sodium ion efflux. Biochim. Biophys. Acta 339:291–302.
Geck, P., Heinz, E., and Pfeiffer, B. (1974): Evidence against direct coupling between amino acid transport and ATP hydrolysis. Biochim. Biophys. Acta 339:419–425.
Goldberg, D. M., Campbell, R., and Roy, A. D. (1971): The interaction of trypsin and chymotrypsin with intestinal cells in man and several animal species. Comp. Biochem. Physiol. 38B:697–706.
Gracey, M., Burke, V., and Oshin, A. (1972): Active intestinal transport of d-fructose. Biochim. Biophys. Acta 266:397–406.
Gray, G. (1970): Carbohydrate digestion and absorption. Gastroenterology 58:96–107.
Gray, G. M., and Ingelfinger, F. J. (1965): Intestinal absorption of sucrose in man: the site of hydrolysis and absorption. J. Clin. Invest. 44:390–398.
Guy, M. J., and Deren, J. J. (1971): Selective permeability of the small intestine for fructose. Am. J. Physiol. 221:1051–1056.
Hamilton, J. D., and McMichael, H. G. (1968): Role of the microvillus in the absorption of disaccharides. Lancet 2:154–157.
Hanke, D. W., and Diedrich, D. F. (1974): Fate of the hydrolyzed glucose moiety from phlorizin in hamster jejunum. Fed. Proc. 33:271.
Heinz, E., and Geck, P. (1974): The efficiency of energetic coupling between Na^+ flow and amino acid transport in Ehrlich cells: A revised assessment. Biochim. Biophys. Acta 339:426–431.
Holmes, R., and Lobley, R. W. (1970): The localization of enterokinase to the brush border membrane of the guinea-pig small intestine. J. Physiol. (Lond.) 211:50–51P.
Holt, J. H., and Miller, D. (1962): The localization of phosphomonoesterase and aminopeptidase in brush borders isolated from intestinal epithelial cells. Biochim. Biophys. Acta 58:239–243.
Honegger, P., and Semenza, G. (1973): Multiplicity of carriers for free glucalogues in hamster small intestine. Biochim. Biophys. Acta 318:390–410.
Hopfer, U., Nelson, K., Perrotto, J., and Isselbacher, K. J. (1973): Glucose transport in isolated brush border membrane from rat small intestine. J. Biol. Chem. 248:25–32.
Hubel, K. A., and Parsons, D. S. (1971): Membrane digestion of starch. Am. J. Physiol. 221:1827–1831.
Jesuitova, N. N., Delaey, P., and Ugolev, A. M. (1964): Digestion of starch in vivo and in vitro in a rat intestine. Biochim. Biophys. Acta 86:205–210.
Jos, J., Frezal, J., Rey, J., Lamy, M., and Wegmann, R. (1967): La localisation histochimique des disaccharidases intestinales par un nouveau procede. Ann. Histochim. 12:53–61.
Kelly, J. J., and Alpers, D. H. (1973): Properties of human intestinal glucoamylase. Biochim. Biophys. Acta 315:113–122.

Kimmich, G. A. (1970): Active sugar accumulation by isolated intestinal epithelial cells: A new model for sodium-dependent metabolite transport. Biochemistry 9:3669–3677.
Kimmich, G. A. (1973): Coupling between Na$^+$ and sugar transport in small intestine. Biochim. Biophys. Acta 300:31–78.
Leese, H. J., and Semenza, G. (1973): On the identity between the small intestinal enzymes phlorizin hydrolase and glycosylceramidase. J. Biol. Chem. 248:8170–8173.
Lojda, Z. (1965): Some remarks concerning the histochemical detection of disaccharidases and glucosidases. Histochemie 5:339–360.
MacDonald, I., and Turner, C. J. (1968): Serum fructose levels after sucrose or its constituent monosaccharides. Lancet 1:841–843.
Malathi, P., and Crane, R. K. (1968): Spatial relationship between intestinal disaccharidases and the active transport system for sugars. Biochim. Biophys. Acta 163:275–276.
Malathi, P., and Crane, R. K. (1969): Phlorizin hydrolase, a β-glucosidase of hamster intestinal brush border membrane. Biochim. Biophys. Acta 173:245–256.
Malathi, P., Ramaswamy, K., Caspary, W. F., and Crane, R. K. (1973): Studies on transport of glucose from disaccharides by hamster small intestine in vitro. I. Evidence for a disaccharidase related transport system. Biochim. Biophys. Acta 307:613–622.
McDougal, D. B., Jr., Little, K. D., and Crane, R. K. (1960): Studies on the mechanism of intestinal absorption of sugars. IV. Localization of galactose concentrations within the intestinal wall during active transport, in vitro, Biochim. Biophys. Acta 45:483–489.
Miller, D., and Crane, R. K. (1960): The concept of a digestive surface in the small intestine: Cellular nature of disaccharide and phosphate ester hydrolysis. J. Lab. Clin. Med. 56:928–932.
Miller, D., and Crane, R. K. (1961a): The digestive function of the epithelium of the small intestine. I. An intracellular locus of disaccharide and sugar phosphate ester hydrolysis. Biochim. Biophys. Acta 52:281–293.
Miller, D., and Crane, R. K. (1961b): The digestive function of the epithelium of the small intestine. II. Localization of disaccharide hydrolysis in the isolated brush border portion of intestinal epithelial cells. Biochim. Biophys. Acta 52:293–298.
Miller, D., and Crane, (1963): Digestion of carbohydrates in the small intestine. Amer. J. Clin. Nutrition. 12:220–227.
Mitchell, P. (1961): Approaches to the analysis of specific membrane transport. In: Biological structure and function, Vol. 2, edited by T. W. Goodwin and L. O. Lindberg, Academic, New York, pp. 581–603.
Nordstrom, C., and Dahlqvist, A. (1971): The cellular localization of enterokinase. Biochim. Biophys. Acta 198:621–622; 242:209–225.
Overton, J., Eichholz, A., and Crane, R. K. (1965): Studies of the organization of the brush border in intestinal epithelial cells. II. Structure of hamster microvilli as revealed by electron microscopic examination of the fractions of Tris-disrupted brush borders. J. Cell Biol. 26L:693–706.
Parsons, D. S., and Prichard, J. S. (1965): Hydrolysis of disaccharides during absorption by the perfused small intestine of amphibia. Nature 208:1097–1098.
Parsons, D. S., and Prichard, J. S. (1968): A preparation of perfused small intestine for the study of absorption in amphibia. J. Physiol. 198:405–434.
Parsons, D. S., and Prichard, J. S. (1971): Relationships between disaccharide hydrolysis and sugar transport in amphibian small intestine. J. Physiol. 212:299–319.
Peters, T. J. (1970): The subcellular localization of di- and tri-peptide hydrolase activity in guinea pig small intestine. Biochem. J. 120:195–203.
Quigley, J. P., and Gotterer, G. S. (1972): A comparison of the (Na$^+$ − K$^+$) − ATPase activities found in isolated brush border and plasma membrane of the rate intestinal mucosa. Biochim. Biophys. Acta 255:107–113.
Ramaswamy, K., Malathi, P., Caspary, W. F., and Crane, R. K. (1974): Studies on the transport of glucose from disaccharides by hamster small intestine in vitro. II.

Characteristics of the disaccharidase-related transport system. Biochim. Biophys. Acta, in press.

Rhodes, J. B., Eichholz, A., and Crane, R. K. (1967): Studies on the organization of the brush border in intestinal epithelial cells. IV. Aminopeptidase activity in microvillus membranes of hamster intestinal brush borders. Biochim. Biophys. Acta *135:*959–965.

Rosenberg, I. H., and Rosenberg, L. E. (1968): Localization and characterization of adenosine triphosphatase in guinea pig intestinal epithelium. Comp. Biochem. Physiol. *24:*975–985.

Ruttloff, H., Friese, R., and Taufel, K. (1965): Zur Spaltung und resorption von oligosacchariden im dunndarm, II Bildung von glucose in gewebeschnitten des Rattendarmes aus maltooligosacchariden. Zeit. Physiol. Chem. *341:*134–142.

Schafer, J. A., and Heinz, E. (1971): The effect of reversal of Na^+ and K^+ electrochemical potential gradients on the active transport of amino acids in Ehrlich ascites tumor cells. Biochim. Biophys. Acta *249:*15–33.

Schmitz, J., Preiser, H., Maestracci, D., Crane, R. K., Troesch, V., and Hadorn, B. (1974): Subcellular localization of enterokinase in human small intestine. Biochim. Biophys. Acta, in press.

Schultz, S. G., and Curran, P. F. (1968): Intestinal absorption of sodium chloride and water. In: *Handbook of Physiology, Alimentary Canal*, Washington, D.C., Am. Physiol. Soc., Sec. 6, Vol. 3, pp. 1245–1275.

Schultz, S. G., and Curran, P. F. (1970): Coupled transport of sodium and organic solutes. Physiol. Rev. *50:*637–718.

Schultz, S. G., and Strecker, C. K. (1970): Fructose influx across the brush border of rabbit ileum. Biochim. Biophys. Acta *211:*586–588.

Schultz, S. G., and Zalusky, R. (1965): Interactions between active sodium transport and active amino acid transport in isolated rabbit ileum. Nature *204:*292–294.

Smyth, D. H. (1972): Peptide transport by mammalian gut. In: *Peptide transport in bacteria and mammalian gut*, A Ciba Foundation Symposium, pp. 59–70.

Stirling, C. E. (1967): High-resolution radioautography of phlorizin-^{3}H in rings of hamster intestine. J. Cell Biol. *35:*605–618.

Stirling, C. E., and Kinter, W. B. (1967): High-resolution radioautography of galactose-^{3}H accumulation in rings of hamster intestine. J. Cell Biol. *35:*585–604.

Stirling, C. E., Schneider, A. J., Wong, M. D., and Kinter, W. B. (1972): Quantitative radioautography of sugar transport in intestinal biopsies from normal humans and a patient with glucose-galactose malabsorption. J. Clin. Invest. *51:*438–451.

Storelli, C., Vogeli, H., and Semenza, G. (1972): Reconstitution of a sucrase-mediated sugar transport system in lipid membranes. Feb. Lett. *24:*287–292.

Ugolev, A. (1960): Influence of the surface of the small intestine on enzymatic hydrolysis of starch by enzymes. Nature *188:*588.

Ugolev, A. M. (1965): Membrane (contact) digestion. Physiol. Rev. *45:*555–595.

Ugolev, A. M. (1972a): Progress report: Membrane digestion. Gut *13:*735–747.

Ugolev, A. M. (1972b): Membrane digestion and peptide transport. In: *Peptide transport in bacteria and mammalian gut*. A Ciba Foundation Symposium, pp. 123–137.

Ugolev, A. M., and Jesuitova, N. N., and DeLaey, P. (1964): Localization of invertase activity in small intestinal cells. Nature *203:*879–880.

DISCUSSION

The available energy for the gradient hypothesis was questioned. One also has to consider the thermodynamic efficiency of coupling. Apparently calculations by Heinz and his group resulted in a rather low value. One has to consider whether sufficient energy is available and how it is utilized. CRANE agreed with the comment but emphasized that the theory of co-transport and gradient coupling should be rejected only on adequate grounds.

FARMANFARMAIAN asked about the source of the energy for accumulation in the case of the hydrolase-related transport. CRANE replied that there are 7,000 calories per mole available in the glycosidic bond. Since the splitting of sucrose is faster than the escape of the products, accumulation occurs.

KESTON mentioned that some years ago he postulated a mechanism for the absorption of glucose in the kidney and intestine consisting of a change in the anomeric form of the sugar into another form involving mutarotation. No energy is needed for this process as it is essentially a downhill transport. CRANE replied that he did not discuss the possible involvement of mutarotase because his topic was the role of the brush border in intestinal transport and Bailey has shown that mutarotase is not a brush border enzyme.

Intestinal Absorption and Malabsorption,
edited by T. Z. Csáky.
Raven Press, New York © 1975

Relationship Between Glycosidase Activity and Sugar Transport in the Intestine

Donald F. Diedrich, Dan W. Hanke, and James O. Evans

Department of Pharmacology, University of Kentucky, College of Medicine, Lexington, Kentucky 40506

I. INTRODUCTION

The characteristics of a complex biological process can be uncovered in a variety of ways. One approach is to gain an understanding of the mechanism by which a specific poison blocks the operation; this knowledge is often tantamount to an understanding of the basic process itself. For a number of years, we have attempted to determine the mechanism by which the inhibitor phlorizin interferes with the transport of sugar across epithelial barriers. We think our search thus far has been an adventurous one. As a natural outgrowth of this early work, we report here some recent findings, which we believe bring us closer to achieving our initial objective—learning something about the sugar transport process itself.

An oversimplified version of the intestinal sugar uptake mechanism is shown in Fig. 1. The cartoon serves to illustrate how free glucose is thought to interact with some external component in the brush border membrane (which for clarity is shown here without the wrinkles). Presumably, as the complex is formed, the protein undergoes some kind of conformational change that causes the receptor site loaded with the sugar to be translocated to the cell interior. It is not surprising that phlorizin acts as a competitive inhibitor in this operation (part of the inhibitor molecule is itself a glucose residue that is connected to the phenolic phloretin portion through a β-glucosidic linkage). Competition with glucose for this receptor site is an effective one since phlorizin is bound tighter than free sugar by many orders of magnitude (Alvarado and Crane, 1962; Diedrich, 1966; Alvarado, 1967; Vick, Diedrich, and Baumann, 1973). This extraordinary affinity is attributable, for the most part, to the formation of a hydrogen bond between one of the phenolic —OHs of the inhibitor and a polar group of the membrane receptor in an exact spatial relationship. This view is derived from work designed to establish the critical structural aspect of the inhibitor molecule (Diedrich, 1963, 1966; Vick et al., 1973). Analogues of phlorizin were synthesized and then tested for their ability to competitively block the active transport of glucose in two separate series of *in vitro* experiments with the hamster intestine. In Fig. 2 the inhibitory constant, K_i, for each

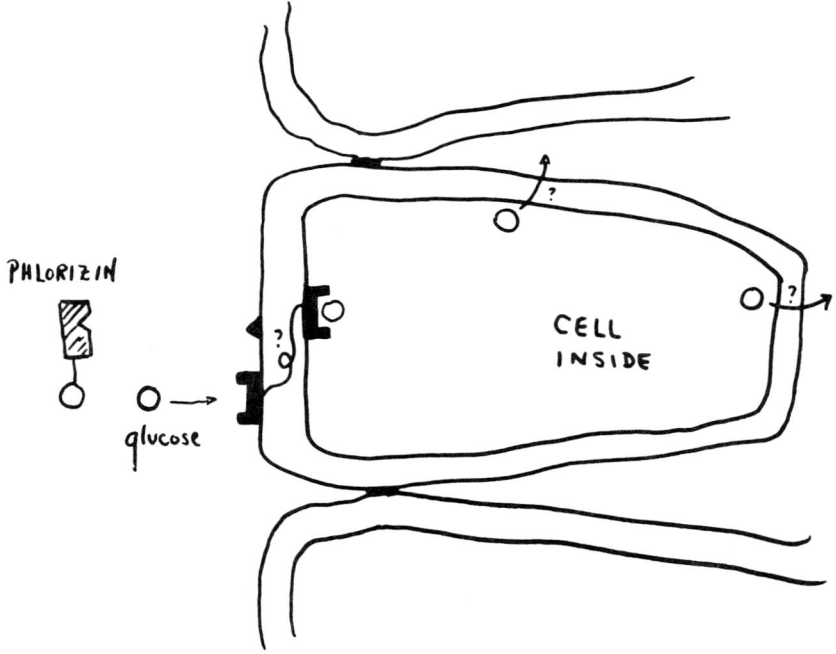

FIG. 1. Abbreviated concept of the intestinal sugar uptake mechanism.

compound is tabulated relative to phlorizin which was assigned an arbitrary value of 100. Subtle differences in structure are seen to have major effects on the apparent affinity of the compounds for the sugar carrier receptor site. Whereas the analogue without the 4'-hydroxyl group fits much better than phlorizin, the critical nature of the phenolic tail is apparent; the 4-methoxy derivative has less affinity and the phloracetophenone glucoside is virtually inactive. The specificity of the sugar residue linked to the aglycone was also clearly demonstrated. When 3-O-methyl glucose and galactose were substituted for glucose, the loss in analogue affinity paralleled the relative attraction each of the free hexoses had for the transport system. With the synthesis of these analogues, we not only have developed tools to partially map the sugar-transport binding site, but we also have a collection of test probes that displays a varying degree of fit for this receptor. They should be useful in identifying this specific portion of the transport system when various membrane components are isolated in future work.

About 6 years ago Crane and his colleagues and Diedrich drew attention to the importance of an enzyme in small intestine brush borders. We both called it phlorizin hydrolase, because it split the β-glucosidic bond of phlorizin (Diedrich, 1968; Malathi and Crane, 1969). It has since been reported that this β-glucosidase bears a relationship to lactase (Semenza,

INHIBITOR STRUCTURE	TRIVIAL NAME	RELATIVE INHIBITORY POTENCY INTESTINAL SUGAR TRANSPORT
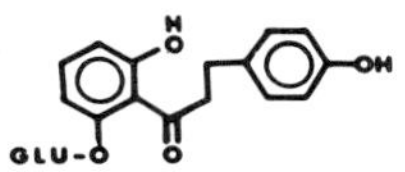	4'-DEOXYPHLORIZIN	155 ; 170
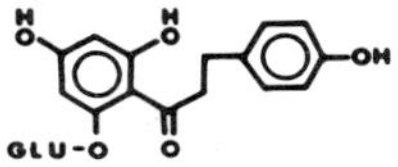	PHLORIZIN	100 ; 100
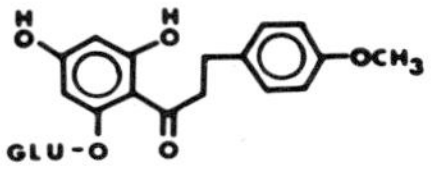	4-METHOXYPHLORIZIN	54 ; 59
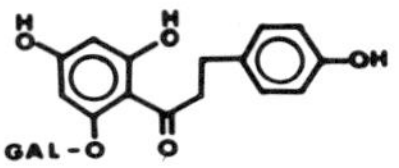	PHLORETIN 2'-GALACTOSIDE	16 ; 6
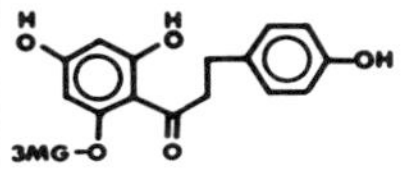	PHLORETIN 2'-(3-METHOXYGLUCOSIDE)	13 ; 8
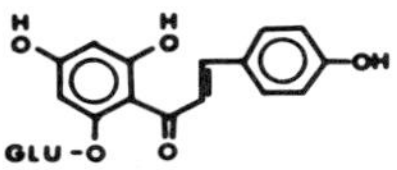	PHLORIZIN CHALCONE	0 ; –
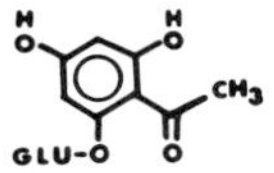	PHLORACETOPHENONE 2'-GLUCOSIDE	2 ; 1
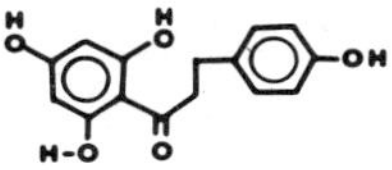	PHLORETIN	4 ; 4
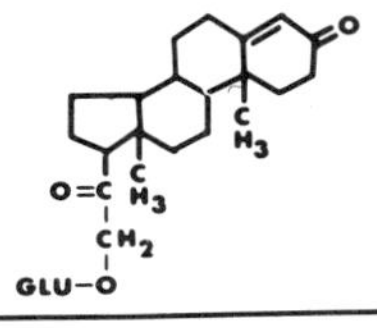	DEOXYCORTICOSTERONE GLUCOSIDE	16 ; 12

FIG. 2. Ranking of phlorizin and analogues as intestinal glucose transport inhibitors.

Auricchio, and Rubino, 1965; Kraml, Kolínská, Ellederová, and Hiršová, 1972) and may serve a nutritional role by hydrolyzing glucosylceramide, a glycolipid component of milk (Leese and Semenza, 1973). In Diedrich's early report on this enzyme he raised the following questions: Since phlorizin was hydrolyzed under conditions in which it was being tested for its potency as a sugar-transport poison, what was the actual inhibitor? Was it phlorizin itself, or was it the phloretin molecule generated in the membrane? Furthermore, were we still justified in equating the potency of the various phlorizin analogues with their affinity for the carrier? Perhaps their inhibitory activity varied because of differences in their rate of cleavage by the so-called phlorizin hydrolase. The first question prompted divergent responses from other workers (Alvarado, 1969; Semenza, 1969), but we felt encumbered to answer the last one ourselves. We therefore set out to measure the apparent affinity of each analogue for the active site of the hydrolase.

II. IDENTITY OF THE ACTIVE SITES ON THE BRUSH BORDER β-GLUCOSIDASE AND GLUCOSE TRANSPORT SYSTEM

We intentionally kept the *in vitro* assay conditions as similar as possible to those used in our transport study. The isolated brush borders, used as our enzyme source in the hydrolase experiments, were purified from the same tissue and same animal source. The incubation buffer pH was identical, and its composition was very similar to that used earlier. Our initial results with a limited number of analogues are summarized in Fig. 3. The data clearly indicate that each phlorizin-like glycoside has the same rela-

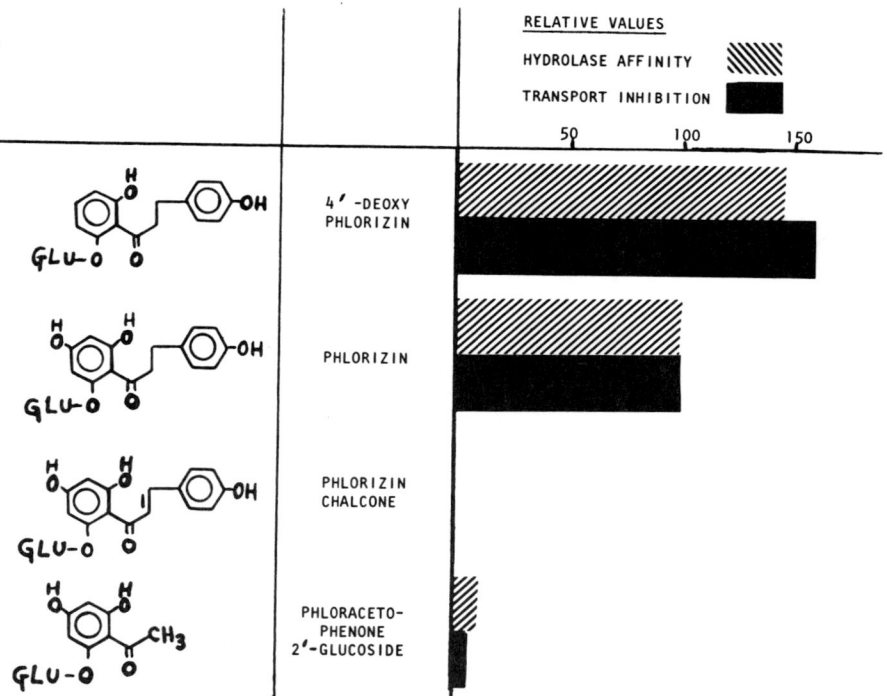

FIG. 3. Comparison of the apparent affinity of phlorizin and some phlorizin analogues for the transport system and the phlorizin hydrolase.

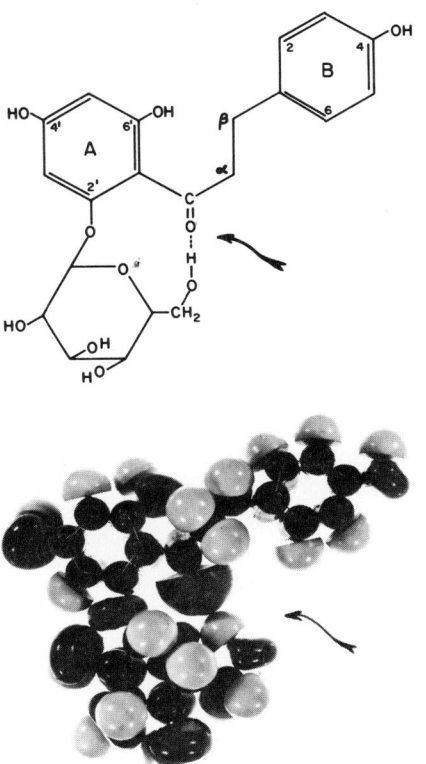

FIG. 4. The structure of phlorizin based on projections from the molecular model.

tive affinity for the active centers of both the β-glucosidase and the sugar binding protein of the carrier system. Specificity of the interaction is apparent; the absence of the 4'-hydroxyl group allows the glucosyl residue a greater opportunity to become fixed into a coplanar position with the aromatic A ring.[1] This appears to be the preferred molecular configuration and gains for the deoxy-derivative the opportunity to fit both receptor sites better than phlorizin itself. The requisite phenolic tail (B ring) is again obvious, inasmuch as phloracetophenone 2'-glucoside has very low binding potential in both systems. However, the most startling finding is the inactivity of the phlorizin chalcone, and this substance forms the most discriminating test of our comparison. The derivative differs from phlorizin only in having a double bond at the α,β position (Fig. 4). What initially

---

[1] The arrow in Fig. 4 points to the intramolecular hydrogen bond formed between the —OH on C-6 of the glucose and the carbonyl oxygen of the phloretin residue. This bond formation is highly favored since the three atoms involved are exactly colinear and the chelation is strain free (Diedrich, 1966).

appears to be a minor structural difference is seen to have major effects on the 3-dimensional structure of the molecule when molecular models of the two compounds are built. Whereas the phenolic tail of phlorizin can swing out of the plane in which the stabilized glucose moiety lies, the chalcone is a rigid and flat molecule; because of the conjugated double bond, both phenolic rings, as well as the glucose moiety, are coplanar. Our data clearly indicate, therefore, that not only are specific chemical groups critical, but, in order for a molecule to fit the receptor site on both the hydrolase and carrier, it must form a nonplanar configuration. From our results with the chalcone this appears to be an *absolute* requirement. Preliminary tests with the other analogues listed in Fig. 2 indicate that the parallelism in affinity for both systems will hold up for the entire series. Our results prompt us to offer the following conclusion: Either (a) two protein molecules exist in the brush border membrane (the β-glucosidase and the sugar-carrier receptor), and they both possess identical construction of the active center which forms the glucose-binding site, or (b) these membrane constituents are identical.

III. DISTRIBUTION OF THE GLUCOSE SPLIT FROM PHLORIZIN

While studying the brush border glycosidase, we were forced to ask the question: what happens to the liberated glucose when phlorizin is split in the membrane? We have recently gained some insight regarding this point which supports the contention that there is indeed a direct relationship between hydrolysis and sugar transport activity in the intestinal brush border.

To study this question we prepared some radioactive phlorizin such that only the glucose moiety at carbon 6 was labeled with tritium. Two selective adsorption steps on small chromatography columns were also developed to permit a separation of unhydrolyzed ^{3}H-phlorizin, tritiated glucose metabolites, and free sugar. This, then, made it easy to selectively follow the distribution of only the split ^{3}H-glucose by conventional radioactivity measurements.

To measure the hydrolytic and transport processes simultaneously we found it convenient to use a technique first described by Wright (1967). Small pieces of jejunum were incubated with the specifically labeled phlorizin in the same medium we had used in all of our other studies. The incubation was terminated by quickly removing the tissue and instantly freezing it in a vial containing bicarbonate buffer. After this tissue is lyophilized, the bulk of adhering salts and substrate can be readily dislodged by tapping the vial—the tissue piece now looks like a porcupine, the quills being the villi, which are brittle, easily chipped off, and with the aid of a stereodissecting microscope can be collected in a clean vial. The muscle layer and other underlying tissue are discarded. We therefore measure only that tritium which enters the tissue through the brush border membrane, and, because of the speed with which we can work, *initial* rates of both phlorizin hydrolysis and glucose uptake can easily be measured. The results of a typical experiment are shown in Fig. 5. Notice that phlorizin (initially present at 100 μM) is hydrolyzed at a constant rate for at least 20 min. We normally conducted our experiments for only 3 min, since the rate of glucose uptake into the tissue was still linear at this time and only about 10% of the phlorizin substrate had been split. A key point can

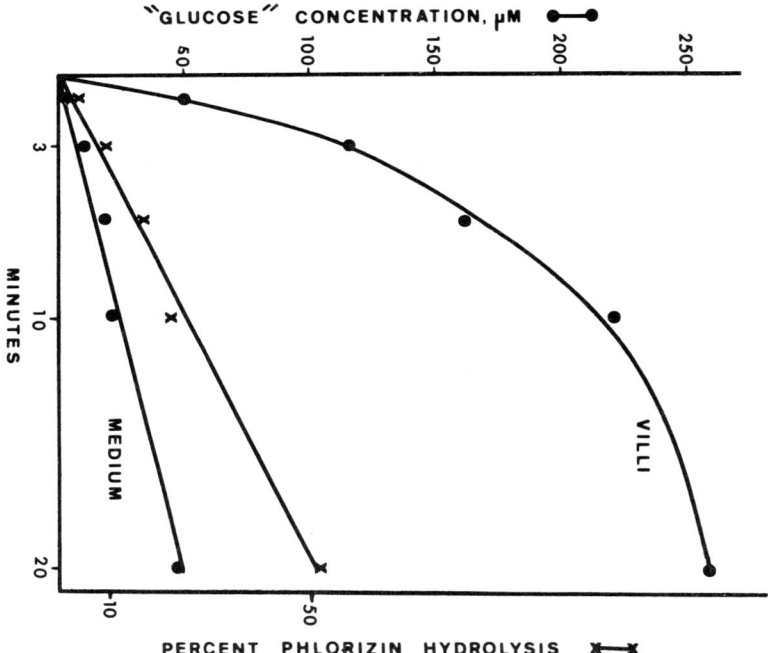

FIG. 5. Distribution of ^{3}H-glucose (plus metabolites) liberated from 100 μM phlorizin.

now be made; even though 60% of the radioactive glucose that entered the tissue has already been converted to metabolites, the liberated, unmetabolized ^{3}H-glucose is still at least four times more concentrated in the villi than in the medium. Since the split glucose is preferentially accumulated into the villi and passive diffusion is an unlikely mechanism, how then does this sugar enter the tissue?

We were attracted to the proposal made by Crane and his colleagues concerning the disposition of sugars liberated from disaccharides such as maltose and sucrose (Miller and Crane, 1961; Crane, 1966; Crane, *this volume*). These investigators suggested that the split monosaccharides had a "kinetic advantage for entry" into the brush border cell over that of free sugar in the medium. In other words, the glucose split from maltose is not simply released into the intestinal lumen but, according to Crane, it is deposited in a compartment from which it is more likely to enter the cell than to diffuse into the medium.

We borrowed this idea and also their test to determine whether the glucose liberated from phlorizin by the brush border hydrolase also had this "kinetic advantage for entry." We added glucose oxidase to the medium containing the specifically labeled phlorizin to see if the liberated glucose was susceptible to attack by the oxidase and what effect there might be on transport of the ^{3}H-sugar. Our experimental results (Table 1) are similar

TABLE 1. *Phlorizin hydrolase and transport of split ^{3}H-glucose: Effect of glucose oxidase in the medium*

Initial medium content	nmoles split/ min/mg dry villi	Free ^{3}H-glucose in medium, μM	Free ^{3}H-glucose in villi, μM
100 μM ^{3}H-Phlorizin	1.09 ± 0.12	10 ± 1	36 ± 5
100 μM ^{3}H-phlorizin + 1% glucose oxidase	0.99 ± 0.05	3 ± 0.2	28 ± 2
100 μM ^{3}H-Phlorizin + 0.33% glucose oxidase	—	1.3 ± 0.1	27 ± 3

Incubations were for 3 min in 3 ml of medium of Krebs-Ringer-phosphate buffer pH 7.4 under 100% oxygen at 37 ± 1° C. Incubations were started by adding two, randomly selected, small pieces of hamster jejunum (about 75 mg wet weight). Termination was accomplished by removing the tissue and freezing in Krebs-Ringer-bicarbonate buffer. The tissue was then handled as described in the test. To ensure proper mixing and to minimize formation of unstirred layers a Dubnoff metabolic incubator was employed shaking at 125 oscillations per min. Means are shown ±1 SEM.

to those observed by Miller and Crane for maltose and sucrose. Notice that glucose oxidase has no effect on the rate of phlorizin hydrolysis. However, the split ^{3}H-glucose that does reach the medium is attacked by the oxidase, and the free sugar at the end of 3 min remains low at 3 μM. We have performed one series of experiments with glucose oxidase in the medium at 0.3% concentration and in this case the glucose content in the medium is reduced about 90%. This is in contrast to the influence of the oxidase on the transport system; the amount of split sugar entering the villi is not compromised very much at all. We think these data are consistent with the idea that the glucose split from phlorizin is indeed released into a compartment that is inaccessible to glucose oxidase. Actually, we wonder whether this hydrolytic step is coupled with the transport process such that as the glycosidic bond is split, the sugar is already in or through the outer membrane barrier. Obviously, however, an important question must be answered before we allow ourselves the privilege of idle speculation. The question is this: Even though phlorizin is present in our experiments at a high level, does a sufficient capacity of the normal glucose carrier remain which could cause the active accumulation of the liberated glucose? We have tested this point and the data in Table 2 indicate that this is not the case. The normal, free glucose transport capacity of our system was first measured by using ^{14}C-labeled glucose at 10 μM with no phlorizin present.[2] The control rate of entry into the tissue was 0.167 nmoles/min/mg dry villi. Furthermore, the free ^{14}C-glucose was actively accumulated and, in 3 min, it reached a tissue concentration of about 2.5 times that in the medium. The experiment was repeated but with phlorizin added in the same concentration at which we studied its hydrolysis (100 μM). Under this condition the carrier is profoundly inhibited and, in fact, so little capacity remains[3] that the rate of glucose entry is reduced to essentially that found for ^{14}C-mannitol,

TABLE 2. *Estimation of sugar carrier capacity with and without 100 μM phlorizin*

Initial medium content	Radioactivity associated with villi nmoles/min/dry mg		Free sugar villi/medium ratio
10 μM ^{14}C-Glucose only	0.167 ± 0.012	(30)	2.48 ± 0.5
10 μM ^{14}C-Glucose + 100 μM phlorizin	0.016 ± 0.0009	(24)	0.18 ± 0.02
10 μM ^{14}C-Mannitol	0.004 ± 0.0004	(12)	0.19 ± 0.004
100 μM ^{3}H-Phlorizin	0.138 ± 0.016	(132)	4.4 ± 0.5

Conditions are as listed for Table 1. Note that the villi/medium ratio of free sugar obtained with 100 μM phlorizin is greater than that for 10 μM glucose only, despite a greater rate of entry for free ^{14}C-glucose. This is the result of 80% metabolism of free ^{14}C-glucose entering as opposed to a 60% metabolism of ^{3}H-glucose split from phlorizin that enters (see text). The rate of association of radioactivity with the villi, therefore, includes glucose plus its metabolites. Numbers in parentheses (n) are the number of experimental observations.

a material we assume enters the tissue by passive leak. Likewise, this amount of phlorizin completely blocks the *accumulating* ability of the glucose carrier; the villi-to-medium concentration ratio is reduced to that attained by the mannitol. We repeat the point made earlier, that our data show the small fraction of glucose carrier which escapes blockade by 100 μM phlorizin under our conditions is (a) incapable of transporting the split ^{3}H-glucose at the rate we have measured (viz., 0.138 nmoles/min or 9 times that attributable to poisoned carrier) and (b) unable to accumulate it to the extent of four times that in the medium.

In an attempt to characterize the new transport system, we continued to

---

[2] We tested glucose transport at this concentration because, at the end of a 3-min incubation with 100 μM phlorizin, the liberated ^{3}H-glucose reaches 10 μM in the medium.

[3] The fraction of carrier that remains unblocked (about 6% when phlorizin is 100 μM and glucose is 10 μM) is predictable on the basis of published affinity values of the competitors for the carrier system under similar incubation conditions (phlorizin K_i, 3–8 μM; glucose K_m, 1–3 mM; Diedrich, 1966; Crane, 1960).

challenge it and tested what effect the addition of a large amount of free, unlabeled glucose to the medium would have on the transport of the sugar split from phlorizin. These results are summarized in Fig. 6. The first two bars represent control values; the cross-hatched column depicts the normal rate at which phlorizin is hydrolyzed in nanomoles per minute per milligram dry villi. The solid bar represents the rate of transport of tritiated glucose equivalents derived from phlorizin expressed in the same units. When unlabeled, free glucose is added to the medium at the 10-mM level (which is 1,000 times the concentration of ^{3}H-glucose liberated into the medium after

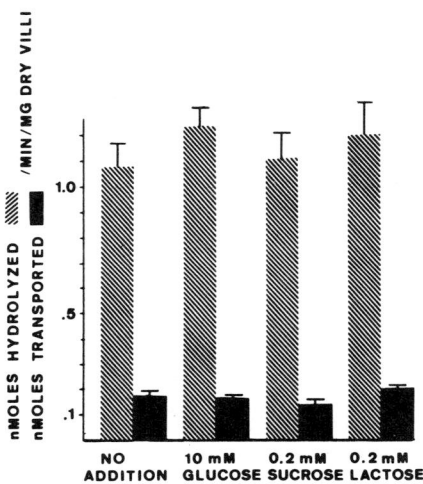

FIG. 6. Transport of glucose hydrolyzed from phlorizin: no effect by other sugars.

3 min), phlorizin hydrolase activity is not decreased nor is the uptake of split glucose blocked. We have extended this experiment and have first preincubated the tissue in the 10-mM unlabeled glucose before exposing it to the phlorizin. Presumably, this preincubation period would allow the free-glucose level in the "fuzzy coat" layer next to the membrane to approach the 10-mM level and give the normal (so-called sodium-dependent) glucose carrier system plenty of sugar to operate on. Even this procedure had no effect on the transport rate or accumulation of the split glucose. We are led to conclude that the liberated glucose from phlorizin does not enter the cell by the same mechanism used by free glucose in the medium.

Sugars liberated from the disaccharides also seem unable to compete with the glucose set free from phlorizin inasmuch as sucrose or lactose at twice the phlorizin concentration had no effect on either hydrolysis or transport activity (Fig. 6)—even 50-mM lactose (data not shown) was ineffective. It appears therefore that our phlorizin-hydrolase coupled transport system is also distinct and separate from the other systems associated with the disaccharidases.

We are left with vital questions. As a result of our structure-activity relationship study, it appears that the phlorizin receptor on the β-glucosidase bears some connection with the phlorizin binding site on the glucose carrier system. What is the relationship, both functional and morphological, between these two brush border membrane components? Furthermore, is it possible that the phlorizin hydrolase, under certain conditions, may act as a transferring enzyme that could cause the translocation of the sugar residue through the membrane at the same time it cleaves the β-glucosyl bond?

REFERENCES

Alvarado, F., and Crane, R. K. (1962): Phlorizin as a competitive inhibitor of the active transport of sugars by hamster small intestine, in vitro. Biochim. Biophys. Acta 56:170–172.

Alvarado, F. (1967): Hypothesis for the interaction of phlorizin and phloretin with membrane carriers for sugars. Biochim. Biophys. Acta 135:483–495.

Alvarado, F. (1969): Effect of phloretin and phlorizin on sugar and amino acid transport systems in small intestine. In: *Symposium on Membranes, Structure and Function*, 6th FEBS Meeting, Madrid, 20:131–139.

Crane, R. K. (1960): Studies on the mechanism of the intestinal absorption of sugars. III. Mutual inhibition, *in vitro*, between some actively transported sugars. Biochim. Biophys. Acta 45:477–482.

Crane, R. K. (1966): Structural and functional organization of an epithelial cell brush border. In: *Symposium of the International Society for Cell Biology*, Vol. 5, edited by K. B. Warren, Academic Press, New York, pp. 71–102.

Diedrich, D. F. (1963): The comparative effects of some phlorizin analogs on the renal reabsorption of glucose. Biochim. Biophys. Acta 71:688–700.

Diedrich, D. F. (1966): Competitive inhibition of intestinal glucose transport by phlorizin analogs. Arch. Biochem. Biophys. 117:248–256.

Diedrich, D. F. (1968): Is phloretin the sugar transport inhibitor in intestine? Arch. Biochem. Biophys. 127:803–812.

Kraml, J. Kolinská, J., Ellederová, D., and Hiršová, D. (1972): β-Glucosidase (phlorizin hydrolase) activity of the lactase fraction isolated from the small intestinal mucosa of infant rats, and the relationship between β-glucosidases and β-galactosidases. Biochim. Biophys. Acta 258:520–530.

Leese, H. J., and Semenza, G. (1973): On the identity between the small intestinal enzymes phlorizin hydrolase and glycosylceramidase. J. Biol. Chem. 248:8170–8173.

Malathi, P., and Crane, R. K. (1969): Phlorizin hydrolase, a β-glucosidase of hamster intestinal brush border membrane. Biochim. Biophys. Acta 173:245–256.

Miller, D., and Crane, R. K. (1961): The digestive function of the epithelium of the small intestine. 1. An intracellular locus of disaccharide and sugar phosphate ester hydrolysis. Biochim. Biophys. Acta 52:281–293.

Semenza, G., Auricchio, S., and Rubino, A. (1965): Multiplicity of human intestinal disaccharidases. I. Chromatographic separation of maltases and of two lactases. Biochim. Biophys. Acta 96:487–497.

Semenza, G. (1969): In search of molecular mechanisms in intestinal sugar absorption. In: *Digestion and Intestinal Absorption*, 7th International Congress of Clinical Chemistry, Geneva/Evian, 4:3–22.

Vick, H., Diedrich, D. F., and Baumann, K. (1973): Reevaluation of renal tubular glucose transport inhibition by phlorizin analogs. Am. J. Physiol., 224:552–557.

Wright, W. (1967): A new *in vitro* method for intestinal active transport studies. Fed. Proc. 26:859.

DISCUSSION

The question was raised as to how phlorizin blocks the sodium-dependent glucose transport mechanism, which is different from the transport system coupled to sucrase and presumably also to phlorizin hydrolase. DIEDRICH expressed difficulty in giving a firm reply and speculated that the two glycosidase-coupled systems may not be quite identical.

KESTON referred to his own studies in which he established a K_i value for phlorizin, for glucose transport, and for mutarotase and found that they were identical: 0.9 mM. DIEDRICH reminded Keston that the relative potency of the phlorizin analogues in the two systems are not similar, e.g., 4'-deoxyphlorizin is the most potent glucose transport inhibitor but has low activity as a mutarotase poison.

CRANE was under the impression that the glucose transfer from phlorizin appears to be very much similar to the glucose transfer from sucrose or maltose and asked if phloretin was also transferred. DIEDRICH replied that he looked for such a transport and for this reason synthesized a phlorizin labeled with ^{14}C in the aglucone portion and followed the label after phlorizin was split: phloretin ended up tightly bound mostly in the brush border membrane and only very small amounts entered the cell.

Intestinal Absorption and Malabsorption,
edited by T. Z. Csáky.
Raven Press, New York © 1975

The Intestinal Brush Border as an Organelle

Robert G. Faust

Department of Physiology, University of North Carolina, School of Medicine, Chapel Hill, North Carolina 27514

I. INTRODUCTION

The digestive and absorptive functions of the brush border or microvilli of mucosal cells in the small intestine have been discussed in this volume. It is known that the final stages of hydrolysis of dietary oligosaccharides and polypeptides to their smallest units, monosaccharides and amino acids, respectively, occur in the brush border (Ugolev and De Laey, 1973). Also, the brush border is the site where these monomers are actively transported against their own concentration gradients into the mucosal cell (Crane, 1962; Kinter and Wilson, 1965).

It has been generally accepted that active monosaccharide and amino acid transport by the small intestine involves an initial Na^+-dependent association or binding of the sugar or amino acid to a component within the brush border to form a ternary complex (Schultz and Curran, 1970). A common brush border binding site may exist for these actively transported sugars (Jorgensen, Landau, and Wilson, 1961), but separate binding sites within the brush border seem to be involved in the active transport of neutral and basic amino acids, as well as for proline and hydroxyproline (Lin, Hagihira, and Wilson, 1962; Newey and Smyth, 1964; Neame, 1965). This initial-binding step apparently requires no metabolic energy (Bihler, Hawkins, and Crane, 1962; Hajjar, Lamont, and Curran, 1970). A second step, however, which is responsible for the intracellular "uphill" accumulation of a sugar or an amino acid and involves the dissociation of the ternary complex, depends on energy. This energy may be derived either indirectly from the "downhill" movement of Na^+ ions across the brush border (Crane, 1964; Curran, Schultz, Chez, and Fuisz, 1967) or directly from cellular metabolism (Kimmich and Randles, 1973). Although competitive inhibitory effects between active intestinal sugar and amino acid transport have been reported by Hindmarsh, Kilby, and Wiseman (1966) and Robinson and Alvarado (1971), the manner by which they occur is uncertain. Furthermore, the precise manner by which sugars and amino acids move across the structurally complex brush border region of the mucosal cell has not been established.

During the past several years my associates and I have been focusing our attention on the absorptive function of the brush border, mainly the mechanism by which sugars and amino acids are actively transported. Our experimental approach has involved the isolation of brush borders from the mucosa of the small intestine and a study of their binding properties in relation to the initial phase of active transport. At the present time our studies have reached a point where we have isolated a binding protein that may be involved in the active transport of both monosaccharides and amino acids by the small intestine. These results have been incorporated into a hypothesis for Na^+-dependent active sugar and amino acid transport by the small intestine which visualizes the intestinal brush border as a digestive-absorptive organelle.

II. MEASUREMENT OF PREFERENTIAL SUGAR AND AMINO ACID BINDING TO ISOLATED BRUSH BORDERS

Epithelial brush borders from the hamster jejunum were obtained by a modification of the methods of Miller and Crane (1961) and Harrison and Webster (1964). These essentially pure preparations of intact brush borders, as well as disrupted brush borders, were used in our binding studies. Since similar data were obtained with both preparations, the disrupted brush borders were used more extensively because eventually they would be fractionated in order to isolate the binding component. Tris (hydroxymethyl) aminomethane was employed to disrupt brush borders at 2°C when sugar binding was to be studied. This disruption procedure, however, seemed to inactivate amino acid binding sites. Consequently, distilled water at 37°C was used to disrupt intact brush borders for the amino acid binding studies.

Sugar and amino acid binding to brush borders was measured by a double-labeling technique. The brush border preparation was incubated at 37°C for at least 30 min in a solution containing a ^3H-labeled sugar or amino acid that is not actively transported and a ^{14}C-labeled sugar or amino acid that is actively transported. After the incubation period, the brush border suspension was centrifuged and the $^3H/^{14}C$ disintegrations per minute (dpm) ratio in the supernatant was compared to the $^3H/^{14}C$ dpm ratio of an incubation solution that did not contain brush borders. An increase in this ratio was indicative of preferential binding of the ^{14}C-labeled actively transported sugar or amino acid to the brush borders. In experiments involving sugar binding 0.01 μM of D-mannose-1-^3H, which is not actively transported by the hamster jejunum was employed, whereas 1.0 μM of D-^{14}C-glucose (uniformly labeled), which is structurally similar to D-mannose, was the representative actively transported compound. DL-Glutamate-3-^3H at 1.0 μM was used as the nonactively transported amino acid and uniformly ^{14}C-labeled L-alanine, L-proline, and L-histidine at 0.5-μM were representative of different types of actively transported amino acids that were employed in the studies involving preferential amino acid binding. The concentrations of the

^{14}C-labeled actively transported compounds were approximately at the K_m for the binding of these substances to the brush borders.

III. PROPERTIES OF PREFERENTIAL D-GLUCOSE BINDING TO BRUSH BORDERS

At first, we established that the actively transported sugar, D-glucose, was bound to brush borders in preference to D-mannose. After this was determined, we studied the nature of D-glucose binding in relation to factors relevant to the first step in its active transport by the small intestine.

Figure 1 illustrates the percentage change in the dpm ratio of D-mannose-1-^{3}H to D-^{14}C-glucose (U.L.) in the presence of Tris-disrupted brush borders under various experimental conditions. Similar results were also obtained with isolated, initially intact brush borders (Faust, Leadbetter, Plenge, and McCaslin, 1968). It can be seen that the preferential binding of D-glucose in plain distilled water was similar to that obtained in a solution containing Na$^+$ (105.8 mM), K$^+$ (30 mM), Mg^{2+} (6 mM), and ATP (6 mM), which Faust and Wu (1966) had shown to stimulate adenosine triphosphatase activity in hamster mucosal homogenates. These data suggest that neither added Na$^+$ ions nor conditions that should have enhanced ATPase activity

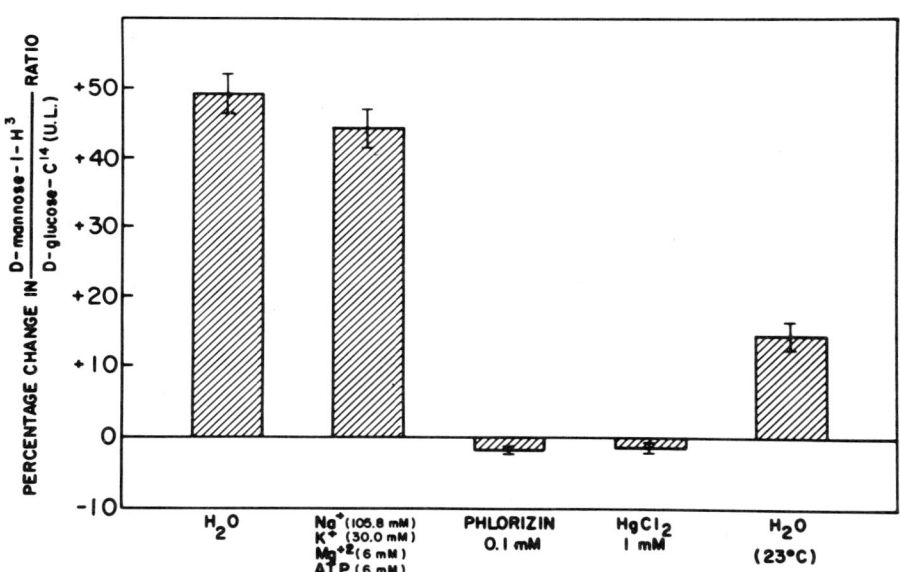

FIG. 1. Percentage change in the dpm ratio of D-mannose-1-^{3}H to uniformly ^{14}C-labeled D-glucose in the supernatant from Tris-disrupted brush borders under various conditions. The suspensions were incubated for 1 hr at 37°C unless noted otherwise. Each bar represents the mean of at least four experiments. The vertical lines represent ±1 SE of mean above and below the bar points (Faust, Wu, and Faggard, 1967).

were required for preferential D-glucose binding. However, the concentration of Na⁺ in the experiments in which Na⁺ was not added was 0.27 mmole/1 as determined by flame photometery. This Na⁺ concentration was greater than the concentration of D-^{14}C-glucose (U.L.) used in these experiments. Since some of these Na⁺ ions may have been closely associated with glucose binding sites, it was impossible to test the Na⁺ dependency hypothesis for D-glucose binding in these experiments, although it was obvious that an increase in the Na⁺ concentration did not produce an increase in D-glucose binding. On the other hand, 0.1-mM phlorizin, a potent competitive inhibitor of intestinal active sugar transport (Alvarado, 1967), completely inhibited the binding of D-glucose, presumably by competing with D-glucose for binding sites within the Tris-disrupted brush borders. The complete inhibition of D-glucose binding in the presence of 1-mM $HgCl_2$ suggested that perhaps protein and sulfhydryl groups within the disrupted microvilli preparation were involved in this process (White, Handler, and

TABLE 1. *Effect of sulfhydryl-reacting compounds on the preferential binding of D-^{14}C-glucose (U.L.) to tris-disrupted brush borders*

Sulfhydryl-reacting compound	Number of experiments	Percentage inhibition
Iodoacetate	3	41.6 ± 5.9
N-Ethylmaleimide	3	54.0 ± 7.6
o-Iodosobenzoate	3	54.2 ± 5.0
p-Hydroxymercuribenzoate	3	90.6 ± 3.2
p-Hydroxymercuribenzoate + L-cysteine (1 mM)	4	−4.6 ± 10.5

All inhibitors are at a concentration of 1 mM. The standard error is given for each mean (Faust et al., 1968).

Smith, 1964). The quantity of D-glucose bound at 23°C in plain distilled water was 70% less than that bound at 37°C, indicating a temperature dependency (temperature coefficient, Q_{10} of 2.4) for this phenomenon.

The importance of SH- groups for preferential binding of D-glucose was investigated more extensively. As shown in Table 1, all of the various sulfhydryl-reacting compounds that were employed reduced the preferential binding of D-glucose to the Tris-disrupted brush borders. A greater reduction was observed with *p*-hydroxymercuribenzoate than with the other inhibitors. However, the SH- groups of an equimolar concentration of L-cysteine protected the Tris-disrupted brush borders from the inhibitory effect of *p*-hydroxymercuribenzoate.

The effects of actively and nonactively transported sugars and amino acids on the preferential binding of D-^{14}C-glucose (U.L.) to Tris-disrupted brush borders are presented in Table 2. Only sugars that are actively transported by the hamster jejunum inhibit the preferential binding of D-^{14}C-glucose (U.L.), although D-galactose was not inhibitory at the lower (1 mM)

TABLE 2. *Effects of sugars and amino acids on the preferential binding of D-^{14}C-glucose (U.L.) to tris-disrupted brush borders*

Compound	Percentage inhibition at the concentration of	
	1 mM	10 mM
Actively transported sugars		
D-Glucose	100.0 (3)	—
3-O-methyl-D-glucose	45.5 ± 6.2(3)	91.7 ± 1.3(3)
D-Xylose	18.8 ± 2.0(4)	46.7 ± 4.9(3)
D-Galactose	1.7 ± 2.2(4)	46.8 ± 0.9(3)
Nonactively transported sugars		
L-Sorbose	−0.5 ± 6.7(3)	6.0 ± 8.2(3)
D-Ribose	7.4 ± 8.5(3)	−10.7 ± 5.4(3)
D-Arabinose	5.5 ± 9.4(6)	−3.3 ± 4.1(3)
L-Arabinose	−1.3 ± 10.0(4)	−2.2 ± 3.4(3)
Actively transported amino acids		
L-Histidine	−10.5 ± 12.5(5)	19.3 ± 5.0(4)
L-Alanine	1.8 ± 5.1(3)	4.5 ± 1.8(4)
L-Hydroxyproline	9.1 ± 10.5(5)	6.1 ± 3.1(3)
L-Proline	0.4 ± 7.2(4)	2.7 ± 2.6(4)
L-Methionine	−10.9 ± 15.7(4)	−5.7 ± 8.8(4)
L-Tryptophan	−1.3 ± 1.3(5)	1.5 ± 3.6(4)
L-Cysteine	6.6 ± 9.2(4)	2.9 ± 2.2(3)
L-Arginine	6.7 ± 8.5(4)	−17.8 ± 6.8(4)
Nonactively transported amino acids		
L-Aspartic acid	−3.3 ± 6.8(6)	−20.7 ± 11.3(3)
L-Glutamic acid	−7.3 ± 8.1(4)	−7.9 ± 19.1(3)

The number of experiments is given in parentheses. The standard error is given for each mean (Faust et al., 1968).

concentration. The ability of these sugars to inhibit preferential binding of D-glucose to Tris-disrupted brush borders corresponds reasonably well with their affinities for intestinal transport. Neither actively transported amino acids nor nonactively transported sugars and amino acids significantly affected the preferential binding of D-^{14}C-glucose (U.L.). The ineffectiveness of actively transported amino acids on this phenomenon was in accord with the observations reported by Munck (1968) who found no competitive inhibition between the intestinal transport of amino acids and sugars. Therefore, factors other than competition for similar binding sites were apparently responsible for the inhibitory effects observed by other investigators (Hindmarsh et al., 1966; Robinson and Alvarado, 1971).

IV. PROPERTIES OF PREFERENTIAL BINDING OF AMINO ACIDS TO BRUSH BORDERS

Our next series of experiments involved amino acid binding to isolated brush borders. In Fig. 2 it is shown that the uniformly ^{14}C-labeled actively

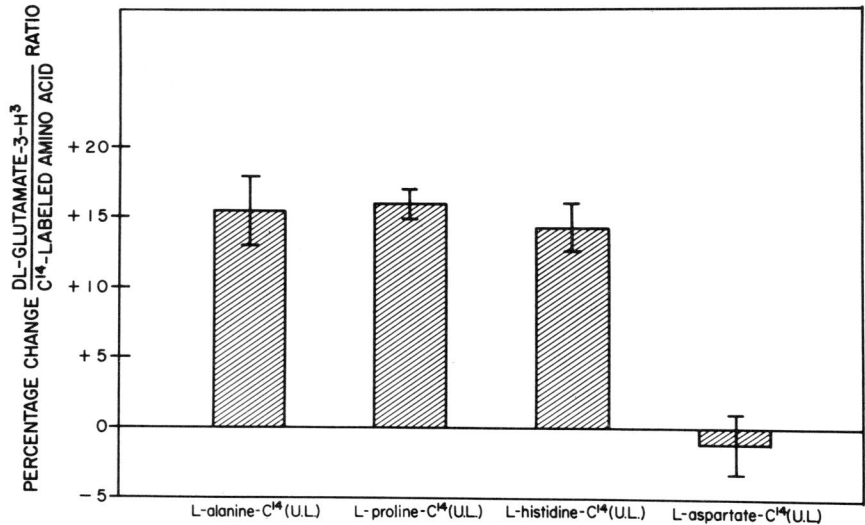

FIG. 2. Preferential binding of uniformly ^{14}C-labeled amino acids to isolated mucosal brush borders. The brush borders were incubated for 30 min at 37°C in 22-mM sodium phosphate buffer (pH 7.2) containing 1-μM DL-glutamate-3-^{3}H and 0.5 μM of a uniformly ^{14}C-labeled amino acid. Each bar point represents the mean of at least seven experiments. The vertical lines represent ±1 SE of the mean above and below the bar points (Burns and Faust, 1969).

transported amino acids, L-alanine, L-proline, and L-histidine, were preferentially bound to initially intact brush borders. In all of these cases there was approximately a 15% increase in the ^{3}H/^{14}C dpm ratios, which indicated that each actively transported amino acid had a similar affinity for binding to the isolated brush borders. When the nonactively transported amino acid, L-^{14}C-aspartate (U.L.), was substituted for one of the actively transported ^{14}C-labeled amino acids, no preferential binding was observed and the ^{3}H/^{14}C dpm ratio was unchanged. In order to establish whether or not uniformly labeled L-^{14}C-alanine, L-^{14}C-proline, and L-^{14}C-histidine were being bound to the same site, the possibility of competition among these amino acids for a common binding site within the brush border was explored. The effects of unlabeled L-alanine, L-proline, L-histidine, and L-aspartate, at the relatively high concentration of 1 mM, on preferential amino acid binding to brush borders are presented in Table 3. Unlabeled L-alanine inhibited the preferential binding of each actively transported ^{14}C-labeled amino acid. Unlabeled L-proline, however, was only inhibitory to the preferential binding of L-alanine ($p < 0.01$) and L-proline; no inhibition of L-histidine binding ($p > 0.3$) was observed in the presence of this amino acid. In the presence of unlabeled L-histidine the preferential binding of L-alanine was unaffected ($p > 0.3$), but L-proline and L-histidine binding to the brush borders was inhibited. The nonactively transported, unlabeled L-aspartate,

TABLE 3. *Effects of unlabeled amino acids on the preferential binding of uniformly ^{14}C-labeled L-alanine, L-proline, and L-histidine to isolated brush borders*

Unlabeled amino acid (1 mM)	Percentage inhibition of binding of		
	L-^{14}C-alanine	L-^{14}C-proline	L-^{14}C-histidine
L-Alanine	50.7 ± 6.0 (6)	99.5 ± 0.5 (3)	22.6 ± 3.4 (5)
L-Proline	21.2 ± 1.7 (5)	83.0 ± 9.8 (4)	−14.4 ± 8.4 (3)
L-Histidine	−21.8 ± 7.5 (3)	91.4 ± 8.2 (4)	63.3 ± 5.3 (4)
L-Aspartate	−14.9 ± 12.0 (7)	−14.4 ± 8.0 (3)	−1.1 ± 0.6 (3)

The concentration of the ^{14}C-labeled amino acids is 0.5 μM. The number of experiments is given in parentheses. The SE is given for each mean (Burns and Faust, 1969).

had no significant effect on the preferential binding of any of the actively transported amino acids that were employed ($p > 0.2$). These results suggest that the binding receptor within the brush border for L-alanine, L-proline, and L-histidine may not be precisely the same. If these amino acids were sharing the same binding site, then unlabeled L-histidine should have inhibited L-alanine binding, unlabeled L-proline should have inhibited the preferential binding of L-histidine, and unlabeled L-proline should have been more inhibitory to the binding of L-alanine. It is possible, however, that the L-alanine, L-proline, and L-histidine binding sites may be in close proximity to each other or they may even be overlapping. The spatial relationship of these binding sites, therefore, may account for the inhibition of L-^{14}C-proline (U.L.) binding by unlabeled L-histidine and L-alanine and for the inhibition of L-^{14}C-histidine (U.L.) binding by unlabeled L-alanine. These observations could be considered to be in accordance with the results of experiments by Lin et al. (1962), Newey and Smyth (1964), and Neame (1965) with the intact small intestine which had demonstrated that a separate instead of a common transport system exists for L-alanine, L-proline, and L-histidine.

Additional information concerning the properties of amino acid binding to isolated brush borders is shown in Table 4. Unlabeled 1 mM D-glucose did not affect preferential amino acid binding ($p > 0.05$) which indicated, once again, that amino acids and sugars do not share the same binding site within the brush border. It can also be seen that neither 100-mM NaCl nor KCl had an effect upon the binding of amino acids. As it has been indicated for preferential sugar binding to brush borders, there were sufficient Na$^+$ ions in our preparation to satisfy a possible Na$^+$-dependent binding requirement for these amino acids. It is obvious from Table 4, however, that protein SH- groups are involved in some manner in the binding of amino acids to isolated brush borders since this phenomenon was inhibited by the sulfhydryl-reacting compound, p-hydroxymercuribenzoate. A similar inhibitory effect on preferential D-glucose binding to brush borders had been previously observed with this compound.

TABLE 4. *Preferential binding of uniformly ^{14}C-labeled amino acids to brush borders in the presence of various compounds*

Amino acid (0.5 μM)	Percentage change in ^{3}H/^{14}C dpm ratio in presence of				
	No addition	D-glucose (1 mM)	NaCl (100 mM)	KCl (100 mM)	p-hydroxymer-curibenzoate (1 mM)
L-^{14}C-alanine	15.5 ± 2.4 (17)	14.4 ± 3.2 (4)	13.3 ± 1.2 (3)	10.4 ± 1.7 (3)	0.4 ± 2.6 (3)
L-^{14}C-proline	15.9 ± 1.0 (12)	16.9 ± 4.5 (4)	18.5 ± 1.8 (5)	14.1 ± 2.1 (3)	−0.2 ± 1.8 (3)
L-^{14}C-histidine	14.4 ± 1.7 (18)	9.5 ± 2.6 (4)	19.2 ± 3.2 (3)	17.7 ± 4.1 (3)	−1.4 ± 3.4 (3)

The number of experiments is given in parentheses. The standard error is given for each mean (Burns and Faust, 1969).

V. SUGAR AND AMINO ACID BINDING TO THE CORE FRACTION OF DISRUPTED BRUSH BORDERS

Up to this point in our investigation of the mechanism of intestinal active sugar and amino acid transport, we had succeeded in demonstrating that (a) isolated brush borders from the intestinal mucosal cell are capable of preferentially binding actively transported D-glucose and actively transported amino acids; (b) the D-glucose binding site is shared by other actively transported sugars, but separate binding sites exist for the three actively transported amino acids that were employed, i.e., L-alanine, L-proline, and L-histidine; and (c) the sugar and amino acid binding sites are associated with protein SH- groups. It had not been demonstrated, however, that preferential D-glucose and amino acid binding were dependent upon Na$^+$. Since sufficient Na$^+$ was bound to the brush borders in our preparations to satisfy a possible Na$^+$ requirement for D-glucose and amino acid binding, experiments were designed to study the Na$^+$-dependent binding of these compounds to a fraction of the brush border which was low in Na$^+$.

In order to identify the fraction containing the sugar or amino acid binding sites, Tris-disrupted or distilled water–disrupted brush borders that had preferentially bound either D-^{14}C-glucose (U.L.) or L-^{14}C-histidine (U.L.), respectively, were fractionated by Ficoll density gradient centrifugation. A discontinuous 10, 20, 30, 35, and 40% Ficoll density gradient, centrifuged at 112,000 × g for 110 min, was used to fractionate the ^{14}C-labeled disrupted brush borders. In both cases the preferentially bound actively transported sugar or amino acid was located in Fraction 1 that floated on the 10% Ficoll layer. It is interesting to note that when these radioactive brush borders were separated by glycerol density gradient centrifugation, the preferentially bound sugar and amino acid were found in the precipitate fraction. Electron photomicrographs of Fraction 1 from the Ficoll density gradient (Faust, Burns, and Misch, 1970) indicated that it contained microvillus core material, which appeared to be similar to that observed in the precipitate of the glycerol density gradient (Overton, Eichholz, and Crane, 1965). In addition, Fraction 1 did not contain sucrase or glycylhistidine peptidase activity, which was found in fractions containing vesicular plasma membranes (Faust, Shearin, and Misch, 1972). The Ficoll gradient proved to be a more useful preparative method because the binding sites were located in a more homogeneous fraction of the disrupted brush borders. Moreover, glycerol seemed to inactivate the core material with respect to Na^+-dependent sugar and amino acid binding.

A. Na^+-Dependent D-Glucose Binding

Figure 3 shows the preferential binding capacity for D-^{14}C-glucose (U.L.) in the presence of Na^+ of each washed fraction of nonradioactive Tris-disrupted brush borders obtained from Ficoll density gradient centrifugation. In addition to 0.01-μM D-[1–^{3}H]-mannose and 1-μM D-^{14}C-glucose (U.L.), the incubation medium contained 100-mM NaCl, 6 mM dithiothreitol (DTT, a protein stabilizer), 10-mM $MgCl_2$, and 20-mM Tris buffer (pH 7.4). The data indicate that only Fraction I, containing core material which had an initially low Na^+ concentration of 10 μM, was capable of preferentially binding D-^{14}C-glucose (U.L.). No binding occurred when either Mg^{2+}, which enhances D-^{14}C-glucose (U.L.) binding to Tris-disrupted brush borders

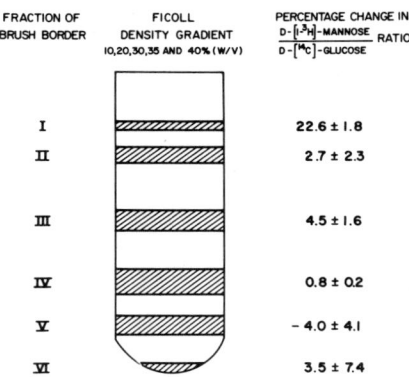

FIG. 3. Schematic diagram of fractions obtained by Ficoll density gradient centrifugation of Tris-disrupted brush borders as visualized by the Tyndall effect. After centrifugation, each fraction was incubated for 30 min at 37°C in a medium containing 0.01-μM D-[1-^{3}H]-mannose, 1-μM D-^{14}C-glucose (U.L.), 100-mM NaCl, 10-mM $MgCl_2$, 6-mM dithiothreitol, and 20-mM Tris buffer (pH 7.4). The percentage change in the ^{3}H/^{14}C ratios in the supernatant from each fraction was observed in five experiments (data from Faust et al., 1972).

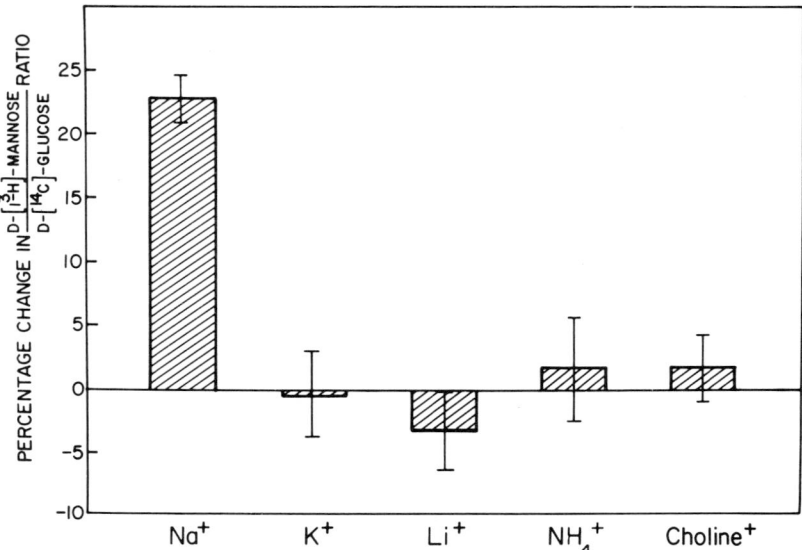

FIG. 4. Preferential binding of D-^{14}C-glucose (U.L.) to brush border Fraction I in 100 mM Na$^+$ and Na$^+$ substituted chloride salts, 6-mM dithiothreitol, 10-mM MgCl$_2$, and 20-mM Tris buffer (pH 7.4). Fraction I was incubated for 30 min at 37°C in the presence of 0.01-μM D-[1-^{3}H]-mannose and 1-μM D-^{14}C-glucose (U.L.). Each bar point represents the mean of at least four experiments. The vertical lines represent ±1 SE above and below the bar points (Faust et al., 1972).

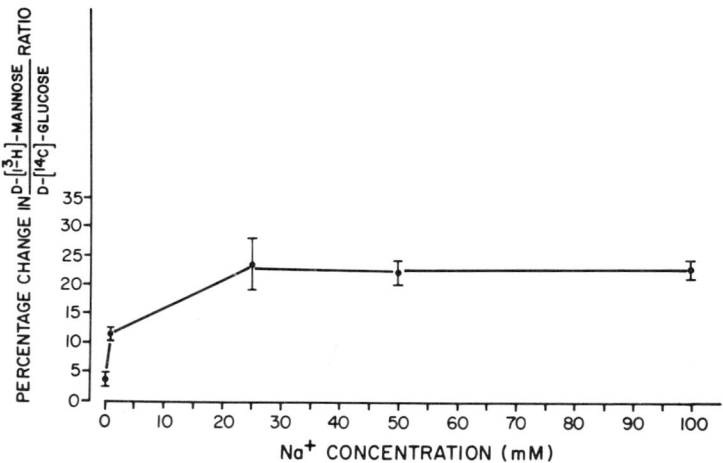

FIG. 5. Effect of various Na$^+$ concentrations on the preferential binding of D-^{14}C-glucose (U.L.) to brush border Fraction I. NaCl was employed. Each point is the average of at least three determinations and the vertical lines indicate ±1 SE of the mean (Faust et al., 1972).

(Faust et al., 1968), or DTT were omitted from the incubation medium.

In order to determine if D-glucose binding to Fraction I was dependent on the presence of Na^+, this cation was replaced in the incubation medium by K^+, Li^+, NH_4^+, and choline. Figure 4 illustrates that D-glucose binding is indeed dependent on Na^+ and that no binding occurs in the presence of the other cations. Preferential D-glucose binding to Fraction I varied with the concentration of Na^+ in the incubation medium as is shown in Fig. 5. Maximum binding occurred at a Na^+ concentration of 25 mM, and there was no increase in this binding even though the Na^+ concentration was elevated to 100 mM.

B. Na^+-Dependent L-Histidine Binding

Na^+-dependent binding of L-^{14}C-histidine (U.L.) was determined with Fraction I from distilled water–disrupted brush borders. Instead of Tris buffer which inhibits amino acid binding, 17.6 mM of Na^+-containing and Na^+-free bicarbonate and phosphate buffers were employed in these studies. The effect of replacing the Na^+ in bicarbonate and phosphate buffers on preferential L-^{14}C-histidine (U.L.) binding to Fraction I is illustrated in Fig. 6. No preferential binding was observed when NH_4^+ and Li^+ were

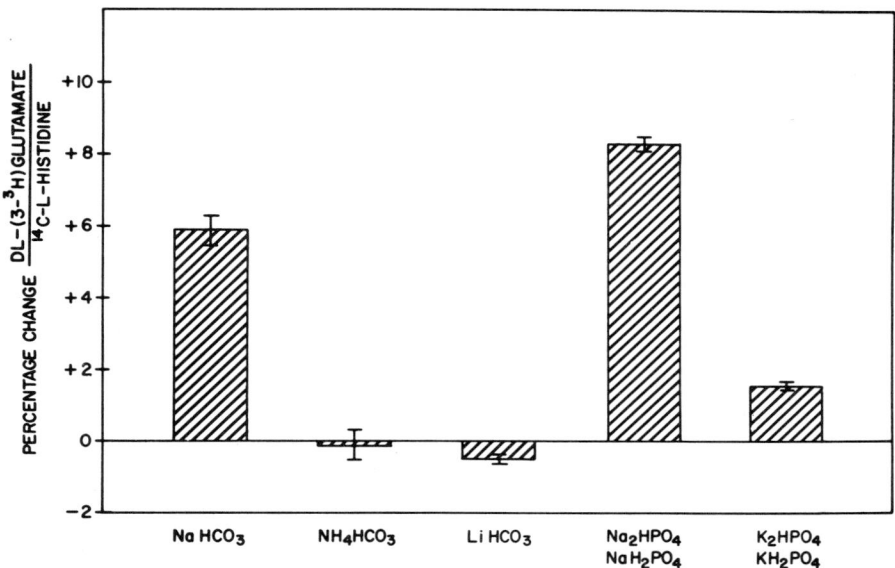

FIG. 6. Preferential binding of L-^{14}C-histidine (U.L.) to brush border Fraction I in Na^+ and Na^+-free buffers. Fraction I was incubated for 30 min at 37°C (pH 7.2) in the presence of 1-μM DL-[3-^{3}H] glutamate and 0.5-μM L-^{14}C-histidine (U.L.). All buffers were at a concentration of 17.6 mM. Each bar point represents the mean of at least four experiments. The vertical lines represent ±1 SE above and below the bar points (Faust et al., 1970).

substituted for Na⁺ in the bicarbonate buffer. The substitution of K⁺ for Na⁺ in the phosphate buffer produced approximately an 81% reduction in the preferential binding of L-^{14}C-histidine (U.L.). The increase in binding ($p < 0.01$) observed when sodium phosphate was substituted for the sodium bicarbonate buffer can be accounted for by the increase in the Na⁺ concentration under these conditions. The Na⁺ concentrations in the sodium bicarbonate and sodium phosphate buffers are 17.6 and 32.3 mM, respectively. A similar increase in the ^{3}H/^{14}C dpm ratio caused by an increase in

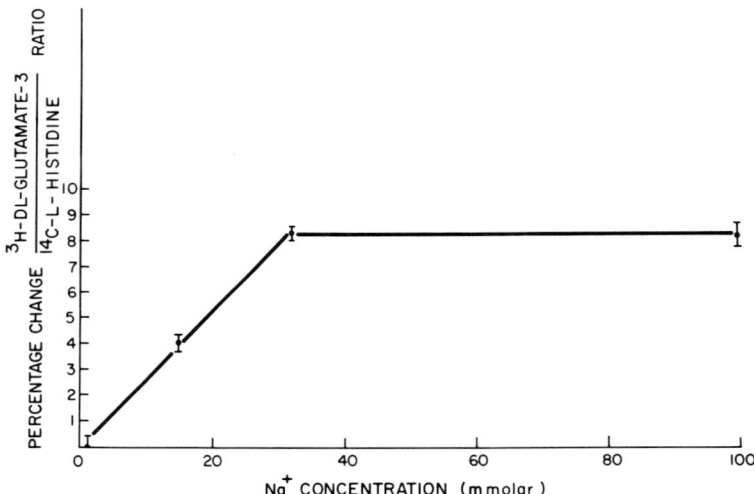

FIG. 7. Effect of various Na⁺ concentrations on the preferential binding of L-^{14}C-histidine (U.L.) to brush border Fraction I. Sodium phosphate buffer (pH 7.2) was employed. Each point is the average of at least three determinations and the vertical lines indicate ±1 SE of the mean (Faust et al., 1970).

the Na⁺ concentration is illustrated in Fig. 7. It can be seen that no binding occurred at a 1-mM Na⁺ concentration, and maximum amino acid binding was observed at 32.3 mM of Na⁺. However, there was no increase in this binding even though the Na⁺ concentration is elevated to 100 mM. These results did not depend on the presence of either Mg^{2+} or DTT as was the case with Na⁺-dependent D-glucose binding to Fraction I.

VI. ISOLATION OF A D-GLUCOSE AND L-HISTIDINE BINDING PROTEIN

Since we had established that both actively transported D-glucose and L-histidine depended on Na⁺ to be preferentially bound to the core fraction of disrupted brush borders, the next phase of our investigation involved the isolation of the binding component. The Fraction I core material, which had been labeled with either D-^{14}C-glucose (U.L.) or L-^{14}C-histidine (U.L.)

in the presence of Na⁺ ions, was extracted with cold acetone. Most of the radioactivity remained in the insoluble precipitate indicating that the ^{14}C-labeled compound was not bound to the lipid-soluble portion of the core material. This observation was supported by experiments in which chloroform:methanol (3:1) was also employed as the lipid extracting solution. The ^{14}C-labeled acetone powder was solubilized by incubation, at 25°C for approximately 12 hr, in 1% sodium dodecyl sulfate (SDS), 25-mM

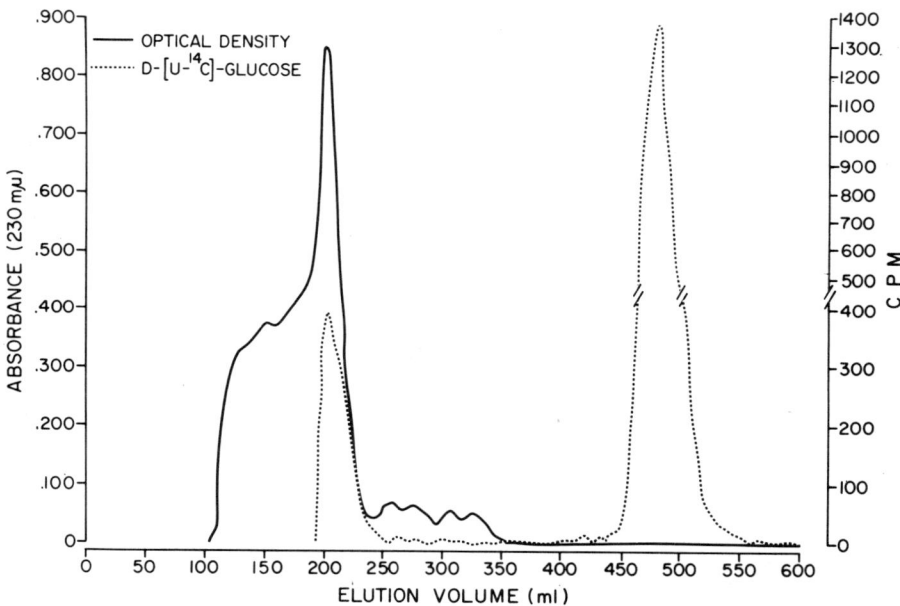

FIG. 8. Elution profile from Sephadex G-75 gel filtration of acetone extracted, SDS solubilized brush border core material labeled with D-^{14}C-glucose (U.L.) in the presence of Na⁺ ions. The column was eluted with 25-mM Na₂HPO₄-NaH₂PO₄ buffer (pH 7.2) containing 0.1% SDS, 10-mM MgCl₂, and 6-mM dithiothreitol. The void volume of the gel bed was 140 ml. After the absorption of the eluant was read at 230 nm to detect peptide bonds, each 5 ml fraction was dried at 80°C in a vial. Then 15 ml of liquid scintillation fluid was added to each vial before it was counted in a Nuclear Chicago Mark I Liquid Scintillation System. ———, absorbance; . . . , D-^{14}C-glucose (U.L.) (Faust and Shearin, 1973).

sodium phosphate buffer (pH 7.2), 10-mM MgCl₂, 6-mM DTT, and the same concentration of the ^{14}C-labeled compound that was used in the binding experiment. Figure 8 illustrates a typical elution profile of this solution obtained by Sephadex G-75 gel filtration. In the experiment illustrated, D-^{14}C-glucose (U.L.) was bound within a sharp peak absorbing at 230 nm. Although there was some absorption before and after the peak, it did not contain any bound D-^{14}C-glucose (U.L.). Free radioactive sugar appeared in the elution volume between 450 ml and approximately 550 ml. This was confirmed by control experiments in which only free D-^{14}C-glucose

(U.L.) was placed on the column. Similar results were obtained when L-^{14}C-histidine (U.L.) was used as the binding compound. Although both D-^{14}C-glucose (U.L.) and L-^{14}C-histidine (U.L.) were bound within the same peak of absorbance, more D-^{14}C-glucose ($4.17 \pm 0.96 \times 10^{-8}$ mmole) than L-^{14}C-histidine ($1.95 \pm 0.07 \times 10^{-10}$ mmole) was bound per mg of protein as determined by four and three experiments, respectively. The amount of the ^{14}C-labeled compound bound was calculated from its measured radioactivity and specific activity, 288 and 240 mCi mmole^{-1} for ^{14}C-labeled D-glucose and L-histidine, respectively. Protein was determined by the Lowry, Rosebrough, Farr, and Randall (1951) method using bovine crystalline serum albumin as standard.

It should be emphasized that the amount of sugar and amino acid dissociated during the solubilization and fractionation procedures was unknown. Consequently, a calculation of the number of sugar and amino acid molecules bound per molecule of protein from the results of this experiment would be meaningless.

A. Na$^+$-Dependent D-Glucose Binding to the Isolated Protein

To verify that the isolated protein was the component involved in Na$^+$-dependent binding of actively transported nutrients by the hamster jejunum, the denaturing SDS adhering to it had to be removed. This was accomplished by precipitating the partially purified binding protein with 30% (NH$_4$)$_2$SO$_4$ and subsequently redissolving this unlabeled precipitate in 50-mM Tris-acetate buffer, pH 7.8, containing 6-mM DDT and 6 M urea. This solution was passed through a SDS-removal column containing Dowex 1-X2 (Weber and Kunter, 1971). The SDS-free effluent was then placed in the hollow bore fibers of Bio-Fiber 50 minibeakers[1] to exchange 25-mM sodium, potassium, or ammonium phosphate buffer, pH 7.2, for the Tris-acetate buffer and to remove urea. The buffer on the outside of the hollow fibers was replaced every 15 min for 1 hr at 5°C. The last replacement contained 0.1 μM of D-^{14}C-glucose (U.L.). Diffusion of the D-^{14}C-glucose (U.L.) across the fiber walls was then allowed to proceed for 1 hr at 37°C. We had previously determined that, in the absence of protein, D-^{14}C-glucose (U.L.) could reach a diffusion equilibrium under these conditions. After this incubation period, ^{14}C in 0.1 ml samples of the solutions inside and outside the hollow fibers was counted. The results from these studies demonstrated that D-^{14}C-glucose (U.L.) was a higher concentration within the hollow fiber compartment containing the binding protein only when Na$^+$ ions were present. When either K$^+$ or NH$_4^+$ were substituted for Na$^+$ in the phosphate buffer, D-^{14}C-glucose (U.L.) was observed to be at the same concentration in both compartments. Therefore, the increase in D-^{14}C-glucose

---

[1] Obtained from Bio-Rad Laboratories, Richmond, California.

(U.L.) within the protein compartment in the presence of Na^+ could only be attributed to the binding of this sugar to the isolated protein. The amount of sugar bound per milligram of protein was similar to that observed in the absorbance peak from the Sephadex G-75 gel filtration column (Fig. 8). Once again, caution should be exercised when interpreting these results. Since we do not know the quantity of protein that has been inactivated with respect to Na^+-dependent binding by our preparative procedures, it is not possible to predict, on a molecule to molecule basis, the number of sugar binding sites on a protein molecule.

B. Molecular Weight of the Binding Protein

The molecular weight of the partially purified binding protein, precipitated by 30% $(NH_4)_2SO_4$ and redissolved in 25-mM sodium phosphate buffer (pH 7.2), was first determined by the Sephadex G-75 gel filtration method of Andrews (1964). In Fig. 9 the selectivity curve for various proteins that were placed on the column is illustrated. The binding protein was estimated to have a molecular weight of 59,000 by this procedure.

SDS-acrylamide gel electrophoresis was then employed to determine the

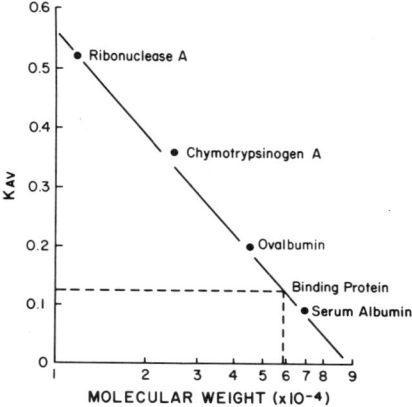

FIG. 9. Molecular weight of the D-glucose and L-histidine binding protein as determined by Sephadex G-75 gel filtration. The K_{av} for each standard protein, calculated from the equation $Ve - Vo/Vt - Vo$ (Ve = the elution volume of protein, Vo = the elution volume of blue dextran, and Vt = the total bed volume), was plotted against the molecular weight of the protein on a semi-logarithmic scale. The molecular weight of the binding protein was determined by comparing its measured K_{av} against this curve (data taken from Faust and Shearin, 1973).

molecular weight of the binding protein (Shapiro, Vinuela, and Maizel, 1967; Weber and Osborn, 1969). As can be seen in Fig. 10, the binding protein has an estimated molecular weight of 56,000 by this method. Only a single discernible band was observed for the binding protein during these experiments, indicating that it was homogeneous under these conditions.

Finally, the molecular weight of the binding protein in 25-mM sodium phosphate buffer (pH 7.2) was estimated by sedimentation velocity analysis at 20°C with a Spinco model E ultracentrifuge equipped with schlieren optics (Schachman, 1959). A sedimentation coefficient of 3.87×10^{-13} sec

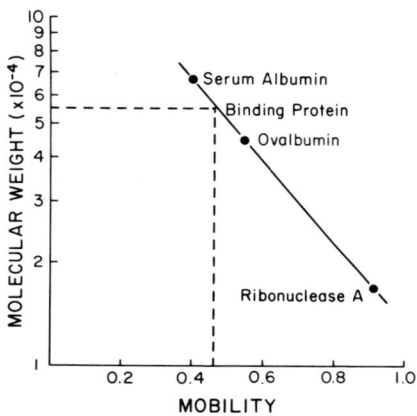

FIG. 10. Determination of the molecular weight of the D-glucose and L-histidine binding protein by SDS-gel electrophoresis (data taken from Faust and Shearin, 1973).

was obtained for the binding protein from the schlieren profiles during centrifugation at 35,000 rpm. The bulk of the material appeared to be homogeneous and of uniform size. The binding protein was calculated to have a molecular weight of 50,934 by the use of the equation M.W. = $RTs/D(1-\bar{v}p)$; M.W. = molecular weight, R = gas constant, T = absolute temperature, s = measured sedimentation coefficient, D = diffusion coefficient (assumed to be 7.4×10^{-7} cm^2/sec), and $(1-\bar{v}p)$ = buoyancy factor [estimated to be 0.25 by assuming a partial specific volume $(\bar{v}p)$ of 0.75].

The results of these studies at the molecular level indicate that protein subunits with a molecular weight of approximately 55,000 daltons are involved in the Na⁺-dependent binding of actively transported D-glucose and L-histidine. These protein subunits are probably constituents of the same macromolecule which seems to be located in the core material of the brush border. However, it is also conceivable that the sugar and amino acid receptor sites could be within or in close proximity to the plasma membrane and that they were retracted from the plasma membrane upon disruption of the brush borders. In any event, the presence of both Na^+-dependent sugar and amino acid binding sites on the same macromolecule could account for some of the observed competitive inhibitory effects between active intestinal sugar and amino acid transport that have been reported (Hindmarsh et al., 1966; Robinson and Alvarado, 1971). It is not known at this time whether or not the sugar and amino acid binding sites exist on the same protein subunit.

VII. ACTIVE SUGAR AND AMINO ACID TRANSPORT BY THE INTESTINAL BRUSH BORDER ORGANELLE: A HYPOTHESIS

In Fig. 11 a hypothesis for active sugar and amino acid transport by the small intestine that takes into consideration the digestive properties of the brush border organelle is presented. Under normal physiological conditions, *in situ,* a major portion of the monosaccharides and amino acids that are actively transported by the small intestine are derived from the final stages of carbohydrate and protein hydrolysis, respectively, on the luminal face of the brush border (Ugolev and De Laey, 1973). The products of this enzymic activity, in contrast to similar dietary monomers in the lumen, have a kinetic advantage for the active transport system (Parsons and Boyd, 1972). According to the hypothesis presented here, the monomers in both cases may move "downhill" through the plasma membrane by facilitated diffusion.

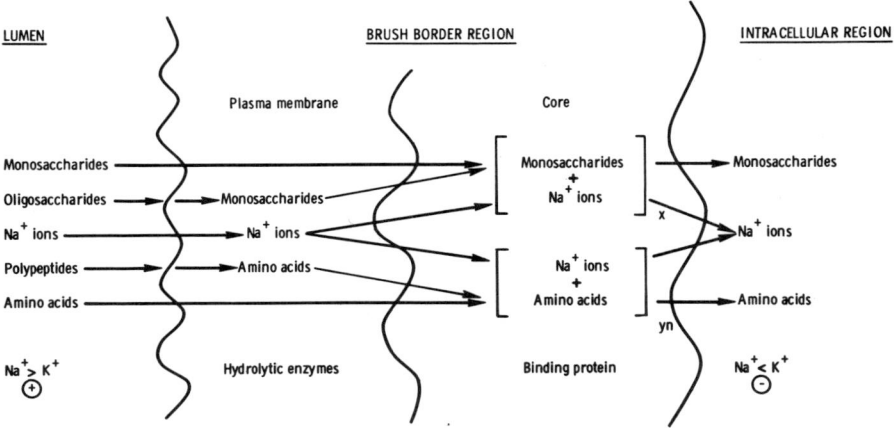

FIG. 11. A hypothesis for active sugar and amino acid transport by the intestinal brush border organelle, *in situ.* (See text for explanation.)

The hydrolysis of oligosaccharides and polypeptides could enhance the movement of monomer products through the membrane to the inner or core region of the brush borders. Monosaccharides that require Na^+ to be actively transported would bind to common sites (x) on a protein macromolecule in the brush border core. This binding would be dependent on Na^+ normally derived from the luminal fluid which has a higher Na^+ activity than the intracellular region of the mucosal cell. Actively transported amino acids dependent on Na^+ would bind to sites (y) on the protein macromolecule in the core that are different from the sugar binding sites. Several amino acid binding sites (n) would be available to accommodate the different types of amino acids that are actively transported.

The movement of sugars, amino acids, and Na^+ ions from the core region of the brush border to the intracellular region of the mucosal cell may be assisted by the contraction of actin filaments that Tilney and Mooseker (1971) have observed to be in the brush border. Perhaps contraction of the microvilli and a change in conformation of the binding protein are coupled. Dissociation of the sugar and amino acid ternary complexes could be triggered by the conformational change in the binding protein caused by the low intracellular Na^+ concentration (Crane, 1964; Curran et al., 1967), the replacement of Na^+ in the ternary complex by K^+ from the high K^+ intracellular region (Crane, 1968), and by a combination of these phenomena with the aid of energy derived directly from cellular metabolism (Kimmich and Randles, 1973). If the normal Na^+ and K^+ gradients across the brush border are reversed, then it is conceivable that sugars and amino acids could be pumped "uphill" from the intracellular to the luminal compartment (Crane, 1964). Under these conditions, however, the Na^+ required to form the ternary complexes would be derived from the intracellular fluid, energy would still be available from cellular metabolism, and the conformational change in the binding protein producing dissociation could be reversed. Consequently, dissociation of the ternary complexes would occur during the relaxation instead of the contraction phase of the actin filaments or binding protein.

In any event, the results from our investigations indicate that the structurally complex intestinal brush border must be considered as a multifunctional organelle in any scheme proposed to explain the molecular basis of active sugar and amino acid transport by the small intestine.

ACKNOWLEDGMENTS

The author gratefully acknowledges the technical assistance of S. M. L. Wu, M. L. Faggard, M. G. Leadbetter, R. K. Plenge, A. J. McCaslin, M. J. Burns, E. F. Therrien, D. W. Misch, and S. J. Shearin.

This investigation was supported by U.S. Public Health Service grant AM 07998 from the National Institute of Arthritis, Metabolism, and Digestive Diseases.

REFERENCES

Alvarado, F. (1967): Hypothesis for the interaction of phlorizin and phloretin with membrane carriers for sugars. Biochim. Biophys. Acta *135*:483–495.
Andrews, P. (1964): Estimation of the molecular weights of proteins by Sephadex gel filtration. Biochem. J. *91*:222–233.
Bihler, I., Hawkins, K. A., and Crane, R. K. (1962): Studies on the mechanism of intestinal absorption of sugars. VI. The specificity and other properties of Na^+-dependent entrance of sugars into intestinal tissue under anaerobic conditions, *in vitro*. Biochim. Biophys. Acta *59*:94–102.
Burns, M. J., and Faust, R. G. (1969): Preferential binding of amino acids to isolated mucosal brush borders from hamster jejunum. Biochim. Biophys. Acta *183*:642–645.
Crane, R. K. (1962): Hypothesis for mechanism of intestinal active transport of sugars. Fed. Proc. *21*:891–895.
Crane, R. K. (1964): Uphill outflow of sugar from intestinal epithelial cells induced by reversal of the Na^+ gradient: Its significance for the mechanism of Na^+-dependent active transport. Biochem. Biophys. Res. Commun. *17*:481–485.
Crane, R. K. (1968): Absorption of sugars. In: *Handbook of physiology*, edited by C. F. Code, Sect. 6, Vol. III, Williams and Wilkins, Baltimore.
Curran, P. F., Schultz, S. G., Chez, R. A., and Fuisz, R. E. (1967): Kinetic relations of the Na-amino acid interaction at the mucosal border of intestine. J. Gen Physiol. *50*:1261–1286.
Faust, R. G., and Shearin, S. J. (1973): Molecular weight of a D-glucose and L-histidine binding protein from intestinal brush borders. Nature *248*:60–61.
Faust, R. G., and Wu, S. M. L. (1966): The effect of bile salts on oxygen consumption, oxidative phosphorylation and ATP-ase activity of mucosal homogenates from rat jejunum and ileum. J. Cell Physiol. *67*:149–158.
Faust, R. G., Burns, M. J., and Misch, D. W. (1970): Sodium dependent binding of L-histidine to a fraction of mucosal brush borders from hamster jejunum. Biochim. Biophys. Acta *219*:507–511.
Faust, R. G., Shearin, S. J., and Misch, D. W. (1972): Sodium-dependent binding of D-glucose to a filamentous fraction of Tris-disrupted brush borders from hamster jejunum. Biochim. Biophys. Acta *255*:685–690.
Faust, R. G., Wu, S. M. L., and Faggard, M. L. (1967): D-glucose: Preferential binding to brush borders disrupted with Tris (hydroxymethyl) aminomethane. Science *155*:1261–1263.
Faust, R. G., Leadbetter, M. G., Plenge, R. K., and McCaslin, A. J. (1968): Active sugar transport by the small intestine. The effects of sugars, amino acids, hexosamines, sulfhydryl-reacting compounds, and cations on the preferential binding of D-glucose to Tris-disrupted brush borders. J. Gen. Physiol. *52*:482–494.
Hajjar, J. J., Lamont, A. S., and Curran, P. F. (1970): The Na-alanine interaction in rabbit ileum: Effect of Na on alanine fluxes. J. Gen. Physiol. *55*:277–296.
Harrison, D. D., and Webster, H. L. (1964): An improved method for the isolation of brush borders from rat intestine. Biochim. Biophys Acta *93*:662–664.
Hindmarsh, J. T., Kilby, D., and Wiseman, G. (1966): Effects of amino acids on sugar absorption. J. Physiol. *186*:166–174.
Jorgensen, C. R., Landau, B. R., and Wilson, T. H. (1961): A common pathway for sugar transport in hamster intestine. Am. J. Physiol., *200*:111–116.
Kimmich, G. A., and Randles, J. (1973): Interaction between Na^+-dependent transport systems for sugars and amino acids. Evidence against a role for the sodium gradient. J. Membrane Biol. *12*:47–68.
Kinter, W. B., and Wilson, T. H. (1965): Autoradiographic study of sugar and amino acid absorption by everted sacs of hamster intestine. J. Cell Biol. *25*:19–39.
Lin, E. C. C., Hagihira, H., and Wilson, T. H. (1962): Specificity of the transport system for neutral amino acids in the hamster intestine. Am. J. Physiol. *202*:919–925.
Lowry, O. H., Rosebrough, N. J., Farr, A. L., and Randall, R. J. (1951): Protein measurement with the folin phenol reagent. J. Biol. Chem. *193*:265–275.

Miller, D., and Crane, R. K. (1961): A procedure for the isolation of the epithelial brush border membrane of hamster small intestine. Anal. Biochem. 2:284–286.

Munck, B. G. (1968): Amino acid transport by the small intestine. Evidence against interactions between sugars and amino acids at the carrier level. Biochim. Biophys. Acta 156:192–194.

Neame, K. D. (1965): Effect of acidic (dicarboxylic) α-amino acids on uptake of L-histidine by intestinal mucosa, testis, spleen, and kidney *in vitro*. A comparison with effect in brain. J. Physiol. 181:114–123.

Newey, H., and Smyth, D. H. (1964): The transfer system for neutral amino acids in the rat small intestine. J. Physiol. 170:328–343.

Overton, J. A., Eichholz, A., and Crane, R. K. (1965): Studies on the organization of the brush border in intestinal cells. II. Fine structure of Tris-disrupted hamster brush borders. J. Cell Biol. 26:693–706.

Parsons, D. S., and Boyd, C. A. R. (1972): Transport across the intestinal mucosal cell: Hierarchies of function. Intern. Rev. Cytol. 32:209–255.

Robinson, J. W. L., and Alvarado, F. (1971): Interaction between the sugar and amino acid transport systems at the small intestinal brush border: A comparative study. Pflügers Arch. 326:48–75.

Schachman, H. K. (1959): *Ultracentrifugation in Biochemistry*, Academic Press, New York.

Schultz, S. G., and Curran, P. F. (1970): Coupled transport of sodium and organic solutes. Physiol. Rev. 50:637–718.

Shapiro, A. L., Vinuela, E., and Maizel, J. V., Jr. (1967): Molecular weight estimation of polypeptide chains by electrophoresis in SDS-polyacrylamide gels. Biochem. Biophys. Res. Commun. 28:815–820.

Tilney, L. G., and Mooseker, M. (1971): Actin in the brush border of epithelial cells of the chicken intestine. Proc. Nat. Acad. Sci. 68:2611–2615.

Ugolev, A. M., and DeLaey, P. (1973): Membrane digestion. A concept of enzymic hydrolysis on cell membranes. Biochim. Biophys. Acta 300:105–128.

Weber, K., and Kunter, D. J. (1971): Reversible denaturation of enzymes by sodium dodecyl sulfate. J. Biol. Chem. 246:4504–4509.

Weber, K., and Osborn, M. (1969): The reliability of molecular weight determinations by dodecyl sulfate-polyacrylamide gel electrophoresis. J. Biol. Chem. 244:4406–4412.

White, A., Handler, P., and Smith, E. L. (1964):*Principles of Biochemistry*, McGraw-Hill, New York, p. 237.

DISCUSSION

The author was asked whether the binding of the amino acids or sugars depended on noncovalent bonds with the protein and how it is that after SDS or 6 M urea treatment the protein still had the right configuration to carry out the selective binding. FAUST answered that binding involved noncovalent bonds and that a lot of the binding capacity was probably lost but that not all the protein was irreversibly denatured; some of it was reversible after removing SDS and urea.

The question was raised whether impurity could have been responsible for the binding; that is, could some cytoplasmic material have still been present in the preparation. FAUST replied that he could not find preferential binding with separated cytoplasmic fractions, microsomal or nuclear, or with the other brush border fractions. To the question as to how he identifies his material as core material, FAUST replied that by its morphological appearance and by the absence of hydrolyzing enzymatic activity.

DIEDRICH asked how the sugar gets through the brush border membrane. FAUST visualized this as similar to the passage of sugar across the red blood cell: at this time he thinks that the passage is mediated by virtue of a spatial configuration of the constituents of the membrane.

CURRAN quoted a recent work by Hopfer et al., in which they showed that the isolated plasma membrane from the brush border contains the whole transport system including the sodium sensitivity. FAUST replied that he visualizes his binding protein as the mechanism by which monomers can be trapped by the brush border and subsequently accumulated against their concentration gradients within the mucosal cell. It could be possible that the plasma membrane has transport properties, but he could never observe preferential binding with the plasma membrane fraction.

Intestinal Absorption and Malabsorption,
edited by T. Z. Csáky.
Raven Press, New York © 1975

Transcellular and Intercellular Intestinal Transport

T. Z. Csáky and Birgit Autenrieth

Department of Pharmacology, University of Kentucky, College of Medicine, Lexington, Kentucky 40506

The gastrointestinal tract represents a highly differentiated barrier between the body and its environment which mediates the efficient uptake of nutrients from the lumen into the circulation while preventing the loss of the same materials by a back-leak. Essentially this barrier consists of the epithelial layer composed of a variety of cells with cuboidal appearance displaying a clear morphological and functional membrane asymmetry: the lumen-facing membrane which with its hundreds of bristles, not unlike a brush, is called the "brush border" and the serosal-facing basal membrane which displays a structure similar to other plasma membranes.

Morphologists when examining the fixed dead epithelial layer under the electron microscope are impressed by the fact that the brush borders of adjacent cells appear to be continuous. Thus, they describe "tight junctions" between the brush borders of neighboring cells. However, as is frequently the case, the dead fixed image of the living tissue does not necessarily reflect the dynamic functional state of the same system. It is by now increasingly evident that functionally the tight junction is anything but tight; it is rather part of a membrane system with specialized permeability properties.

Consequently the overall permeability of the epithelial layer is a composite of the transcellular as well as intercellular permeabilities. Selectivity is one of the most significant functions of the intestinal epithelial layer; therefore it is important to assess the contribution to selectivity of both the cells and the intercellular junctions.

The kinetics of the transcellular permeation of polar nutrients indicate a likely combination with receptor sites of limited number. These receptors are called "carrier." With the help of the carrier the substrate enters the epithelial cell and is transported from there into the intercellular space and finally into the circulation. The relatively high degree of substrate specificity of various carriers is responsible for the selectivity of the brush border.

Another type of regulation of the across-the-cell permeability is presented by the osmotic flow of water. In the isolated small intestine of the frog we found an osmotic flux asymmetry of water, the flux being greater in the mucosal-to-serosal than in the opposite direction (Loeschke, Bentzel, and Csáky, 1970). This flux asymmetry could be explained by the fact that when water flows osmotically in the mucosal-to-serosal direction the intercellular spaces open up, resulting in an enlargement of the area of permeation. It should be noted however that, whereas the intercellular channels are wide open, the tight junctions still appear morphologically quite tight (Fig. 1). This suggests that the preferential path of the osmotic water flow is across the cells.

The mentioned mechanisms provide the logical basis for selectivity in the transcellular transport; however no such mechanisms are known to exist in the permeability of the intercellular junction. Admittedly this area has not yet been explored as extensively as the brush border; but so far there is no evidence for a specific carrier mechanism in the intercellular junction. The morphological changes causing the transcellular osmotic water flow asymmetry do not apply to the junctions either. Yet there appears to be some selectivity even in the permeability of the intercellular junctions, as is evident from the following experiments performed in our laboratory.

In urethan-anesthetized rats (15 g/kg subcutaneously) a segment of the small intestine was perfused *in situ* with a warm isosmotic solution of different composition, according to the method described earlier (Csáky and Ho, 1965). Glucose was added to the perfusate in varying concentrations and the rate of its disappearance from the lumen was measured. If the glucose concentration in the lumen is kept below that in the plasma, one can assume that the absorption proceeds against a concentration gradient by active transport. If the concentration in the lumen is considerably higher than in the plasma, the absorption can proceed as a downhill passive diffusion mediated nevertheless by the function of the carrier.

With this experimental setup, the effect of the increased proton concentration in the lumen upon the active uphill transport of glucose was examined. As reported earlier (Csáky, 1971), even a slight increment of the hydrogen-ion concentration depresses considerably the rate of the apparent active glucose transport from the intestine. Since it has been known that an increased proton concentration inhibits the function of the epithelial sodium pump, the above finding was considered as one of many which support our thesis that the primary, if not the only, pump in the intestine is the sodium pump.

A subsequent finding was that the high intraluminal proton concentration influences only the active, uphill absorption of glucose but not the carrier-mediated, downhill, nonactive transport. This was derived from the following observations.

In our earlier studies (Csáky and Ho, 1966), we found that the presence of sodium ions in the lumen is essential for the active but not for the carrier-mediated nonactive glucose transport. The later proceeds without sodium, as for instance, when the gut lumen is perfused with a solution containing potassium as the sole cation. Quantitatively at lower intraluminal glucose concentration, when the transport is due to an active, uphill process, the inhibition due to the lack of sodium is almost complete, whereas at higher

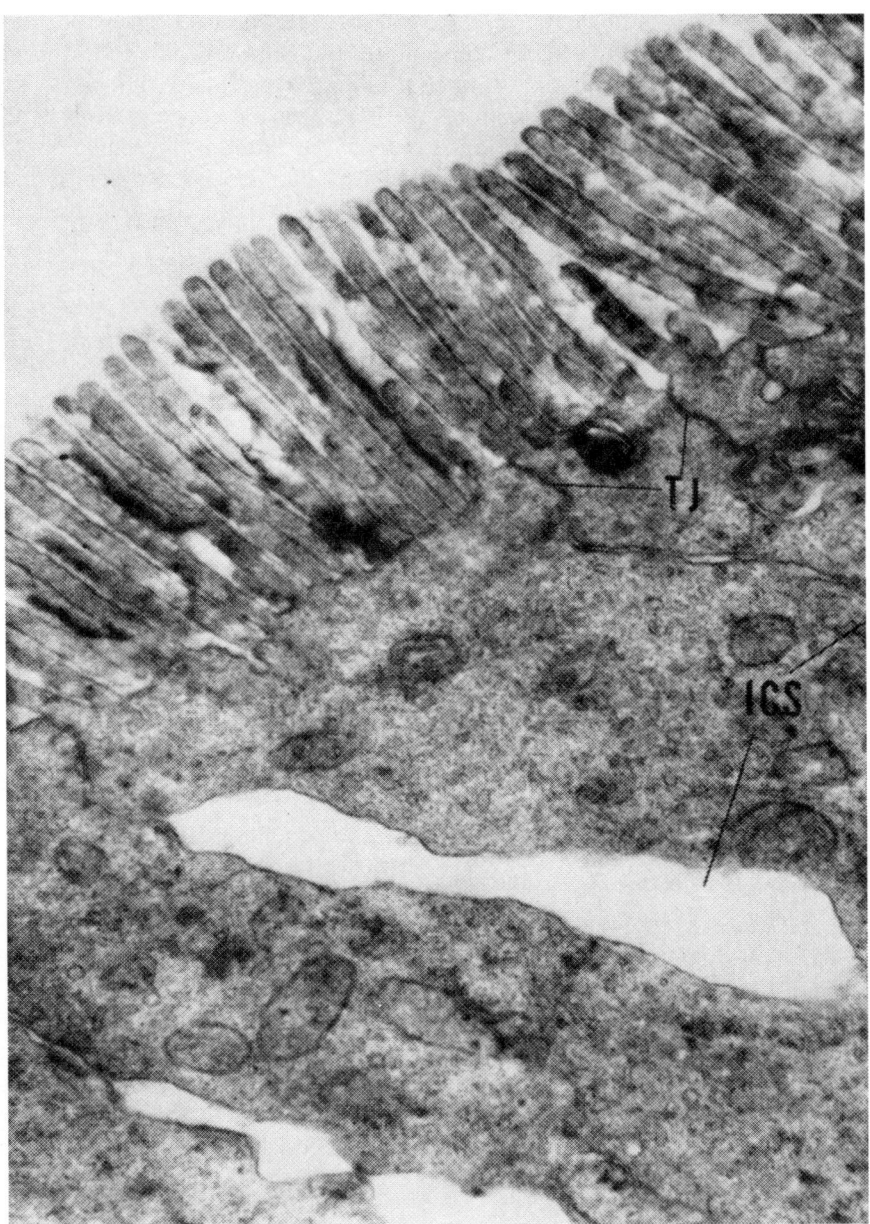

FIG. 1. Electromicroscopic section of apical portion of epithelial cell border of the bullfrog intestine fixed during a mucosal-to-serosal osmotic water flow. The dilated intercellular spaces (ICS) extend up to tight junction (Tj) which remain closed. Magnification 16,000× (from Loeschke, Bentzel, and Csáky, 1970, l.c.).

initial glucose concentrations the inhibition due to the lack of sodium disappears. The transition occurs at an initial concentration in the neighborhood of 100 mM; above this glucose concentration the pump effect disappears and the absorption becomes essentially a carrier-mediated diffusion. The data presented in Fig. 2 show that 10^{-4} M hydrogen ion concentration in the lumen inhibits the glucose absorption only if the latter is presented in the lumen in low initial concentrations. At higher glucose concentrations there was no inhibition. Significantly the transition occurred in the neighborhood

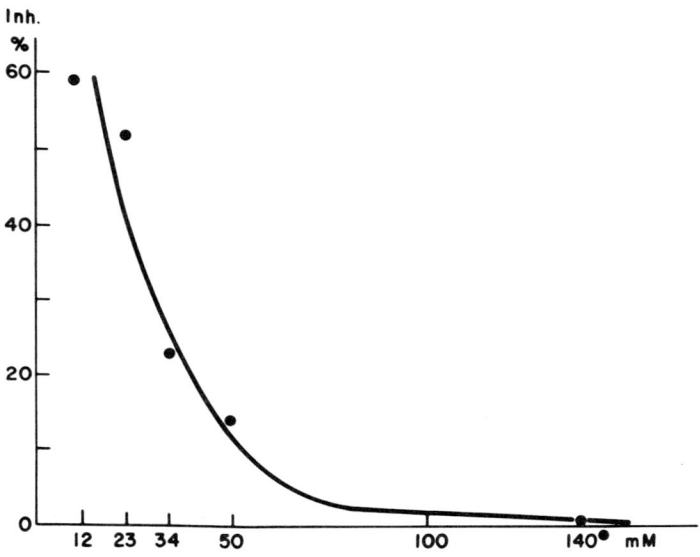

FIG. 2. High luminal proton concentration inhibits the intestinal glucose transport only at low initial (<100 mM) sugar concentration. Ordinate: % inhibition; abscissa: initial glucose concentration in mM.

of 100 mM of glucose. Thus, it is clear that the higher intraluminal proton concentration does not affect the sugar carrier but only the pump.

If the luminal hydrogen-ion concentration is decreased, at pH values above 7.0, the picture is quite different. The pH of the luminal fluid can be considerably increased without any apparent effect upon the active sugar transport. However, when approaching pH 10, an abrupt change occurs: not only does the net glucose absorption cease but occasionally it becomes negative; in other words, the concentration of the glucose in the lumen increases in the course of the experiment (Fig. 3).

The effect is fully reversible; if the pH of the perfusate is readjusted to about 7.0, the net uphill transport is completely restored. Figure 4 shows that when the lumen of the gut was perfused with an isosmotic solution of pH 10 containing 10^{-3} M phlorizin the net glucose outflux into the lumen further increased. Phlorizin inhibits the absorption of glucose by competing with it at the carrier level; therefore, it is reasonable to assume that at high intraluminal pH the absorption still proceeds but cannot compensate for the large leak, hence the net glucose outflux. The fact that at high pH the outflux of the intravenously administered inulin increased at a rate parallel to

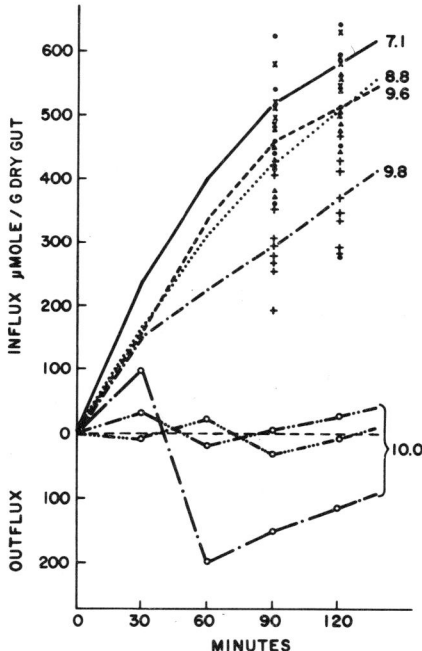

FIG. 3. Disappearance of glucose from the lumen of the intestine perfused with an isosmotic $NaHCO_3$–Na_2CO_3 solution of varying pH (indicated at the right end of the curve). Initial glucose concentration in the lumen: 2.8 mM. Ordinate: glucose disappeared in μmole/g gut dry wt. Abscissa: time in minutes. Note that at high luminal pH the values are negative viz. net glucose outflux occurs.

that of glucose is a strong indication that the site of the leak is not the cell membrane but the intercellular cement at the tight junction.

At pH 10.0 the bicarbonate-carbonate buffer, which was used in these experiments, consists of almost pure carbonate. Also at this pH the soluble calcium bicarbonate is converted to insoluble calcium carbonate. Consequently it can be assumed that the increase of the permeability of the tight junction is related to the chelation of calcium ions by carbonate. This as-

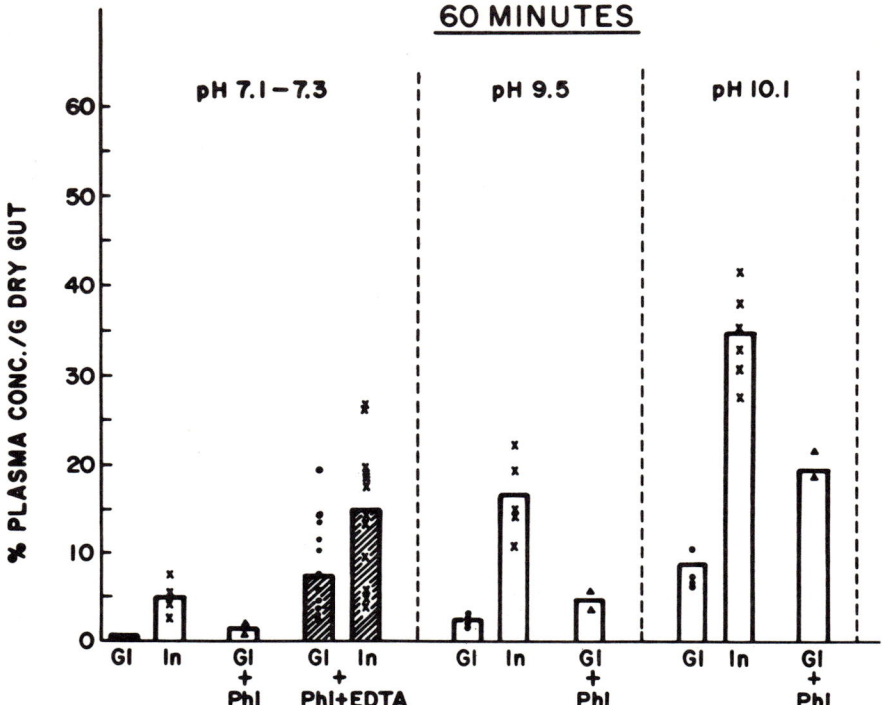

FIG. 4. Outflux of glucose (GL) and inulin (In) from the blood into the lumen at different luminal pH values. Phlorizin (Phl) enhances the glucose outflux. Ethylenediamine tetraacetate (EDTA) mimics the effect of high pH.

sumption is corroborated by the finding that the blood-to-lumen leak can be increased even at pH 7.0 by adding ethylenediamine tetraacetate (EDTA) in a concentration 10^{-3} M to the perfusate. The exact role of the ionized calcium in the permeability of the tight junction is not clear. However, because the above-described permeability changes are fully reversible by readjusting to pH 7.0, it follows that chelating the calcium does not produce a drastic, irreversible change.

It appears as if at high pH, perhaps because of the chelation of the ionized calcium, the tight junction opens up into a permeable channel through which even large colloidal particles can flow from the blood into the intestinal lumen. However, even this flow is not completely unrestricted. We compared the outflux of polyethylene glycol (PEG) and sodium ions at two luminal pH's: 7.0 and 10.0. In both instances the buffer with which the gut lumen was perfused was initially sodium free: $KHCO_3$ and K_2CO_3. The outflux of PEG was determined by injecting the ^{14}C-tagged marker intravenously and measuring its appearance in the lumen. Since the plasma-to-lumen ratio remained rather high during the entire experiment, the rate of appearance of the radioactivity in the lumen was a good measure of the outflux of PEG. In the case of sodium, which is rapidly reabsorbed across the brush border, the following approach was employed: the lumen was perfused with an essentially sodium-free bicarbonate-carbonate buffer, adjusted to a pH of either 7.0 or 10.0. A trace of ^{22}Na was added to the perfusate. From time to time samples were withdrawn from the lumen in which the sodium was determined with the flame photometer, and the ^{22}Na concentration was

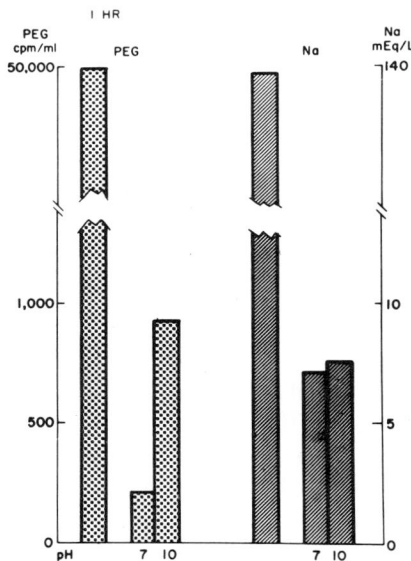

FIG. 5. Blood-to-lumen flux of polyethylene glycol (PEG) and Na at pH 7 and 10 in 1 hr. (First columns: plasma concentrations.)

measured by counting; thus the specific activity of the sodium in the perfusate could be calculated. This way the net luminal gain of sodium and the influx could be measured, which allowed the calculation of the sodium outflux. Figure 5 shows that whereas the outflux of PEG increased almost fivefold when the pH was increased from 7.0 to 10.0, the sodium outflux remained essentially unchanged.

The results concerning the fluxes of glucose and PEG at high intraluminal pH can be explained by assuming an opening up of the tight junctions allowing the outflux of solutes even of such molecular size as PEG which does not enter the cellular water. The outflux of glucose follows the same route because the lumen-to-blood sugar absorption, as was shown, apparently continues to function; consequently the flux across the cell is in an uphill direction and is not an outflux.

It is more difficult to explain why the outflux of sodium was not changed during the apparent opening-up of the junctions. Several speculative reasons can be offered:

(a) The sodium outflux proceeds mainly across the cells, therefore the intercellular route or shunt is insignificant. At present there is no direct evidence justifying this assumption (see Ussing, Erlij, and Lassen, 1974).

(b) In case of a solute, such as sodium, which after leaking into the lumen is rapidly reabsorbed, a complication possibly arising from an unstirred layer effect cannot be neglected (see Dietschy and Westergaard, *this volume*). Generally speaking such an effect can be demonstrated, at least qualitatively, by varying the rate of the luminal perfusion and assuming that the rate is inversely proportional to the size of the unstirred layer. The described effects on the calculated sodium outflux were not substantially altered by varying the rate of perfusion from moderate (2 ml/min) to rapid (30 ml/min). This seems to indicate that it is unlikely, that the unstirred layer effect is fully responsible for the observed phenomenon.

(c) At pH 7 when the junction is relatively tight, the intercellular sodium channel is already functioning at maximum capacity and opening it up does not enlarge considerably the functional channel. In view of the small size and relatively high permeability of a hydrated sodium ion this explanation appears to be more feasible.

(d) There exists a possibility that the flux of the charged-sodium ion is not completely unrestricted in the intercellular space but is influenced by an interaction between the sodium ion and the negatively charged intercellular cement of the tight junction. Such an interaction would not be strongly modified by a widening of the channel.

Although the above experiments clearly indicate a mechanism different from the carrier function that produces a substrate-selective transjunctional permeation, we cannot offer conclusive evidence of the properties of this mechanism at the present time. Their elucidation should be the goal of further research.

ACKNOWLEDGMENTS

The valuable technical assistance rendered by Mrs. Jan Carpenter and Mr. Timothy Nolan is acknowledged with thanks. This research was supported by grants from the U.S. Public Health Service.

REFERENCES

Csáky, T. Z. (1971): Physiological considerations of the relationship between intestinal absorption and electrolytes and nonelectrolytes. In: *Intestinal transport of electrolytes, amino acids and sugars,* edited by W. M. Armstrong and A. S. Nunn, Jr., Charles C Thomas, Springfield.

Csáky, T. Z., and Ho, P. M. (1965): Intestinal transport of D-xylose. Proc. Soc. Exp. Biol. Med. *120:*403–408.
Csáky, T. Z., and Ho, P. M. (1966): The effect of potassium on the intestinal transport of glucose. J. Gen. Physiol. *50:*113–128.
Loeschke, K., Bentzel, C. J., and Csáky, T. Z. (1970): Asymmetry of osmotic flow in frog intestine: Functional and structural correlation. Am. J. Physiol. *218:*1723–1731.
Ussing, H. H., Erlij, D., and Lassen, U. (1974): Transport pathways in biological membranes. Ann. Rev. Physiol. *36:*17–49.

DISCUSSION

KESTON suggested that in these experiments there appears to be a system which transports glucose independently of sodium. CSÁKY remarked that there is no evidence that the passage of glucose across the tight junction is mediated by a specific transport system. Noncharged particles, such as glucose or polyethylene glycol, can leak out while positively charged ions, such as sodium, may be involved in a reaction with the negatively charged intercellular cement.

ARMSTRONG referred to a recent analysis of the shunt pathway by Schultz and co-workers and asked Frizzell to talk about it. FRIZZELL pointed out that they did not examine a perturbation of the tight junction permeability as was done in the present work. In their study the leak of potassium could be expressed by a simple diffusion.

Another comment dealt with the dilemma that puzzles radiation biologists who find that, after radiation, plasma proteins can leak out into the gut without an increase in the sodium leak-out. CSÁKY responded that this may be a situation similar to the one described in his chapter and perhaps the chelation of calcium creates circumstances similar to that after irradiation.

HENDRIX raised the question that, if the channel opens up to accommodate the outflow of such a large particle as polyethylene glycol, how much charge would be required to restrict the movement of sodium. CSÁKY answered that he doesn't know of such calculations but that it is known that the intercellular cement and mucus represent most highly charged colloids.

The question was raised that by increasing the pH would the chelation of calcium be a step-by-step process and how could that be reconciled with the results of the present study. CSÁKY responded that he did not actually measure the chelation of calcium at different pH's therefore he can refer only to the experimental data in which one has to increase the pH to about 9.5 to observe a sudden change of permeability. The similarity of the results obtained at pH 7.0 with EDTA suggests, but does not necessarily prove, that the high pH acts by the same mechanism.

Intestinal Absorption and Malabsorption,
edited by T. Z. Csáky.
Raven Press, New York © 1975

Comparative Biological Aspects of Intestinal Absorption

K. C. Huang and T. S. T. Chen

University of Louisville, School of Medicine, Department of Pharmacology, Louisville, Kentucky 40201

Over the past few years, our group has been very much interested in comparative studies on the intestinal transport of amino acids, sugars, and electrolytes. Our intention has been to show that knowledge on the evolutional or embryonic development of intestinal transport systems may shed some light on the problem of how the transport mechanisms for amino acids and sugars are formed.

Abundant evidence is available in the literature that there is a structural specificity in the intestinal absorption of amino acids and sugars. Wilson (1962) and Lin, Hagihira, and Wilson (1962) used the everted sac technique and demonstrated with few exceptions that L-amino acids were transported across the intestine of mammals whereas most D-isomers were not. Using the same technique, our group also found that the intestine of the golden hamster, guinea pig, and mouse can transport L-tyrosine, L-tryptophan, and monosubstituted derivatives of tyrosine across the mucosa against a concentration gradient, but that D-tryptophan and the disubstituted derivatives of tyrosine were not transported (Huang, 1962; Cohen and Huang, 1964). These results are summarized in Table 1. Since L-tryptophan and L-tyrosine transport are competitively inhibited by L-phenylalanine, it appears that there is a common transport system for aromatic amino acids. The transport system is stereoselective for the L-configuration. Also, the finding that the rabbit ileum transported L-tyrosine, but not L-tryptophan, further suggests that there may be a flat area on the transport receptor, which preferentially interacts with the benzene ring in comparison with the indole ring.

Questions have been raised, such as when is the structural specificity of transport systems developed in the animal and is such selectivity in transport systems also present in the fetal intestine or the intestine of lower vertebrates. A former associate in this laboratory (Sells, 1969) surveyed the intestinal transport of aromatic amino acids in several vertebrates during their early stages of development, including the rabbit and guinea pig fetus, chick embryo, and tadpole. It was found that the intestine of the 25-day-old rabbit fetus transported both L- and D-tryptophan and L- and D-tyrosine; the transport of the D-isomers was temperature dependent and susceptible to inhibition by L-phenylalanine. As shown in Fig. 1, *o*-tyrosine was also trans-

TABLE 1. *Structural specificity in mammalian intestinal transport of aromatic amino acids*

Mammal	Actively transported	Rate μmole/g-hr	Nonactively transported[a]
Golden hamster	L-tryptophan	14.6	D-tryptophan
	4-CH$_3$-DL-tryptophan	1.46	5-OH-DL-tryptophan
	5-CH$_3$- "	1.11	5-OH-tryptamine
	6-CH$_3$- "	3.78	tryptamine
	L-tyrosine and its mono-substituted derivatives		3,5-disubstituted tyrosine derivatives
Mice (over 24 days old)	L-tryptophan	0.77	D-tryptophan
Guinea pig	L-tryptophan	0.21	D-tryptophan
	L-tyrosine	1.82	o-tyrosine
	D-tyrosine	0.90	
	m-tyrosine	0.97	
Rabbit	L-tyrosine	0.27	D-tyrosine
			m- and o-tyrosine
			L- and D-tryptophan

[a] Nonactively transported means that the test compound is not transported from mucosal-to-serosal side against a concentration gradient.

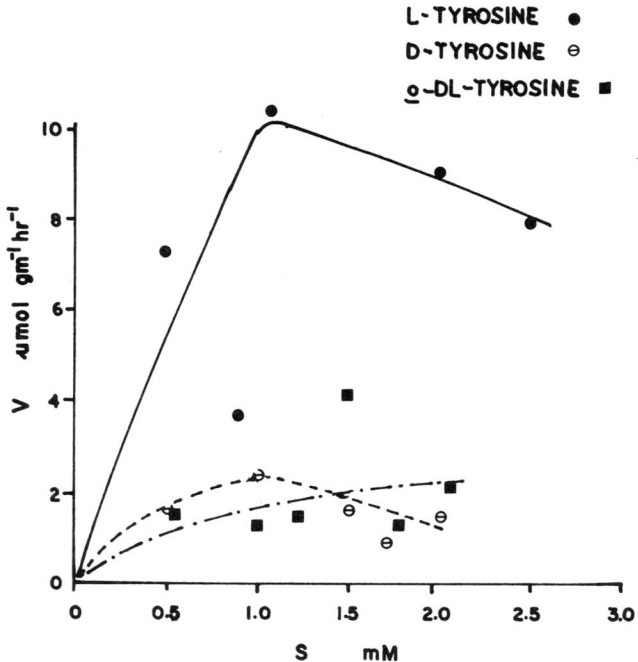

FIG. 1. Transport of tyrosine isomers by 30-day-old rabbit fetal intestine. The ordinate is the net transport rate calculated from the concentration difference of the final and initial serosal solution. The abscissa is the substrate concentration (initial).

ported by the fetal rabbit intestine. In contrast to the fetus, the adult rabbit ileum did not transport D-tyrosine or o-tyrosine. The 55-day-old guinea pig fetal intestine also showed a lack of structural specificity in the transport of tryptophan and tyrosine; the fetal intestine transported both the L- and D-isomers against a concentration gradient. This lack of stereospecificity was also found in the intestines of 19- to 20-day-old chick embryos and tadpoles. An interesting finding was that the intestine of the 19-day-old mouse, as illustrated in Fig. 2, transported D-tryptophan against a concentration gradient by an L-phenylalanine inhibitable system, but, by 24 days of age, the ability to transport D-tryptophan had disappeared and the capacity for L-tryptophan transport had increased.

Holdsworth and Wilson (1967) studied the development of active sugar

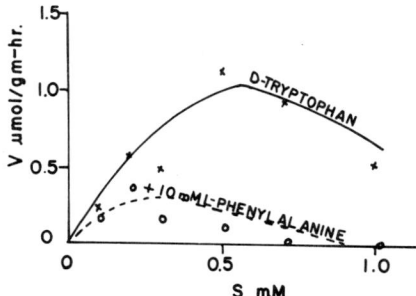

FIG. 2. Transport of D-tryptophan by 19-day-old mouse intestine in the presence or absence of 10-mM L-phenylalanine.

and amino acid transport in the yolk sac and intestine of the chicken and reported a very interesting observation. They showed that the intestine of chick embryo accumulated glycine against a concentration gradient; this capacity for accumulation decreased as the age of the chicken increased. A similar phenomenon was observed in the yolk sac of the chick embryo. As in the chick cecum, the transport mechanism for glycine had disappeared by the age of 5 to 8 days. The ability to transport sugars appeared gradually with increasing age, both in the small intestine and yolk sac of the chick.

Batt and Schachter (1969) studied the intestinal transport of L-proline in newborn rats and mice and found that the transport mechanism was widespread throughout the small intestine shortly after birth and was also detected in the colon. By the third week after birth, the transport mechanism in the small intestine was fully developed, but at this time the colon had lost its amino acid transport ability. This was confirmed by our studies on D-tryptophan transport by the mouse intestine (Sells, 1969).

Bogner (1961), Bogner and Haines (1961), and Bogner, Braham, and

McLain (1966) found that glucose uptake was negligible in the chick embryonic intestine but increased significantly with age. Glucose uptake was inhibited by phlorizin.

It might be concluded from the data reported by these investigators that the intestinal transport of glucose gradually develops with age; simultaneously the intestine may lose its ability to transport certain amino acids due to the development of structural specificity in the transport system.

It may then be postulated that the evolutionary development of the intestinal transport system duplicates the pattern seen in embryonic development. For more than 15 years, Csáky and his colleagues have extensively studied sugar transport by the frog intestine and the interaction between sugar transport and sodium ion transport. We have examined the transport systems of other adult vertebrates to determine whether there is species variation in the intestinal transport of amino acids and/or sugars. The results of these studies are summarized in Table 2. The intestine of both garter snake and frog was found to transport both the L- and D-isomers of tryptophan and tyrosine against a concentration gradient, although the transport rates for the D-isomers were smaller than those for the L-isomers. As also shown in Fig. 3, the

TABLE 2. Intestinal transport of aromatic amino acids and sugars in the lower vertebrates

Vertebrates	Actively transported	Nonactively transported
Chicken (14 days old)	L- and D-tyrosine o-tyrosine	
Garter snake	L- and D-tryptophan	
Frog (R. pipens)	L- and D-tryptophan L- and D-tyrosine o- and m-tyrosine	
Fish Marine: Winter flounder	L-tryptophan L- and D-tyrosine o- and m-tyrosine	D-tryptophan tryptamine D-glucose and galactose
Fundulus heteroclitus	L-tryptophan L-tyrosine o- and m-tyrosine 3-NH$_2$-tyrosine D-glucose and 3MG	D-tryptophan N-acetyl-L-tyrosine α-methylglucoside
Freshwater: Catfish	L-tyrosine o- and m-tyrosine D-glucose and galactose	D-tyrosine 3MG
Elasmobranch: Dogfish	L-tryptophan D-glucose and galactose	

intestine of chick embryo and 14-day-old chick can transport all tyrosine analogues against a concentration gradient. If the lack of structural specificity in intestinal transport of amino acids is considered a sign of underdevelopment during the evolutional stage, then one would expect the fish intestine to show a pattern similar to that observed in the reptile and amphibian intestine. As shown here, the intestine of winter flounder, a marine euryhaline fish, does not transport D-glucose, D-galactose, or 3-O-methyl-D-glucose (3MG) against a concentration gradient. The flounder intestine was found to transport both L- and D-tyrosine, m- and o-tyrosine, and L-tryptophan, but not D-tryptophan (Rout, Lin, and Huang, 1965). In contrast, it was found

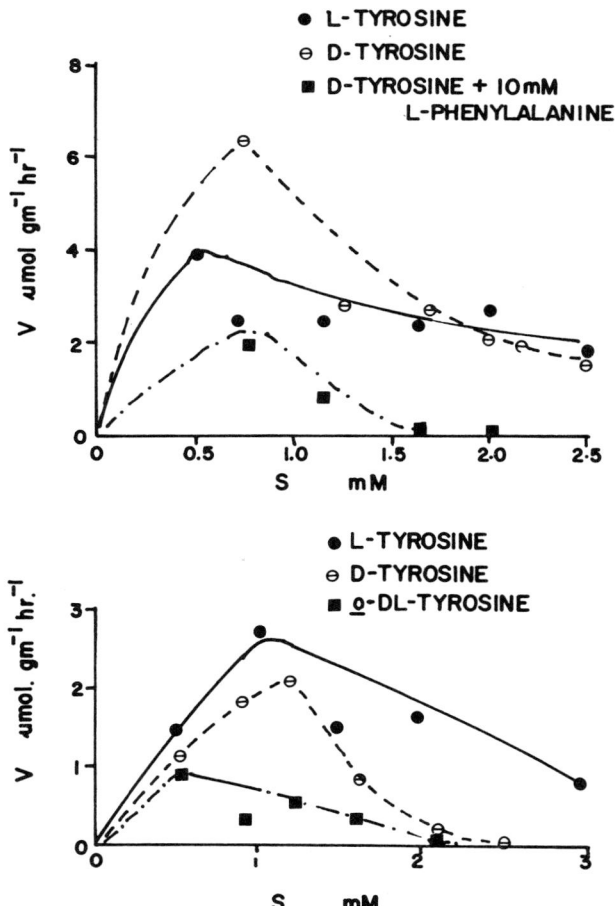

FIG. 3. Transport of tyrosine isomers by 20-day-old chick embryo intestine (top) or by 14-day-after-hatched chick intestine (bottom).

that the intestine of freshwater catfish transported L-tyrosine but not the D-isomer, and transported D-glucose and D-galactose, but not 3MG (Chen and Huang, 1972).

Based on these data, it appears that even among different fish there is a high degree of species variation with respect to the extent of development of intestinal transport systems. It is also true that selectivity in the amino acid transport system can be developed in some fish, but not in the amphibian or reptile intestine.

To pursue further the evolutionary development of transport mechanisms, we have investigated the electrolyte transport and electrical properties of the intestine of various species. Investigations concerning the electrolyte fluxes and electrical properties of the mammalian intestine have been reported by Curran, Schultz, Field, and their colleagues. These investigators, using the Ussing chamber technique, demonstrated a potential difference (PD) across the intestine of the rat, rabbit, and guinea pig, with the serosa electropositive to the mucosal side. The addition of glucose increased both the PD and short-

TABLE 3. Comparative studies on electrical properties of vertebrate intestines

Vertebrate	PD^a (mV)	I_{sc} (μA)	Resistance (Ohm)	Glucose effect
Mammals:				
Monkey, adult	+2.6	22	118	inc.[b]
fetus	+0.5	9.5	50	inc.
Dog	+0.3	3.5	86	inc.
Hamster	+2.3	30	77	inc.
Mouse, albino	+1.5	16	94	inc.
Avians (chicken)	+1.8	12	146	inc.
Reptiles (turtle)	+5.1	14	351	no
Amphibians:				
Frog (R. pipens)	+1.5	12	125	no
Bullfrog (1) (R. catesbeiana)	+1.2	8	150	inc.
Toad colon (2)	+28.0			
Fish:				
Freshwater:				
Goldfish (3)	+2.0			inc.
Catfish	−1.7	10	170	no
Seawater:				
Flounder	−2.9	24	120	no
Fundulus	+1.5	15	100	
Eel (stripped)	−2.8	18	156	
Cottus scorpius (4)	0			

[a] +PD means that the serosal side is electropositive to the mucosal side.
[b] inc. = increased.

(1) Quay and Armstrong (1969). (2) Ussing and Andersen (1956). (3) Smith (1966).
(4) House and Green (1963).

circuit current (I_{sc}) across the intestine; phlorizin or ouabain abolished this augmentation. We have extended the study to include other mammals and lower vertebrates. The results are summarized in Table 3. As shown here, each mammalian intestine studied, including that of the monkey, dog, hamster, and mouse, as well as the chicken, turtle, and frog intestine, was found to have a serosa-positive PD across the membrane. Augmentation of the PD and I_{sc} by glucose was observed in the mammalian and chicken intestine but not in the frog or turtle intestine.

The fish intestine demonstrated a quite different pattern (Huang and Chen, 1971; Chen and Huang, 1972). There was a serosa-negative PD across the flounder intestine. Figure 4 illustrates the change of I_{sc} in varying bathing solutions. When the NaCl bathing fluid was replaced with Na_2SO_4 Ringer, the PD and I_{sc} changed from negative to positive values. A similar phenomenon was observed in the catfish intestine. Isotopic flux measurements indicated a simultaneous net mucosal-to-serosal flux of Na and Cl ions; the Cl flux was bicarbonate dependent. Species differences in electrical properties of the fish intestine have been observed. For example, in goldfish and fundulus, positive PDs have been demonstrated (Smith, 1964, 1966).

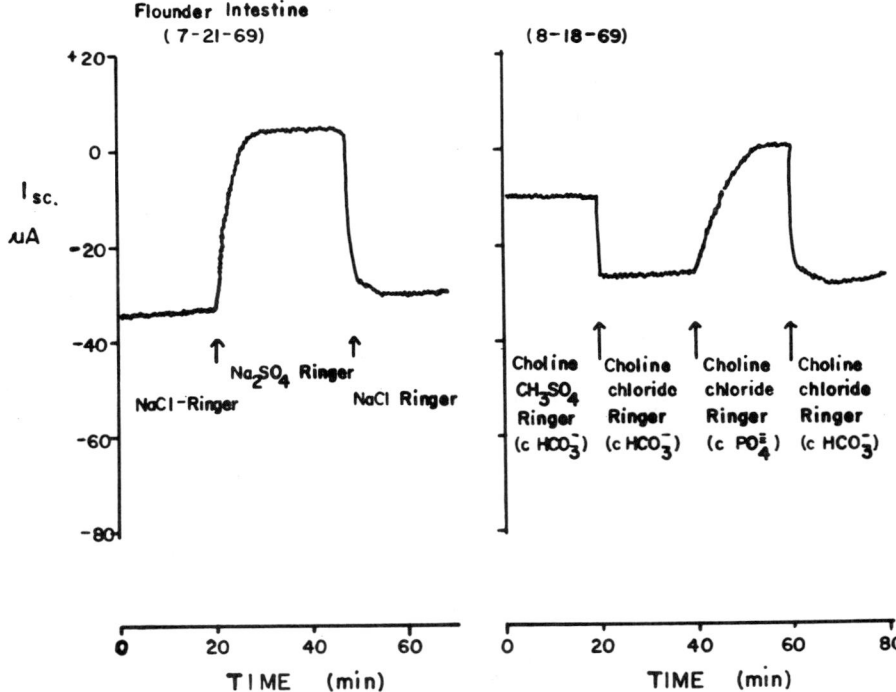

FIG. 4. Electrical measurements across flounder intestine. The ordinate is short-circuit current (I_{sc}) with orientation in respect to serosal side (reproduced from Huang and Chen, 1971).

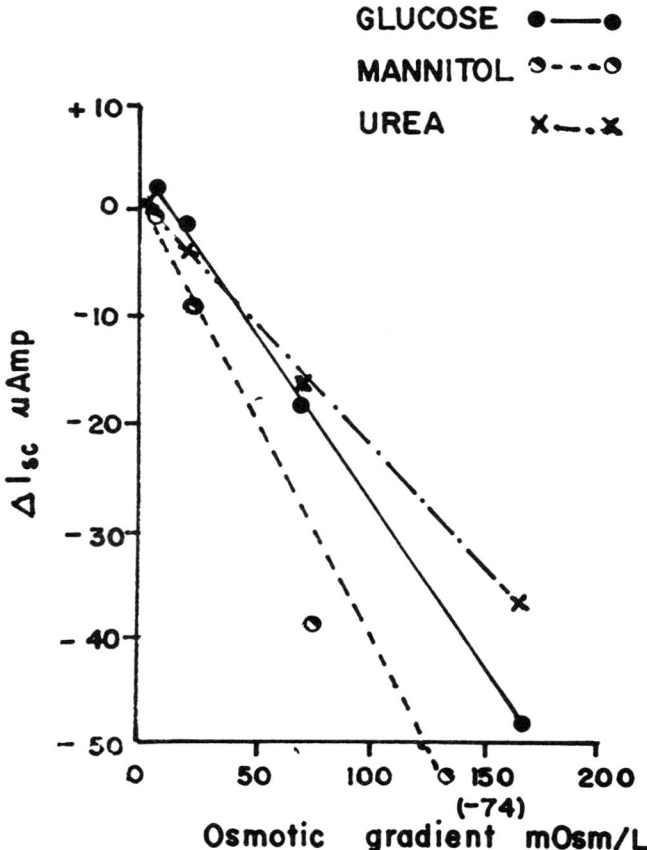

FIG. 5. Effect of osmotically active substances on short circuit current measurement across flounder intestine. The ordinate is ΔI_{sc} (observed I_{sc} − control I_{sc}); the abscissa is osmotic gradient added to the mucosal bathing solution.

Recently, Oide and Utida (1967) and Hirano and Utida (1968) reported that changes in the environment greatly influenced water and Na fluxes across the intestinal mucosa of the eel. When they placed the Japanese cultured eel, *Angilla japonica*, in a seawater medium, the water and Na fluxes from mucosal-to-serosal side were greatly increased. This increase was abolished by hypophysectomy and then restored by the injection of adrenocorticotrophin (ACTH) or cortisol.

The active absorption of Cl by the fish intestine is clearly in contrast to findings in the mammalian intestine (Huang and Chen, 1971; Chen et al., 1972; Chang et al., 1974). We have also studied the effect of D-glucose on the electrical properties of the flounder and catfish intestine. There was no augmentation of PD or I_{sc}; rather, as shown in Fig. 5, there was a shift

TABLE 4. Effect of ouabain and bicarbonate ion on intestinal transport of L-tyrosine and D-glucose

Bathing solution	Inhibitor	Rate of Transport (μmole g^{-1}hr^{-1})	
		D-Glucose	L-Tyrosine
Hamster			
Bicarbonate Ringer	None	26.74 ± 2.17	7.32 ± 0.87
	Ouabain 2 × 10^{-4}M	8.06 ± 0.46	5.20 ± 0.44
Phosphate Ringer	None	17.26 ± 1.32	8.32 ± 0.56
	Ouabain	1.30	5.59
Catfish			
Bicarbonate Ringer	None	12.54 ± 1.03	9.00 ± 1.76
	Phlorizin 2 × 10^{-4}M	0	9.60 ± 1.09
	Ouabain	0.12 ± 0.08	4.15 ± 1.42
Phosphate Ringer	None	0	14.10 ± 2.54
Bicarbonate choline Chloride Ringer	None	0	4.93 ± 0.40

toward more negative values in the presence of glucose. Similar changes occurred on the addition of mannitol or urea, indicating an osmotic effect. The glucose effect was not blocked by ouabain or phlorizin.

Finally, we wish to report an interesting observation on the interaction between amino acid and sugar transport systems and bicarbonate. As shown in Table 4, glucose absorption in freshwater catfish was found to be dependent on not only Na but also bicarbonate. In contrast, the transport of L-tyrosine was not influenced by bicarbonate but was reduced to half of control values in the presence of ouabain. These data indicate that amino acid and glucose transport are not mediated by a common system as has been suggested for other species (Chen and Huang, 1972).

ACKNOWLEDGMENT

This research was supported by U.S. Public Health Service Grant Am-2217 and National Science Foundation Grant GB 27495.

REFERENCES

Batt, E. R., and Schachter, D. (1969): Developmental pattern of some intestinal transport mechanisms in newborn rats and mice. Amer. J. Physiol. *216*:1064–1068.
Bogner, P. H. (1961): Alimentary absorption of reducing sugars by embryos and young chicks. Proc. Soc. Exp. Biol. Med. *107*:263–265.
Bogner, P. H., Braham, A. H., and McLain, P. L., Jr. (1966): Glucose metabolism during ontogeny of intestinal active sugar transport in the chick. J. Physiol. *187*:307–321.

Bogner, P. H., and Haines, I. A. (1961): Development of intestinal selective absorption of glucose in newly-hatched chicks. Proc. Soc. Exp. Biol. Med. *107:*265–267.

Chang, L. R., Chen, T. S. T., and Huang, K. C. (1974): Electrolyte transport across the mouse small intestine. Proc. Soc. Exp. Biol. Med. *145:*1220–1224.

Chen, T. S. T., and Huang, K. C. (1972): Structural specificity in the intestinal transport of hexoses, tyrosine derivatives and electrolytes in freshwater catfish. J. Pharmacol. Exp. Ther. *180:*777–783.

Cohen, L. L., and Huang, K. C. (1964): Intestinal transport of tryptophan and its derivatives. Amer. J. Physiol. *206:*647–652.

Hirano, T., and Utida, S. (1968): Effects of ACTH and cortisol on water movement in isolated intestine of the eel, *Anguilla japonica.* Gen. Comp. Endocr. *11:*373–380.

Holdsworth, C. D., and Wilson, T. H. (1967): Development of active sugar and amino acid transport in the yolk sac and intestine of the chicken. Amer. J. Physiol. *212:*233–240.

House, C. R., and Green, K. (1963): Sodium and water transport across isolated intestine of a marine teleost. Nature *199:*1293–1294.

Huang, K. C. (1962): Intestinal transport of L-tyrosine and its derivatives. J. Pharmacol. Exp. Ther. *136:*361–365.

Huang, K. C., and Chen, T. S. T. (1971): Ion transport across intestinal mucosa of winter flounder, *Pseudopleuronectes americanus.* Amer. J. Physiol. *220:*1734–1738.

Lin, E. C., Hagihira, H., and Wilson, T. H. (1962): Specificity of the transport system for neutral amino acids in the hamster intestine. Amer. J. Physiol. *202:*919–925.

Oide, M., and Utida, S. (1967): Changes in water and ion transport in isolated intestines of the eel during salt adaptation and migration. Marine Biol. *1:*102–106.

Quay, J. F., and Armstrong, W. M. (1969): Sodium and chloride transport by isolated bullfrog small intestine. Amer. J. Physiol. *217:*694–702.

Rout, W. R., Lin, D. S. T., and Huang, K. C. (1965): Intestinal transport of amino acids and glucose in flounder fish. Proc. Soc. Exp. Biol. Med. *118:*933–938.

Sells, G. D. (1969): Studies of the development of intestinal transport. Ph.D. thesis, University of Louisville Graduate School.

Smith, M. W. (1964): Electrical properties and glucose transfer in the goldfish intestine. Experientia *20:*613–614.

Smith, M. W. (1966): Influence of temperature acclimatization on sodium-glucose interactions in the goldfish intestine. J. Physiol. *182:*574–590.

Ussing, H. H., and Andersen, B. (1956): The relation between solvent drag and active transport of ions. In: *Proceedings of the Third International Congress of Biochemistry,* Brussels, 1955, Academic Press, New York, pp. 434–440.

Wilson, T. H. (1962): *Intestinal Absorption.* Saunders, Philadelphia.

DISCUSSION

ARMSTRONG wondered whether in the flounder gut, when the osmotic gradient was increased and a so-called short circuit current applied, if this can really be called "short circuit current" in the classical sense. CURRAN commented that if the current applied reduced the potential to zero it can be called short circuit current and perhaps Armstrong's objection is more academic than practical. HUANG commented that his results indicate that sodium probably goes through the tight junction pathway more easily than chloride with which ARMSTRONG agreed.

The Effect of Unstirred Water Layers on Various Transport Processes in the Intestine

John M. Dietschy and Henrik Westergaard

Gastrointestinal-Liver Unit, Department of Medicine, University of Texas Southwestern Medical School, Dallas, Texas 75235

Adjacent to all biological membranes there exists a layer of relatively unstirred water through which solute molecules must move by simple diffusion (Dainty, 1963). In the case of the small intestine this unstirred water layer presumably consists of a series of water lamellae extending outward from the mucosal cell membrane, each progressively more stirred, until they blend imperceptibly with the bulk water phase of the intestinal contents. Although the boundary between the bulk water phase and the unstirred water layer is not sharply defined, the unstirred water layer can be assigned a finite, functional thickness knowledge of which is critical for dealing with various transport phenomena. Thus, during absorption into the intestinal mucosa solutes must penetrate both an unstirred water "membrane" and the lipid membrane of the microvillus surface. Both of these membranes may exert significant resistance to absorption and, therefore, it is commonly necessary to correct transport data for unstirred layer effects in order to obtain true values for such kinetic parameters as permeability coefficients for passively transported molecules and K_m and J^{max} values for actively transported substances.

The flux rate, J, for a substance across the unstirred water layer is given by the expression (Diamond, 1969; Dietschy, 1973)

$$J = (C_1 - C_2)\left(\frac{D}{d}\right), \qquad (1)$$

where C_1 and C_2 are the concentrations of the probe molecule in the bulk water phase and at the aqueous-lipid interface, respectively, D is its free diffusion coefficient, and d is the effective thickness of the unstirred layer. The mathematical expression for the unidirectional flux rate across the lipid membrane varies depending upon whether the substance is passively or actively absorbed. For molecules that passively permeate the microvillus border the flux rate equals

$$J = (C_2)(P), \qquad (2)$$

where P is the passive permeability coefficient for the molecule. For molecules that are absorbed by an energy-linked, carrier-mediated process the rate of absorption across the cell membrane equals

$$J = (J^{max})\left(\frac{C_2}{K_m + C_2}\right), \quad (3)$$

where J^{max} and K_m, respectively, represent the true maximal transport rate and true Michaelis constant for the transport process.

For any transport mechanism, it is apparent that the rate of absorption across the unstirred water layer must equal the rate of absorption across the lipid cell membrane. For example, for a substance that is absorbed by passive means

$$J = (C_1 - C_2)\left(\frac{D}{d}\right) = (C_2)(P). \quad (4)$$

The same would be true for an actively transported substance except Eq. 3 would be substituted for the right-hand term in Eq. 4.

In both of these instances it is apparent that J is dependent on the concentration of the probe molecule at the aqueous-membrane interface, C_2, not the concentration present in the bulk phase of the perfusate, C_1. However, by rearranging Eq. 1 the values of C_2 can be expressed in terms of C_1; thus

$$C_2 = C_1 - J\frac{d}{D}. \quad (5)$$

Substituting this expression for C_2 into Eq. 2 yields the following expression which gives the passive unidirectional flux rate for a probe molecule across the microvillus membrane in terms of its concentration in the bulk aqueous perfusate.

$$J = \frac{PC_1}{1 + \frac{dP}{D}}. \quad (6)$$

Similarly, substituting Eq. 5 into Eq. 3 gives a second expression that defines the unidirectional flux rate for a probe molecule that is actively transported across the microvillus membrane in terms of its bulk phase concentration (Wilson, 1972, 1974; Winne, 1973).

$$J = 0.5\frac{D}{d}\left[K_m + C_1 + \frac{J^{max}d}{D} \pm \sqrt{\left(K_m + C_1 + \frac{J^{max}d}{D}\right)^2 - 4\left(\frac{d}{D}\right)(J^{max}C_1)}\right]. \quad (7)$$

Thus, Eqs. 6 and 7 should provide a means for describing the flux, J, of a solute molecule into the mucosal epithelial cell by either passive diffusion or active, carrier-mediated mechanisms taking into consideration the thickness of the unstirred water layer external to the microvillus membrane. However, there is one other problem associated with the application of these two equations to the transport of solutes across a membrane of so complex anatomy as the small intestine. In these equations, the flux term J must have the units of mass crossing the diffusion barrier per unit time per square centimeter of unstirred water layer. Experimentally determined flux rates, J_d, however, are commonly normalized to wet or dry weight of tissue and centimeter length of intestine or square centimeter of intestine exposed in a particular transport chamber. Experimentally determined flux rates, J_d, therefore, must be normalized to the effective surface area of the unstirred water layer through which a particular flux occurs. If S_w is defined as the effective surface area of the diffusion barrier in a particular experimental situation then the term J can be calculated from J_d using the relationship

$$J = \frac{J_d}{S_w}. \tag{8}$$

The units of S_w will be determined by the units of J_d. For example, if J_d is measured in terms of the nmoles of a particular solute absorbed per second per gram wet weight of intestine, then S_w must have the units of square centimeter of unstirred water layer per gram wet weight of intestine. In this case J_d divided by S_w yields values of J with the units nmoles absorbed per second per square centimeter of unstirred water layer.

It is evident from these latter considerations that Eqs. 6 and 7 must be further modified in order to be applicable to studies of transport in the intestine. The experimental flux rate J_d divided by S_w, i.e., the term J_d/S_w, must be substituted for J in each of the above equations. Furthermore, J_d^{max}/S_w must be substituted for J^{max} in Eq. 7.

In summary, unstirred water layers may introduce significant errors into the determination of values for various parameters of the kinetics of active and passive solute transport. The magnitude of these errors in a particular experimental circumstance will be directly proportional to the effective thickness of the unstirred water layer (d) and to the velocity of transport across the diffusion barrier (as determined by P or J^{max}) and will be inversely related to the diffusivity of the solute (D) and to the effective surface area of the unstirred water layer (S_w).

On the basis of these general considerations it is possible to discuss in more detail the effect of unstirred water layers on four specific problems associated with the passive and active transport of solutes into the intestinal mucosal cell. These include (a) the effect of unstirred layers on obtaining an accurate appraisal of the volume of adherent mucosal fluid during determination of unidirectional flux rates, (b) the influence of these aqueous diffusion barriers on determination of passive permeability coefficients, (c) the identification of the special circumstance in which unstirred water layers may be totally rate limiting to passive uptake, and (d) the complex effects of unstirred water layers on the kinetics of active transport processes.

The Effects of Unstirred Layers on the Accurate Measurement of Adherent Mucosal Fluid Volumes

Many recent studies dealing with transport in the intestine have been undertaken using techniques in which essentially unidirectional uptake of various solutes into the intestinal mucosal cell was quantitated by exposing the mucosal surface of the gut to a perfusate for very brief periods of time. In such studies it is often necessary to include a volume marker in the perfusate in order to correct the apparent flux rates for the mass of probe molecules present in the layer of fluid adherent to the external surface of the mucosal cells. Because of the barrier to diffusion presented by the unstirred water layer, the tissue must be incubated sufficiently long to allow the volume marker to uniformly label this layer. The time required to accomplish this can be calculated from the formula (Diamond, 1966)

$$t_{1/2} = \frac{(d)^2(0.38)}{D}, \tag{9}$$

where $t_{1/2}$ is the time required for the concentration of the marker compound to achieve half of its bulk phase concentration at the aqueous-membrane interface, i.e., the time required for C_2 to equal 0.5 C_1.

As shown in Table 1, the values of $t_{1/2}$ for various marker compounds vary

TABLE 1. *Time required to achieve half the bulk-phase concentration at the aqueous-membrane interface for various markers of the adherent mucosal fluid volume*

Volume marker	$t_{1/2}$ (sec)	
	$d = 150\ \mu M$	$d = 400\ \mu M$
Mannitol	10	69
Sucrose	12	87
Inulin	30	209
Dextran	43	304

Using the equation $t_{1/2} = (d)^2 (0.38)/D$ the time required for the concentration of various volume markers to achieve half the bulk phase concentration at the aqueous-membrane interface, i.e., the time required for C_2 to equal 0.5 C_1, was calculated (Diamond, 1966). These values were derived for two conditions of stirring of the bulk mucosal solution in which the mean value of d was assumed to equal either 150 or 400 μM: these two extremes represent reasonable values for the thickness of the unstirred water layer in the intestine in a highly stirred and unstirred situation, respectively. Assuming a linear gradient between C_1 and C_2, the volume of the adherent mucosal solution will equal 75% of its maximum value at a time of incubation equal to the $t_{1/2}$.

markedly depending upon their particular molecular weight, and, therefore, their particular free-diffusion coefficient and the effective thickness of the unstirred water layer. In an experimental setting with a high degree of stirring of the bulk solution where d might equal approximately 150 μM the $t_{1/2}$ varies from 10 sec for mannitol to 43 sec for dextran. In a very unstirred situation where d may approach 400 μM these two values would increase markedly to 69 sec and 304 sec, respectively. Assuming that the concentration gradient between C_1 and C_2 is linear, the apparent volume of the adherent mucosal fluid layer will have achieved 75% of its maximum value at the time equal to $t_{1/2}$. Thus, it is apparent that significant periods of time are required to label fully the unstirred water layer, particularly when using relatively large volume markers such as inulin or dextran or where measurements are made under relatively unstirred conditions in which d is large.

That these theoretical calculations coincide reasonably well with experimental findings in the intestine is shown in Fig. 1. As seen in the left panel, when d is very large because the bulk perfusate is unstirred, mannitol, but not the much larger inulin, achieves an essentially constant value for the adherent fluid volume within about 2 min. Alternatively, as shown in the right panel, when the same marker compound is used but the stirring rate is varied, much less time is required to achieve a constant value for the adherent fluid volume at the high stirring rate than in the unstirred condition. Thus, experimentally the time required to fully label the adherent

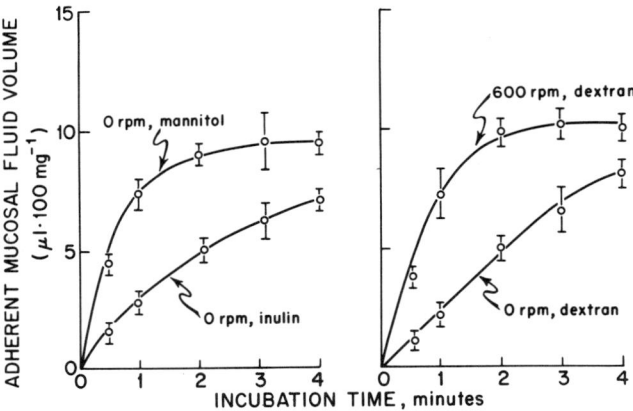

FIG. 1. Time course for labeling of the adherent mucosal fluid volume in the rabbit small intestine. Using a chamber described in detail in Lukie et al. (1974), the rabbit jejunum was exposed to mucosal perfusates containing various radiolabeled volume markers and the volume of the adherent mucosal fluid was determined as a function of the time of incubation. The units given in this figure are the μl of adherent mucosal fluid contained in an amount of jejunal tissue with a dry weight of 100 mg ($\mu l \cdot 100$ mg^{-1}). In the left panel the bulk perfusate was totally unstirred, whereas in the right panel the mucosal solution was either unstirred or was stirred at a rapid rate by a magnetic stirring bar driven at 600 rpm.

mucosal fluid volume varies with d and D, and, therefore, these findings agree reasonably well with the predictions shown in Table 1.

The significance of these findings derives from the fact that unidirectional uptake rates of various probe molecules into the intestinal mucosal cell cannot be accurately corrected for the mass of probe molecules in the adherent fluid layers unless the marker compound has fully equilibrated with the unstirred layers. Hence, as we have reported (Sallee, 1972, 1973), unidirectional flux rates measured at incubation times of only 1 or 2 min lead to overestimation of uptake rates for such compounds as monosaccharides, amino acids, and various fatty acids. The magnitude of this error will depend upon the rate of uptake of a particular compound and upon the free-diffusion coefficient of the probe molecule relative to that of the marker compound (Sallee, 1972). It is apparent, therefore, that one important effect of unstirred layers in the intestine is to introduce potentially significant errors into the determination of unidirectional uptake rates.

The Determination of Passive Permeability Coefficients in the Presence of Unstirred Layers

It is well known that the presence of a significant aqueous diffusion barrier leads to gross underestimation of passive permeability coefficients since P equals J_d divided by C_2 rather than by C_1. By making the appropriate substitutions from Eqs. 5 and 8, this expression may be rewritten

$$P = \frac{J_d}{C_1 - \frac{(J_d)(d)}{(S_w)(D)}}. \quad (10)$$

It is evident that the magnitude of the error introduced into calculations of passive permeability coefficients if unstirred layer resistance is ignored is directly proportional to J_d and d and inversely proportional to S_w and D.

That these predictions are again borne out by experimental data derived from studies in the intestine is shown by the data presented in Fig. 2. These data are derived from experiments performed in the rabbit jejunum (Westergaard, 1974), where passive permeability coefficients were determined for a homologous series of saturated alcohols with chain lengths varying from 6 to 12 carbons. In this diagram P^* represents apparent permeability coefficients, i.e., values not corrected for unstirred layer resistance, whereas P equals true permeability coefficients, i.e., values corrected for the presence of this aqueous diffusion barrier using Eq. 10. Two points warrant emphasis. First, at either stirring rate the deviation of P^* from P becomes proportionately greater with increasing chain length, i.e., as predicted, unstirred layer resistance is proportional to the rate of flux across the aqueous diffusion barrier. Second, for any given chain length the deviation of P^* from P is greater in the unstirred condition than when the

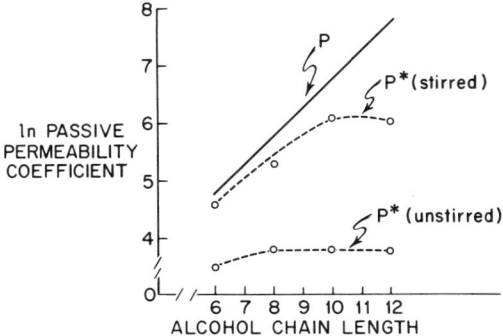

FIG. 2. The effect of the unstirred water layer in the intestine on the determination of passive permeability coefficients for several alcohols across the intestinal microvillus border. Uptake rates for the saturated alcohols 6:0, 8:0, 10:0, and 12:0 into the jejunal mucosa of the rabbit were determined under two different conditions of stirring of the bulk mucosal perfusate as described by Westergaard and Dietschy (1974). In this diagram these values are normalized to a constant mucosal perfusate concentration of 1.0 mM and are plotted as apparent passive permeability coefficients, P^*, i.e., uptake rates normalized to a constant bulk phase concentration but not corrected for unstirred layer resistance. In addition, true passive permeability coefficients, P, i.e., uptake rates normalized to a constant bulk-phase concentration and corrected for unstirred-layer resistance, also are shown by the solid line.

mucosal perfusate is rapidly mixed, i.e., also as predicted, the magnitude of the term in Eq. 10 denoting unstirred layer resistance is proportional to d.

From these and other published results it is evident that unstirred layers constitute a significant barrier to diffusion of solute molecules up to the microvillus border of the intestine. Measurement of passive permeability coefficients in this organ, therefore, requires correction for unstirred layer resistance in order to obtain reliable values denoting the passive permeability characteristics of the microvillus membrane.

Unstirred Layers as the Rate-Limiting "Membrane" for the Mucosal Cell Uptake of Certain Highly Permeant Molecules

As discussed earlier, during the passive uptake of a solute molecule into the intestinal mucosa, it must penetrate both the unstirred water layer and the microvillus membrane of the cell. The rate of penetration of the aqueous diffusion barrier is proportional to D/d, whereas the velocity of movement across the lipid cell membrane is determined by the passive permeability coefficient, P, of the particular molecule. In one extreme circumstance molecules with very large passive permeability coefficients may penetrate the cell membrane much more rapidly than they are capable of diffusing across the unstirred water layer, i.e., $P \gg D/d$. Under these conditions the rate of movement across the unstirred diffusion barrier becomes rate limiting to the overall rate of absorption into the mucosal cell. In this special circumstance C_2 essentially equals zero so that the observed rate of uptake into the cell will be given by the expression

$$J_d = \frac{C_1 D S_w}{d}. \tag{11}$$

If unstirred layers become totally rate limiting to uptake of highly permeant molecules in the intestine then this equation predicts, first, that J_d would be proportional to D so that the quantity J_d/D would equal a constant and, second, that the value of J_d/D would vary inversely with d.

As shown in Table 2, these two findings have been demonstrated in at

TABLE 2. *Evidence that unstirred water layers in the intestine are rate limiting to the passive mucosal cell uptake of certain highly permeant solutes*

Solute	$\frac{J_d}{D} \times 10^{-3}$ (nmoles · min^{-1} · 100 mg^{-1})	
	Unstirred	Stirred
Fatty acid 8:0	21.1	48.2
Fatty acid 9:0	29.4	84.0
Fatty acid 10:0	49.4	127.0
Fatty acid 12:0	71.5	276.5
Alcohol 6:0	46.1	144.7
Alcohol 8:0	72.7	347.6
Alcohol 10:0	71.3	830.9
Alcohol 12:0	76.1	800.4

These values are derived from experiments dealing with passive uptake of various probe molecules into the rabbit jejunum as described in detail by Westergaard and Dietschy (1974). Uptake rates, J_d, were determined from solutions containing 0.25- to 1.0-mM concentrations of the test molecules but all values are normalized to a bulk phase concentration of 1.0 mM. The observed value of J_d for each probe molecule found when the mucosal perfusate was either stirred or unstirred has been divided by its appropriate free-diffusion coefficient, D.

least one study dealing with the passive uptake of a number of saturated fatty acids and alcohols into the small intestinal mucosa (Westergaard, 1974). First, as seen in both the unstirred and stirred situations, the quantity J_d/D approaches a constant value when uptake of the longer chain-length members of the series was measured. Thus, in the unstirred situation the aqueous diffusion barrier is rate limiting for the absorption of the 12:0 fatty acid and the 8:0, 10:0, and 12:0 alcohols. In the stirred situation, however, uptake of only the two longer chain-length alcohols are diffusion limited. Second, it is also evident that the mean value of J_d/D in the diffusion-limited situation is increased by nearly 11-fold by vigorous stirring—a change that would be anticipated if stirring reduced the effective value of d.

Hence, these and other published data would strongly suggest that unstirred layers in the intestine may exert so much resistance to the passive absorption of certain highly permeant molecules that this diffusion barrier represents, for practical purposes, the rate-limiting step to mucosal uptake. It follows from this conclusion that the precise role of such structures as bile acid micelles in facilitating the mucosal uptake of compounds such as fatty acids and sterols must be explained in terms of overcoming unstirred layer resistance.

The Effect of Unstirred Layers on the Kinetic Parameters of Active Transport

Heretofore, most kinetic data dealing with active transport of solutes across the intestine have been derived using double-reciprocal plots of experimental data to estimate values of K_m and J^{max}. Such a method assumes that the relationship between J for an actively transported molecule and C_1 is described by a curve having the form of a rectangular hyperbole. This assumption clearly is incorrect, particularly in the intestine where relatively thick unstirred water layers are interposed between the bulk perfusate and the transport sites on the microvillus membrane. Equation 7, therefore, properly defines the relationship between the active transport of a solute molecule and its bulk phase concentration since this formulation takes into account unstirred layer resistance in terms of d, D, and J^{max}.

Three points warrant emphasis concerning the characteristics of the curves relating J to C_1 derived from this expression. First, if C_1 is taken to a sufficiently high level, J^{max} will be achieved. That is, in contrast to the situation described above for passive uptake, unstirred layers will never become rate limiting for an active transport process; rather, J^{max} will be determined by the characteristics of the membrane carrier. Second, the presence of the diffusion barrier shifts the midportion of the kinetic curve to the right so that apparent K_m values derived from such data may be gross overestimations of the true K_m values of the membrane carrier. Third, as recently emphasized by Winne (1973), curves derived from Eq. 7 are not rectangular hyperboles; therefore, analysis of the data using double-reciprocal plots leads to an artifactual overestimation of J^{max} values.

Again, data derived experimentally on the active transport of various sugars and amino acids into the intestinal mucosa confirm the presence of significant unstirred layer effects as predicted by Eq. 7. For example, the apparent K_m values for these molecules are markedly reduced by vigorous stirring of the bulk perfusate, i.e., by a reduction of d. In contrast, increasing the viscosity of the mucosal solution increases the apparent K_m value presumably by reducing D for the test molecule. Finally, it has also been shown that the change in the K_m value brought about by stirring is directly proportional to the J^{max} value for the active transport of a given solute (Wilson, 1972, 1974).

Thus, there is little doubt that unstirred layers may significantly influence experimentally determined values of J^{max} and K_m for various active transport processes. Correction of such data for unstirred-layer effects ultimately will require utilization of mathematical expressions based upon Eq. 7; however, as discussed earlier such mathematical manipulations require knowledge not only of appropriate values for the mean thickness of the unstirred water layer, d, but also require information concerning the effective surface area of this diffusion barrier, S_w. Neither of these values currently is available for the active transport of solutes across the intestine so that such calculations are not now possible.

In summary, it is obvious that the presence of significant unstirred water layers in the intestine profoundly influence the kinetics of both passive and active transport processes. Acceptable experimental determination of these various transport parameters, therefore, must take into consideration these important unstirred layer effects.

ACKNOWLEDGMENTS

This work was supported by U.S. Public Health Service Research Grants RO1 AM16386 and RO1 HL09610. During the period of time when these studies were carried out, Dr. Westergaard was a postdoctoral research fellow supported by an award from the Fogarty International Fellowship Grant FO5 TW01808.

REFERENCES

Dainty, J. (1963): Water relations of plant cells. Adv. Botan. Res. *1*:279–326.

Diamond, J. M. (1966): A rapid method for determining voltage-concentration relations across membranes. J. Physiol. *183*:83–100.

Diamond, J. M., and Wright, E. M. (1969): Biological membranes: The physical basis of ion and nonelectrolyte selectivity. Ann. Rev. Physiol. *31*:581–646.

Dietschy, J. M. (1973): Mechanisms of bile acid and fatty acid absorption across the unstirred water layer and brush border of the intestine. Helv. Med. Acta. *37*:89–102.

Lukie, B. E., Westergaard, H., and Dietschy, J. M. (1974): Validation of a chamber that allows measurement of both tissue uptake rates and unstirred layer thicknesses in the intestine under conditions of controlled stirring. Gastroenterology *67*:652–661.

Sallee, V. L., Wilson, F. A., and Dietschy, J. M. (1972): Determination of unidirectional uptake rates for lipids across the intestinal brush border. J. Lipid Res. *13*:184–192.

Sallee, V. L., and Dietschy, J. M.: Determinants of intestinal mucosal uptake of short- and medium-chain fatty acids and alcohols. J. Lipid Res. *14*:475–484.

Westergaard, H., and Dietschy, J. M. (1974): Delineation of the dimensions and permeability characteristics of the two major diffusion barriers to passive mucosal uptake in the rabbit intestine. J. Clin. Invest. *54*:718–732.

Wilson, F. A., and Dietschy, J. M. (1972): The effect of unstirred layers on the kinetics of active transport in the rat intestine. Clin. Res. *20*:783 (Abstr.).

Wilson, F. A., and Dietschy, J. M. (1974): The intestinal unstirred layer: Its surface area and effect on active transport kinetics. Biochim. Biophys. Acta *363*:112–126.

Winne, D. (1973): Unstirred layer, source of biased Michaelis constant in membrane transport. Biochim. Biophys. Acta *298*:27–31.

DISCUSSION

DIETSCHY commented that in several flat membranes which he examined the unstirred layer varied from approximately 90 to 400 μm. However, *in vivo* the unstirred layer may be much thicker due to, among other things, the presence of mucus. When questioned about the possible influence of intestinal motility (peristalsis and villus movements) upon unstirred layers, DIETSCHY speculated that such movements may not be vigorous enough to significantly alter the functional thickness of the aqueous barrier. He did comment, however, that in studies reported from Dr. Ernest Wright's laboratory that movement of cilia in the choroid plexus apparently resulted in a significant reduction in unstirred layer thickness.

KESTON questioned whether, in view of the complication due to the unstirred layer, one should reexamine the kinetic data obtained in transport studied over a very short period of time. DIETSCHY thinks that the unstirred layer problem will definitely enter into the studies with regard to transport. Much depends on how fast the substance moves across the unstirred layer: if the transport across this layer is slow, the unstirred resistance term can be eliminated; however, if it is fast, such as in the case of glucose, it certainly will have to be taken into account in measuring transport.

BANWELL asked whether, besides the mechanical stirring, could osmotic stirring, such as osmotic drag or water or fluid movement, influence the unstirred layer. DIETSCHY answered that the diffusion across the water layer is usually relatively fast so that the rate of the water movement will probably have less drastic influence upon the unstirred layer.

Intestinal Absorption and Malabsorption,
edited by T. Z. Csáky.
Raven Press, New York © 1975

Action Mechanisms of Antiabsorptive and Hydragogue Drugs

W. Rummel, G. Nell, and R. Wanitschke

Institut für Pharmakologie und Toxikologie der Universität des Saarlandes, D-6650 Homburg, Germany

When studying the effects of drugs on epithelial membranes, drugs are used by physiologists as tools to elucidate the mechanisms of transport. The pharmacologist, however, is obliged to focus attention on mechanism of action of drugs. Sometimes these two approaches lead to identical lines of experimental inquiry. Most of the drugs used by physiologists do not have any pharmacologic or therapeutic relevance with regard to the intestine. Therefore, it does not appear reasonable to enumerate all the drugs used for inhibition or activation of transfer processes in the intestinal mucosa. Cardiac glycosides, e.g., are useful experimental tools, of course, but their action on the intestinal mucosa is only of toxicological interest under extreme conditions. Therefore, it is justified to restrict this chapter to drugs whose site of therapeutic and pathophysiologic action is located in the gut. Laxatives, mainly the dihydroxiphenylmethan derivatives, and bile acids, the dihydroxicholanoic acid derivatives, are representatives of this type of compound. They have in common an "antiabsorptive" and "hydragogue" action on the intestinal mucosa. These terms were used to describe the main actions, when they were originally observed in intestinal preparations *in vitro* and *in vivo* (Forth, Baldauf, and Rummel, 1963, 1966; Forth, Rummel, Glasner, and Andres, 1966).

The main phenomenon was observed in isolated jejunal segments (Fisher and Parsons apparatus) under the influence of deoxycholate. Water, sodium, and chloride absorption are inhibited approximately 50% when applying deoxycholate in a concentration of 2×10^{-4} M, whereas the glucose absorption is already diminished by about 80%. In addition, it should be mentioned that the amounts of potassium and calcium appearing on the serosal side are diminished by deoxycholate by about 25 and 15%, respectively (Forth, Rummel, and Glasner, 1964; Forth, Rummel, Glasner, and Andres, 1966; Forth and Rummel, 1967).

We shall, therefore, use the word "antiabsorptive" to describe this property of deoxycholate. (It is always very easy for a pharmacologist to create a new category of drugs, simply, by combining a word with the prefix "anti".)

One is tempted to explain this effect of deoxycholate by an inhibition of

Na⁺-K⁺-ATPase (Pope, Parkinson, and Olson, 1966). In support of this hypothesis it could be shown that oxyphenisatin, which has an action very similar to that of deoxycholate, inhibits the activity of the Na⁺-K⁺-ATPase of mucosal cells (Chignell and Titus, 1968). Under *in vitro* conditions the predominant driving force for the sodium and water transport is evidently the sodium pump. Therefore, this hypothesis appears reasonable.

For further information the results obtained with *in vivo* experiments will be examined. In tied-off jejunal segments, the absorption of Na^+, K^+, Ca^{2+}, and fluid is inhibited by oxyphenisatin (10^{-5} M) *in vivo* as well. In colon segments, however, not only an inhibition of absorption but also a reverse movement of fluid into the intestinal lumen is observed (Forth et al., 1963; Forth, Rummel, and Baldauf, 1966). Corresponding results were obtained with deoxycholate (Forth, Rummel, Glasner, and Andres, 1966). Consequently, it can be stated that these drugs exert an "hydragogue" action.

More detailed information was obtained using bisacodyl in a concentration too low to induce fluid secretion and large enough to inhibit fluid absorption completely (Fig. 1). Under these conditions, the net transfer of sodium and potassium does not cease. Although the sodium absorption is diminished by

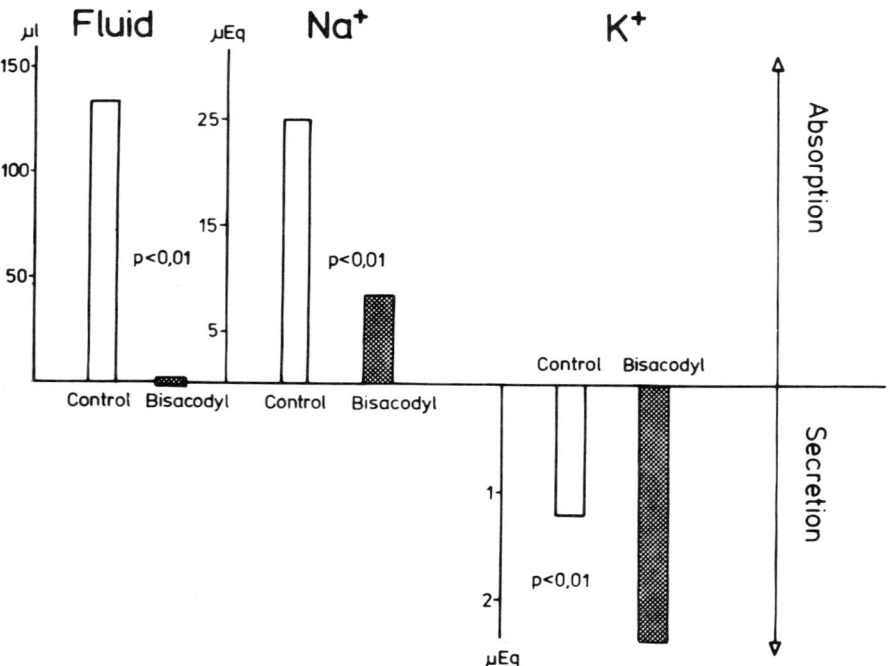

FIG. 1. Influence of bisacodyl on absorption and secretion of the colon *in vivo*. The loops were filled with Tyrode solution (concentration of bisacodyl $1.4 \cdot 10^{-5}$ M), values given are amounts absorbed per hour and centimeter length, columns represent the mean values of $n = 20$ (Forth, Rummel, and Baldauf, 1966).

about 60%, nevertheless, a net transfer of sodium from the luminal fluid against a chemical gradient continues in the presence of bisacodyl. Simultaneously, the secretion of potassium into the luminal fluid is increased by about 50%. Taking into account the difference in the potassium concentration between plasma and lumen, it can be stated that this secretion occurs against a chemical gradient. After 1 hr, the potassium concentration in the lumen is more than three times higher than in the plasma.

The question of whether morphological changes can be correlated with the hydragogue action can be denied. With the exception of an apparent increase in the number of empty goblet cells, no changes could be observed in these tied-off colon segments after experiments with deoxycholate (Forth et al., 1964; Forth, Rummel, Glasner, and Andres, 1966; Mekhjian and Phillips, 1970; Sladen and Harries, 1972; Teem and Phillips, 1972) and oxyphenisatin (Nell, Overhoff, Forth, Kulenkampff, Specht, and Rummel, 1973). Particularly, the integrity of the epithelial cell layer was preserved.

The antiabsorptive activity of the diphenolic laxatives (Table 1) and bile acids (Table 2) has since been noted in many studies of the active transport of several substrates in different species.

The results obtained in animal experiments were confirmed and completed also by investigations in man. Hart and McColl (1968) measured glucose absorption in clamped-off segments of the small intestine in man and rat. By varying the concentration of oxyphenisatin from 3×10^{-6} to 3×10^{-4} M they obtained a dose-dependent inhibition of glucose absorption.

During human perfusion studies of the colon it was shown by Ewe that bisacodyl did not only cause the expected inhibition of sodium and water absorption but that it also reversed the direction of net transfer (Fig. 2). After continuing the perfusion with a bisacodyl-free solution, this effect

TABLE 1. *Inhibition of absorption by diphenolic laxatives*

Substrate	Intestinal area	Species	References
Na$^+$, water	jejunum colon	rat	Forth, Baldauf, and Rummel (1963) Forth, Rummel, and Baldauf (1966) Hart and McColl (1968)
	ileum	rabbit	Phillips, Love, Mitchell, and Neptun (1965)
Glucose	jejunum	rat	Forth, Baldauf, and Rummel (1963) Forth, Rummel, and Baldauf (1966) Hand, Sanford, and Smyth (1966) Hart and McColl (1967, 1968)
3-O-Methyl glucose	jejunum	hamster	Adamic and Bihler (1967)
α-Amino butyric acid	jejunum	hamster	Adamic and Bihler (1967)

TABLE 2. *Inhibition of transport of various substances across intestinal mucosa by deoxycholic acid*

Substances	References
Acetate	Parkinson and Olson (1963), Pope, Parkinson, and Olson (1966)
Glucose	Dawson and Isselbacher (1960), Rummel and Stupp (1962), Parkinson and Olson (1963), Faust (1964), Forth, Rummel, and Glasner (1964), Faust and Wu (1965a,b), Forth, Rummel, Glasner, and Andres (1966), Pope, Parkinson, and Olson (1966), Gracey, Burke, and Oshin (1971), Harris and Sladen (1972)
L-Leucine	Parkinson and Olson (1963), Pope, Parkinson, and Olson (1966)
L-Lysine	Pope, Parkinson, and Olson (1966)
Sodium	Forth, Baldauf, and Rummel (1963), Forth, Rummel, and Glasner (1964), Forth, Rummel, Glasner, and Andres (1966), Pope, Parkinson, and Olson (1966), Mekhjian and Phillips (1970), Harries and Sladen (1972)
Urea	Pope, Parkinson, and Olson (1966)
Water	Rummel and Stupp (1962), Forth, Baldauf, and Rummel (1963), Forth, Rummel, and Glasner (1964), Faust and Wu (1965a,b), Forth, Rummel, Glasner, and Andres (1966), Mekhjian and Phillips (1970), Harries and Sladen (1972), Teem and Phillips (1972)

disappeared although the function is not restored completely after 2 hr. In accordance with animal experiments, potassium secretion is also increased in man by bisacodyl. These results are of interest with respect to the disturbances of electrolyte balance as the consequence of chronical abuse of laxatives. The deficit of sodium and potassium may partially be due to gastrointestinal electrolyte loss which is usually associated with secondary hyperaldosteronism (Meulengracht, 1939; Schwartz and Relman, 1952, 1953; Wolff, Henne, Krück, Roscher, Vecsei, Brown, Düsterdieck, Lever, and Robertson, 1968; Wolff, Krück, Brown, Lever, Vecsei, Roscher, Düsterdieck, and Robertson, 1968; Fleischer, Brown, and Graham, 1969).

A few years ago, Alan Hofmann and his group obtained in principle similar results for dihydroxy bile acids in careful and extensive experiments (Mekhjian, Phillips, and Hofmann, 1971). It is to their credit that they used these experimental results for a conclusive explanation of the pathogenesis of several gastrointestinal diseases associated with diarrhea (Hofmann, 1967, 1968; Phillips, 1972). Summing up, several drugs with laxative properties such as diphenolic compounds, bile acids, and fatty acids (Ammon and Phillips, 1973, 1974; Bright-Asare and Binder, 1973), which can be included here, exert an antiabsorptive and hydragogue action on the intestinal mucosa.

The next question to be answered is whether these properties are actually

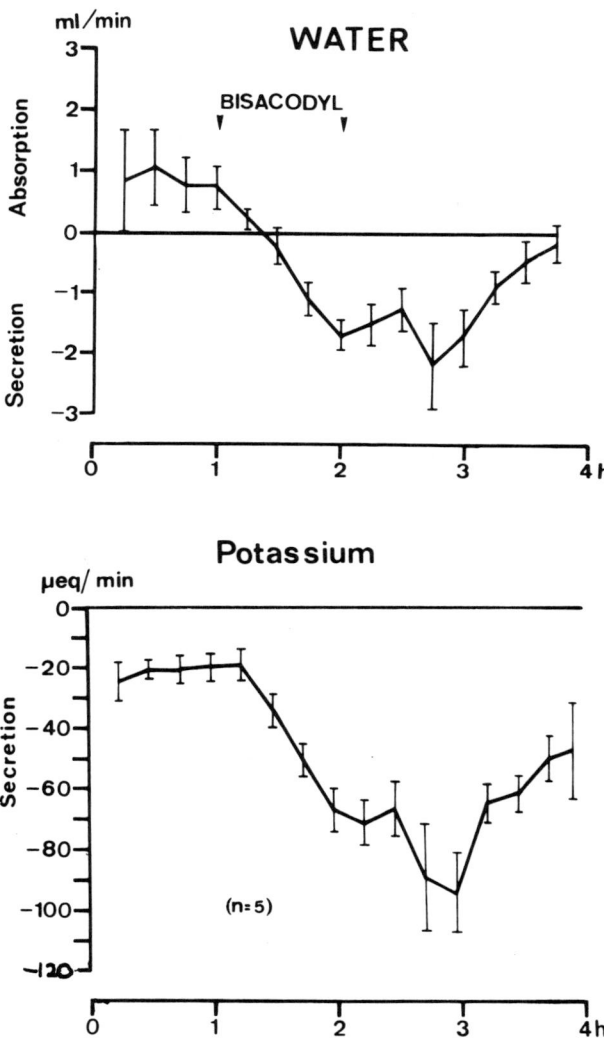

FIG. 2. The effect of bisacodyl on the transfer of water and potassium in the human colon. Colon perfusion was performed according to the method of Devroede and Phillips (1969); values are given with the standard deviation, n = 5 (Ewe, 1974).

responsible for the laxative effect of these drugs. The antiabsorptive activity of five compounds chemically related to bisacodyl were compared with their laxative activity (Forth and Rummel, 1974). The results yielded an unequivocal correlation: only those three compounds that proved to be laxatives inhibited water absorption by jejunal segments *in vitro*. This correlation supports the assumption that antiabsorptive and hydragogue activity are responsible for the laxative capacity of this type of compound.

In Table 3, all drugs proven to have antiabsorptive and hydragogue activity are listed. The list comprises the main representatives of the commonly used laxatives, including ricinoleic acid. Conventionally, the mode of laxative action of these drugs is explained in text books by stating, that they increase the motility of the gut, particularly of the colon. On the basis of the findings described, it can be supposed that this increase of motility is partially due to the increase in fluid volume within the gut lumen.

The question, which change at the cellular or subcellular level is responsible for the action of these drugs, cannot yet be answered. Nevertheless, it can be stated that an inhibitory action on the Na^+-K^+-ATPase cannot account for the observed net transfer of sodium and water into the intestinal lumen.

The net transfer of water and sodium is the result of two unidirectional fluxes, one from the lumen to the blood, and the other from the blood to the lumen. First of all, we must know whether drugs acting like diphenolic laxatives inhibit the unidirectional transfer from the lumen to the blood and/or increase the transfer in the opposite direction from the blood to the lumen. Either effect could lead to an inhibition of absorption. When measuring the unidirectional fluxes by means of double tagging with ^{22}Na and ^{24}Na it can be shown, that the unidirectional fluxes change with increasing doses of oxyphenisatin. The largest change is the increase of unidirectional flux from plasma to lumen (Table 4). Between the calculated (i.e., the difference of the unidirectional fluxes) and the measured values (by flame photometry) a satisfactory agreement exists.

Consequently, it can be stated that the increase of the unidirectional flux from the blood to the gut lumen is mainly responsible for the inhibition of absorption as well as for the secretion. In this connection, it is important to note, that under similar conditions inducing the same effect by deoxycholate instead of oxyphenisatin neither the extracellular space nor the cellular Na^+- and K^+-content changes significantly (Table 5).

TABLE 3. Laxatives with antiabsorptive and hydragogue effect

Substance	References
Senna	Straub and Triendl (1934)
Bisacodyl, oxyphenisatin	Forth, Baldauf, and Rummel (1963), Forth, Rummel, and Baldauf (1966), Ewe (1972, 1974)
Phenolphthalein, cascara sagr. Podophyllum	Phillips, Love, Mitchell, and Neptune (1965)
Hydroxy fatty acids	Phillips, Love, Mitchell, and Neptune (1965), Ammon and Phillips (1973), Bright-Asare and Binder (1973), Ammon and Phillips (1974)

TABLE 4. Transfer of sodium across the mucosa of rat colon under the influence of oxyphenisatin

		Unidirectional sodium flux $\mu Eq \cdot cm^{-1} \cdot min^{-1}$		Calculated net transfer of sodium $\mu Eq \cdot cm^{-1} \cdot min^{-1}$	Measured net transfer of sodium $\mu Eq \cdot cm^{-1} \cdot min^{-1}$
		lumen to plasma	plasma to lumen		
control		0.52 ± 0.05	0.17 ± 0.02	+0.35 ± 0.04	+0.21 ± 0.05
oxyphenisatin trial concentration	7.9 · 10⁻⁶ M	0.37 ± 0.03	0.35ᵃ ± 0.05	+0.02ᵃ ± 0.04	+0.05ᵃ ± 0.05
	6.3 · 10⁻⁵ M	0.39 ± 0.04	0.88ᵃ ± 0.05	−0.38ᵃ ± 0.08	−0.43ᵃ ± 0.05

Tied off segments; ^{24}Na-(NaCl) was administered in the lumen, ^{22}Na-(NaCl) in the plasma; + signifies net transfer from lumen to plasma, − signifies net transfer from plasma to lumen.
ᵃ $p < 0.05$ as compared with the control group, $n = 5$. Values are given with the standard error of the mean (modified from Nell, Overhoff, Forth, Kulenkampff, Specht, and Rummel, 1973).

What is the driving force responsible for the increased unidirectional flux from the blood to the gut lumen? It must be suspected that the capillary pressure is involved as a hydrodynamic force. But under *in vivo* conditions, a satisfactory control of this parameter is obviously not possible. An *in vitro* preparation, the everted sac of isolated colon mucosa (Parsons and Paterson, 1965), offers the advantage of being able to change the hydrostatic pressure on the serosal side in a precisely controlled fashion.

Figures 3 and 4 show a piece of a stripped colonic mucosa (rat). We are looking at the luminal surface by means of a scanning electron microscope. The capacity of such an isolated preparation of colon mucosa can be characterized briefly by two facts (a) it transports sodium uphill and establishes a sodium gradient by about 20 mEq/l during 2 hr if buffered electrolyte solution is presented on both sides; (b) it produces a potential difference of about 18 mV.

When measuring the net transport of sodium and water from the mucosal to the serosal side, the following values per hour and per gram dry weight are obtained: 1.4 mEq sodium and 7.3 ml water. The resulting tonicity in the fluid absorbed is 1.5 times that of isotonicity.

If 10^{-5} M oxyphenisatin is added to the mucosal side, net transport ceases completely and the values no longer differ significantly from zero (Table 6).

TABLE 5. Effect of sodium deoxycholate on intracellular concentrations of sodium and potassium in rat colonic mucosa in vivo

	^{51}CrEDTA space % of w.w.	Sodium $\mu Eq/g$ water	Potassium $\mu Eq/g$ water
Control	20.4 ± 0.8	40 ± 3	151 ± 7
Na deoxycholate 3 · 10⁻³M	19.5 ± 1.2	33 ± 9	141 ± 7

Values are given with the standard error of the mean, w.w. = wet weight, $n = 5$ (modified from Nell, Forth, Rummel, and Wanitschke, 1972).

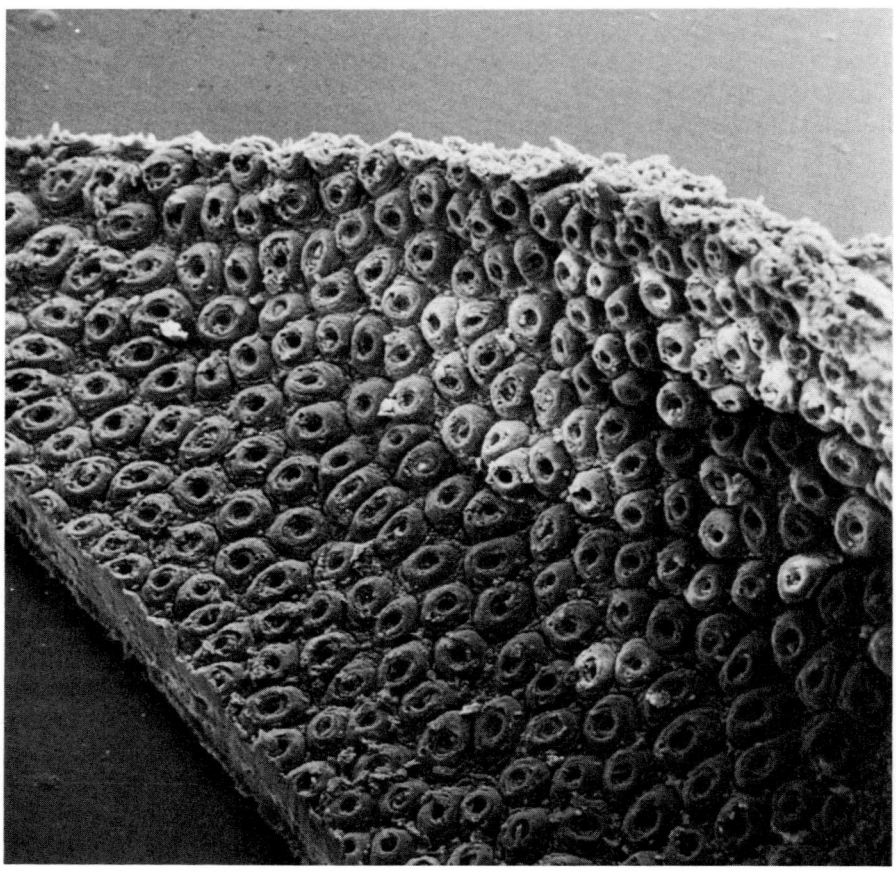

FIG. 3. Colon mucosa (rat) seen from the luminal side in the scanning electron microscope. In the center of the circular walls are the mouths of the Lieberkühn glands. Magnification 130:1. Published with the permission of Prof. B. Lindemann, Abteilung für Membranforschung an Epithelien, 2nd Dept. of Physiology, 665 Homburg (Saar), West Germany.

In the presence of oxyphenisatin no change occurred in the tissue content of potassium or in the size of the extracellular space. This observation is of high importance for the further discussion. (With respect to the difference of the extracellular space in comparison to Table 5 it must be taken into account, that in isolated mucosal preparations the integrity of the submucosal tissue is no longer preserved.)

The part contributed by the unidirectional fluxes to the change in the net transport induced by oxyphenisatin can be determined when measuring the unidirectional fluxes by means of ^{22}Na (Fig. 5).

The unidirectional flux from the serosal to the mucosal side increases about

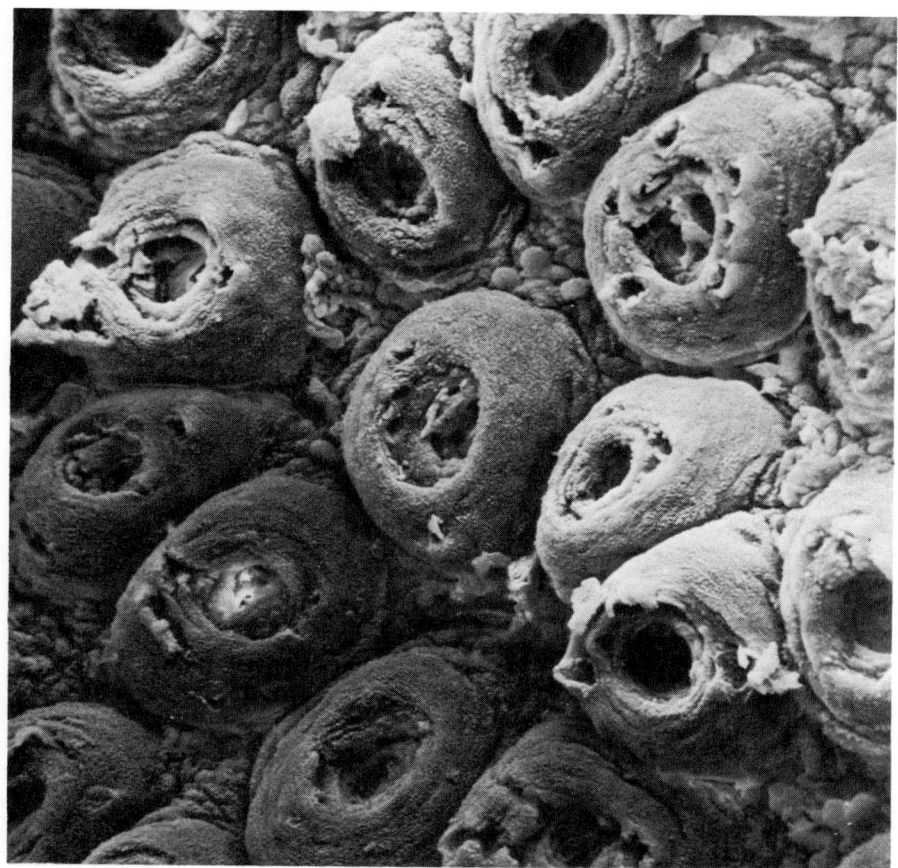

FIG. 4. Detail of Fig. 3. Magnification 650:1. (Also from Lindemann.)

fourfold due to oxyphenisatin. The unidirectional flux from the mucosal to the serosal side is also increased. The calculated values for net transport do not differ from zero. Evidently, the increase in the unidirectional flux from the serosal to the mucosal side is responsible for the cessation of the net transport.

It is important to note that in contrast to the results *in vivo,* a secretion, i.e., a net transport from the serosal to the mucosal side, can not be observed in these experiments *in vitro.* Therefore, we must ask whether the reason for this difference between the *in vivo* and the *in vitro* experiments is the absence of the hydrodynamic force due to the absence of capillary pressure.

The main subject of the following data is to characterize the influence of the hydrodynamic force on the movement of sodium and water across the epithelial layer (Fig. 6). At low pressure differences between the serosal

TABLE 6. *Influence of oxyphenisatin on absorption and tissue potassium content in isolated rat colonic mucosa*

	Absorption		Tissue	
	Sodium mEq[a]	Water ml[a]	Potassium mEq[b]	Extracellular space %[c]
Controls (n = 19)	1.4 ± 0.06	7.3 ± 0.3	278 ± 16	60 ± 2.8
Oxyphenisatin (10^{-5}M on the mucosal side) (n = 16)	0.1 ± 0.07	0.1 ± 0.3	270 ± 11	59 ± 2.3

[a] Per gram dry weight and hour.
[b] Per gram dry weight.
[c] In % of wet weight.
Values are given with the standard error of the mean, method according to Parsons and Paterson (1965), the extracellular space was measured with ^{51}CrEDTA (Wanitschke, Nell, and Rummel, 1974)

and mucosal side a net transport of sodium and water from the mucosal to the serosal side takes place against the hydrostatic pressure. The net transport of sodium is relatively higher than that of water. Therefore the remaining mucosal solution becomes hypotonic as already known (Parsons and Paterson, 1965; Forth, Rummel, and Baldauf, 1966). The intercept between the abscissa and the sodium and the water curve occurs at different points.

A mean hydrostatic pressure of 5.8 cm water suffices to suppress the net water transport from the mucosal to the serosal side, whereas for the suppression of the net transport of sodium twofold higher hydrostatic pressure is needed. These two values—they can be called "compensating pressures" —are a physical measure of the transport capacity of this isolated mucosa for sodium and water.

The difference between these compensating pressures for the sodium and water net transport can be used as a measure for the characterization of the discriminating capacity of the colonic mucosa for sodium and water.

By applying hydrostatic pressures higher than the compensating pressure for the net transfer of water, a filtrate appears at the luminal side and increases the volume. This filtrate is a hypotonic fluid. (The difference between the sodium and the water curve indicates the degree of hypotonicity; isotonicity is present only when the two curves are superimposed.)

The divergence of the sodium and of the water curve is proved to be statistically significant ($0.05 > p > 0.01$). Therefore it can be stated that with increasing hydrostatic pressures the discriminating effect of the colonic mucosa for sodium and water increases. This discriminating capacity disappears when oxyphenisatin 10^{-5} M (Wanitschke and Nell, 1974) is present in the mucosal fluid. Then the filtrate becomes isotonic.

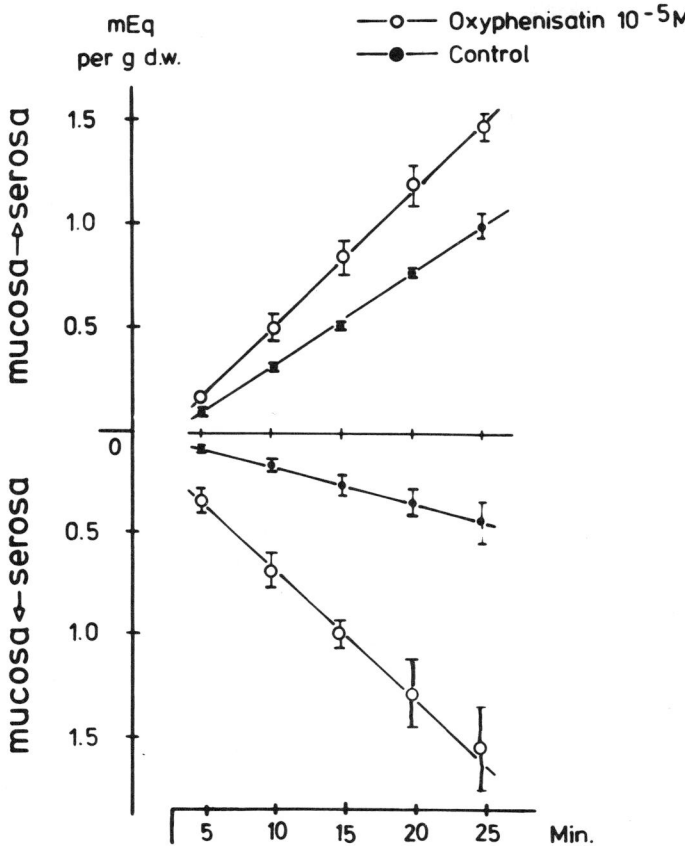

FIG. 5. Unidirectional sodium flux across the isolated colonic mucosa. Method according to Parsons and Paterson (1965), the fluxes are measured as appearance or disappearance rate at the serosal side by ^{22}Na, the vertical bars indicate the standard error of the mean, n = 4 (Wanitschke and Nell, 1974).

Under these conditions a pressure of 5 cm at the serosal side suffices to reverse the net transfer of sodium and water (Fig. 6). Under normal conditions more than the twofold hydrostatic pressure would have been necessary to move the same amount of water from the serosal to the mucosal side and more than the fourfold pressure for sodium.

Summing up these results it can be stated that *in vitro*, in contradistinction to the *in vivo* experiments, neither oxyphenisatin nor deoxycholate induce secretion of sodium and water into the gut lumen. *In vitro* they only stop the net transport from the mucosal to the serosal side. If, however, a pressure of about 5 cm water is applied on the serosal side, a pressure which can not suppress the absorption of sodium under normal conditions, then sodium and water are secreted into the lumen. The height of the pressure applied is in

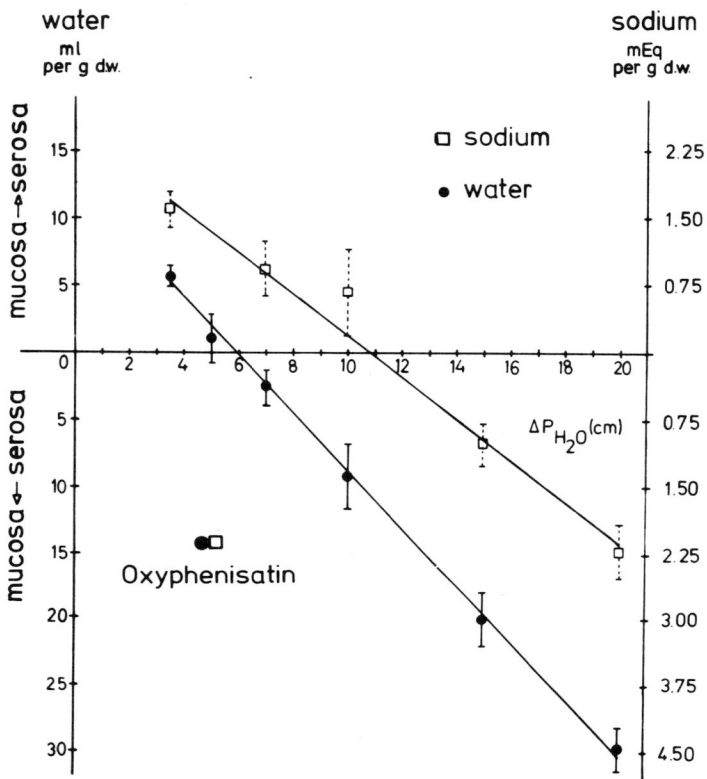

FIG. 6. Net transfer of sodium and water in dependence on hydrostatic pressure at the serosal side of the isolated colonic mucosa. Method according to Parsons and Paterson (1965), n = 5 to 19, vertical bars indicate the standard error of the mean, duration of the experiment: 2 hr (Wanitschke and Nell, 1974).

the same range as would be expected to exist at the basal poles of the epithelial cells due to the capillary filtration pressure.

Which property of the epithelium is changed by deoxycholate or oxyphenisatin respectively? When an isotonic choline chloride solution is administered to a tied-off colonic segment *in vivo*, the osmotic pressure on both sides of the epithelium is equal, whereas there obviously exists a steep concentration gradient for sodium. The concentration of sodium in the lumen equals 6.3 ± 0.3 mEq/l and that of choline 156 ± 2 mEq/l. In spite of the steep gradient, no net transfer of sodium and choline occurs during 30 min under control conditions (Fig. 7).

Oxyphenisatin, however, causes a net transfer of sodium into the lumen together with an osmotically equivalent amount of water, whereas a net transfer of choline does not occur.

In the presence of deoxycholate, in contrast to oxyphenisatin, the amount

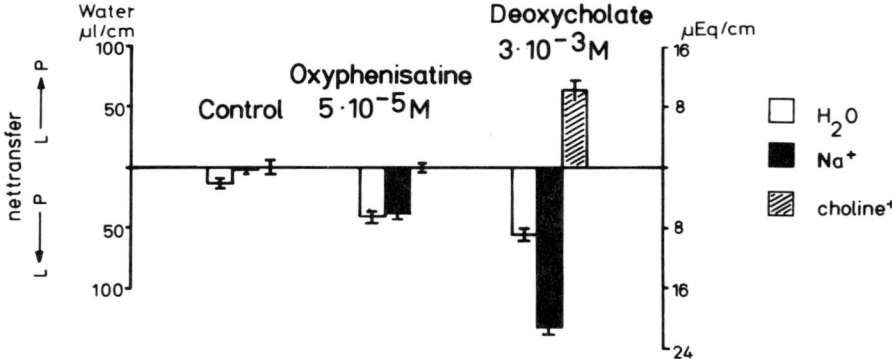

FIG. 7. Comparison of the effects of deoxycholate and oxyphenisatin on the transfer of water and electrolytes in the rat colon *in vivo*. The loops are filled with isotonic choline chloride solution, vertical bars indicate the standard error of the mean, n = 5, duration of the experiment: 30 min (modified from Nell, Forth, Rummel, and Wanitschke, 1972; Nell, Overhoff, Forth, and Rummel, 1973).

of sodium moved into the lumen is about three times higher. Simultaneously, choline leaves the gut lumen and appears in the blood.

Based on these results the change in the respective properties of the epithelium induced by oxyphenisatin and deoxycholate can be described as follows. Since under control conditions, no net movement of sodium or of choline can be observed, it must be stated that the mucosa of the colon shows an "apparent impermeability" for sodium and choline. Under the influence of oxyphenisatin or deoxycholate, this "apparent impermeability" for sodium and for choline, respectively, disappears.

During a 30-min period the sodium crossing the mucosa from the blood to the gut lumen due to the changed permeability under the influence of deoxycholate or oxyphenisatin is about 30-fold higher than the intracellular sodium content of the epithelial cells.

What is the pathway for this sodium moving across the epithelium? Does it move in a trans- or an intercellular way? If the transcellular route is involved, deoxycholate and oxyphenisatin should influence either the active sodium-potassium transport or the sodium-potassium permeability of the cell membranes. In both cases an appreciable change in the concentrations of intracellular electrolytes should occur. But this did not happen (*cf.* Table 5 and 6). Furthermore, when comparing the ratio of the specific activity of the mucosal tissue and the plasma, after intravenous injection of ^{22}Na, no difference between the control group and the oxyphenisatin group can be observed (Table 7). The calculated distribution space of ^{22}Na and of the extracellular marker ^{51}Cr-EDTA is the same without and with oxyphenisatin. However, the specific activity measured simultaneously in the lumen differs considerably. It is about 2.5 times higher in the presence of oxyphenisatin.

Therefore the conclusion can be drawn that the main pathway for the

TABLE 7. Specific ^{22}Na activity in the rat colonic mucosa and lumen under the influence of oxyphenisatin

	Control	Oxyphenisatin $3 \cdot 10^{-5}$ M
Spec. ^{22}Na-activity mucosa / Spec. ^{22}Na-activity plasma	0.68 ± 0.04	0.71 ± 0.03
Spec. ^{22}Na-activity lumen	7.4 ± 0.4	17.9 ± 0.9

Tied off segments, duration of the experiment: 2 min, $n = 8$, values are given with the standard error of the mean (Nell, Rummel, Forth, and Wanitschke, 1972).

sodium secreted into the lumen under the influence of deoxycholate and oxyphenisatin is located between the epithelial cells across the nexus or the so-called tight junctions.

This interpretation is supported by the fact that under the influence of oxyphenisatin and deoxycholate the amount of extracellular markers such as ^{14}C-inulin and ^{51}Cr-EDTA, which crosses the colonic mucosa, increases severalfold (Table 8).

Are these effects reversible? Functional reversibility is proved for deoxycholate (Mekhjian and Phillips, 1970; Mekhjian et al., 1971; Harries and Sladen, 1972), bisacodyl (Ewe, 1972), and also for ricinoleic acid (Ammon and Phillips, 1973, 1974; Bright-Asare and Binder, 1973) *in vivo*. It should not be surprising that the reversion to the normal state is not complete in every case during the observation period, because the completeness of the removal of these drugs can not be guaranteed. For deoxycholate *in vitro* it could also be demonstrated that the increased flux of ^{22}Na from the serosal

TABLE 8. Appearance of extracellular markers administered i.v. in the colonic lumen

	^{51}CrEDTA cpm/ml · 10^{-2}	^{14}C-Inulin cpm/ml
Controls ($n = 6$)	6.2 ± 0.3	298 ± 31
Oxyphenisatin $3 \cdot 10^{-5}$ M ($n = 6$)	15.7 ± 2.5	558 ± 37
Deoxycholate $3 \cdot 10^{-3}$ M ($n = 5$)	703 ± 90	

Tied off loops, duration of the experiment: 1 hr, plasma concentration of ^{51}CrEDTA and ^{14}C-Inulin after 1 hr: 100,000 cpm/ml, values are given with the standard error of the mean, $p < 0.001$ as compared with the controls (Nell, Forth, Rummel, and Wanitschke, 1974).

to the mucosal side on isolated colonic mucosa returns approximately to normal after washing out of the deoxycholate (Wanitschke, Nell, and Rummel, 1973). The conclusions, which can be drawn, are speculative, but they might simultaneously provoke new experiments.

The main site of action of these antiabsorptive and hydragogue drugs is the intercellular cement, which is responsible for the tightness of the so called tight junctions (Tidball, 1964). When comparing the different parts of the intestinal epithelium it can be stated, that the highest degree of tightness can be ascribed to the colonic mucosa. Not even urea is able to penetrate in an appreciable amount across the epithelial layer (Billich and Levitan, 1969). These drugs apparently loosen the junctions and make them leaky. Thereby the efficiency of the pumping system is decreased in spite of the fact that the sodium pumps at the cellular membranes are working or are at least not inhibited to a greater extent. This is apparently so because, in contradistinction to ouabain (Schultz, Fuisz, and Curran, 1966; Ehrenthal, 1974), these drugs did not change the normal distribution of sodium and potassium. A very simplified model may illustrate the situation (Fig. 8).

It seems permissible to assume, that the reason for the disappearance of the transporting activity of the epithelial unit is the loss of the anisotropy of the pumping system. The pumping system responsible for the net transfer of sodium and water consists of two essential parts: of the junction between the cells with a relatively high sodium resistance (Frömter and Diamond, 1972) and of the sodium pumps distributed along the lateral membranes of

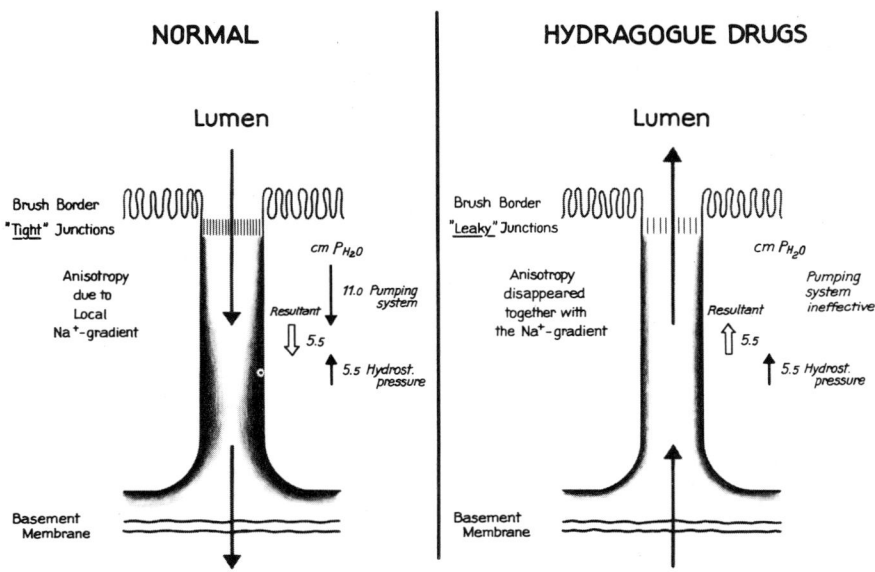

FIG. 8. A simplified model.

the cells. When the resistance of the junctions decreases, i.e., they become leaky, then the standing osmotic gradient (Diamond and Tormey, 1966; Diamond and Bossert, 1967; Tormey and Diamond, 1967; Diamond, 1971) can not be maintained further.

The performance of the pumping system measured as net transfer of sodium in the direction of the serosal side can be expressed in equivalents of hydrostatic pressure determined by the compensating pressure. Using these terms, it can be stated that the pumping system can produce a pressure of 11 cm water and is therefore able to overcome a pressure of 5.5 cm water administered from the opposite direction. If, however, the prerequisite for the anisotropy of the system, the high resistance for sodium of the junctions, is abolished, then the hydrostatic pressure applied at the serosal side determines the net transfer of sodium and water.

The particular property of these hydragogue drugs appears to be the ability in certain concentrations to make the intercellular junctions leaky. The confirmation of this hypothesis needs further experiments.

ACKNOWLEDGMENT

This research was supported in part by a grant of the Sonderforschungsbereich 38, Membrane Research at the Universität des Saarlandes.

REFERENCES

Adamic, S., and Bihler, I. (1967): Inhibition of intestinal sugar transport by phenolphthalein. Molec. Pharmacol. *3:*188–194.

Ammon, H. V., and Phillips, S. F. (1973): Inhibition of colonic water and electrolyte absorption by fatty acids in man. Gastroenterology *65:*744–749.

Ammon, H. V., and Phillips, S. F. (1974): Inhibition of ileal water absorption by intraluminal fatty acids. Influence of chain length, hydroxylation and conjugation of fatty acids. J. Clin. Invest. *53:*205–210.

Billich, C. O., and Levitan, R. (1969): Effects of sodium concentration and osmolality on water and electrolyte absorption from the intact human colon. J. Clin. Invest. *48:*1336–1347.

Bright-Asare, P., and Binder, H. J. (1973): Stimulation of colonic secretion of water and electrolytes by hydroxy fatty acids. Gastroenterology *64:*81–88.

Chignell, C. F., and Titus, E. O. (1968): The inhibition of rat small intestinal $(Na^+ + K^+)$ − ATPase by phenolphthalein and other purgative drugs. Fed. Proc. *27:*831.

Dawson, A. M., and Isselbacher, K. J. (1960): Studies on lipid metabolism in the small intestine with observations on the role of bile salts. J. Clin. Invest. *39:*730–740.

Devroede, G. J., and Phillips, S. F. (1969): Studies of the perfusion technique for colonic absorption. Gastroenterology *56:*92–100.

Diamond, J. M. (1971): Standing-gradient model of fluid transport in epithelia. Fed. Proc. *30:*6–13.

Diamond, J. M., and Bossert, W. H. (1967): Standing-gradient osmotic flow. A mechanism for coupling of water and solute transport in epithelia. J. Gen. Physiol. *50:*2061–2083.

Diamond, J. M., and Tormey, J. M. (1966): Studies on the structural basis of water transport across epithelial membranes. Fed. Proc. *25:*1458–1463.

Ehrenthal, W. (1974): Der Phosphatstoffwechsel des Meerschweinchendünndarmes unter der Einwirkung von Ouabain. Thesis, Mathematisch-Naturwissenschaftliche Fakultät der Universität des Saarlandes, BRD.
Ewe, K. (1972): Effect of laxatives on intestinal water and electrolyte transport. Europ. J. Clin. Invest. 2:283.
Ewe, K., and Hölker, B. (1974): Klin. Wochenschr. 52:827–833.
Faust, K. (1964): Effects of bile salts, sodium deoxycholate, strophantin-G and metabolic inhibitors on the absorption of D-glucose by the rat jejunum *in vitro*. J. Cell. Comp. Physiol. 63:55–64.
Faust, R. G., and Wu, S. L. (1965a): The effect and mechanism of action of bile salts on fluid and glucose movement by rat jejunum *in vitro*. Fed. Proc. 24:652.
Faust, R. G., and Wu, S. L. (1965b): The action of bile salts on fluid and glucose movement by rat and hamster jejunum *in vitro*. J. Cell. Comp. Physiol. 65:435–448.
Fleischer, M., Brown, H., and Graham, D. Y., et al. (1969): Chronic laxative induced hyperaldosteronism and hypokalemia simulating Bartter's syndrome. Ann. Intern. Med. 70:791–798.
Forth, W., Baldauf, J., and Rummel, W. (1963): Ein Beitrag zur Klärung des Wirkungsmechanismus einiger Laxantien. Naunyn-Schmiedebergs Arch. Pharmak. Exp. Path. 246:91–92.
Forth, W., and Rummel, W. (1967): Resorptionshemmung, eine physiologische Wirkung von Gallensäuren. In: *Radioisotope in der Gastroenterologie,* edited by G. Hoffmann and B. Delaloye, F. K. Schattauer Verlag, Stuttgart (Germany), pp. 141–146.
Forth, W., and Rummel, W. (1974): Activation and inhibition of intestinal absorption by drugs. In: *Pharmacology of intestinal absorption: Gastrointestinal absorption of drugs,* edited by W. Forth and W. Rummel, Vol. I, International Encyclopedia of Pharmacology and Therapeutics; Pergamon Press, Oxford, Sec. 39 b, pp. 171–244.
Forth, W., Rummel, W., and Baldauf, J. (1966): Wasser- und Elektrolytbewegung am Dünn- und Dickdarm unter dem Einfluss von Laxantien, ein Beitrag zur Klärung ihres Wirkungsmechanismus. Naunyn-Schmiedebergs Arch. Pharmak. Exp. Path. 254:18–32.
Forth, W., Rummel, W., and Glasner, H. (1964): Zur resorptionshemmenden Wirkung von Gallensäuren. Naunyn-Schmiedebergs Arch. Pharmak. Exp. Path. 247:382.
Forth, W., Rummel, W., Glasner, H., and Andres, H. (1966): Zur resorptionshemmenden Wirkung von Gallensäuren. Naunyn-Schmiedebergs Arch. Pharmak. Exp. Path. 254:364–380.
Frömter, E., and Diamond, J. (1972): Route of passive ion permeation in epithelia. Nature New Biol. 235:9–13.
Gracey, M., Burke, V., and Oshin, A. (1971): Influence of bile salts on intestinal sugar transport *in vivo*. Scand. J. Gastroent. 6:273–276.
Hand, D. W., Sanford, P. A., and Smyth, D. N. (1966): Polyphenolic compounds and intestinal transfer. Nature 209:618.
Harries, J. T., and Sladen, G. E. (1972): The effects of different bile salts on the absorption of fluid, electrolytes and monosaccharides in the small intestine of the rat *in vivo*. Gut 13:596–603.
Hart, S. L., and McColl, I. (1967): The effect of purgative drugs on intestinal absorption of glucose. J. Pharm. Pharmac. 19:70–71.
Hart, S. L., and McColl, I. (1968): The effect of the laxative oxyphenisatin on the intestinal absorption of glucose in rat and man. Brit. J. Pharmacol. Chemotherap. 32:683–686.
Hofmann, A. F. (1967): The syndrome of ileal disease and the broken enterohepatic circulation: Cholerheic enteropathy. Gastroenterology 52:752–757.
Hofmann, A. F. (1968): Functions of bile in the alimentary canal, In: *Handbook of physiology,* edited by C. F. Code, sec. 6, Vol. V. Amer. Physiol. Soc., Washington, D.C., pp. 2507–2533.
Mekhjian, H. S., and Phillips, S. F. (1970): Perfusion of the canine colon with unconjugated bile acids: effect on water and electrolyte transport, morphology and bile acid absorption. Gastroenterology 59:120–129.
Mekhjian, H. S., Phillips, S. F., and Hofmann, A. F. (1971): Colonic secretion of water

and electrolytes induced by bile acids: Perfusion studies in man. J. Clin. Invest. *50:* 1569–1577.

Meulengracht, E. (1939): Osteomalacia of the spinal column from deficient diet or from disease of the digestive tract. III. Osteomalacia e abuse laxantium. Acta Med. Scand. *101:*187–210.

Nell, G., Forth, W., Rummel, W., and Wanitschke, R. (1972): Abolition of the apparent Na^+ impermeability of the colon mucosa by deoxycholate. In: *Bile acids in human diseases,* edited by P. Back and W. Gerok, F. K. Schattauer Verlag, Stuttgart, pp. 263–267.

Nell, G., Forth, W., Rummel, W., and Wanitschke, R. (1974): *Manuscript in preparation.*

Nell, G., Overhoff, H., Forth, W., Kulenkampff, H., Specht, W., and Rummel, W. (1973): Influx and efflux of sodium in jejunal and colonic segments of rats under the influence of oxyphenisatin. Naunyn-Schmiedebergs Arch. Pharmacol. *277:*53–60.

Nell, G., Overhoff, H., Forth, W., and Rummel, W. (1973): The influence of water gradients and oxyphenisatin on the net transfer of sodium and water in the rat colon. Naunyn-Schmiedebergs Arch. Pharmacol. *277:*363–372.

Nell, G., Rummel, W., Forth, W., and Wanitschke, R. (1972): Abolition of the apparent Na^+ impermeability of the colon mucosa by oxyphenisatin. Naunyn-Schmiedebergs Arch. Pharmacol. *274:* Suppl. R 81.

Parkinson, T. M., and Olson, J. A. (1963): Inhibitory effects of bile acids on the uptake, metabolism and transport of water-soluble substances in the small intestine of the rat. Life Sci. *2:*393–398.

Parsons, D. S., and Paterson, C. R. (1965): Fluid and solute transport across rat colonic mucosa. Quart. J. Physiol. *50:*220–231.

Phillips, S. F. (1972): Diarrhea: A current view of the pathophysiology. Gastroenterology *63:*495–518.

Phillips, R. A., Love, A. H. G., Mitchell, T. G., and Neptune, E. M., Jr. (1965): Cathartics and the sodium pump. Nature *206:*1367–1368.

Pope, J. L., Parkinson, T. M., and Olson, J. A. (1966): Action of bile salts on the metabolism and transport of water-soluble nutrients by perfused rat jejunum *in vitro.* Biochim. Biophys. Acta *130:*218–232.

Rummel, W., and Stupp, H. F. (1962): The influence of diuretics on the absorption of salt, glucose and water from the isolated small intestine of the rat. Experientia *18:*303–309.

Schultz, S. G., Fuisz, R. E., and Curran, P. F. (1966): Amino acid and sugar transport in rabbit ileum. J. Gen. Physiol. *49:*849–866.

Schwartz, W. B., and Relman, A. S. (1952): Balance studies in two remarkable instances of "pure" chronic potassium depletion resulting from the overuse of laxatives. J. Clin. Invest. *31:*660.

Schwartz, W. B., and Relman, A. S. (1953): Metabolic and renal studies in chronic potassium depletion resulting from overuse of laxatives. J. Clin. Invest. *32:*258–271.

Sladen, G. E., and Harries, J. T. (1972): Studies on the effects of unconjugated dihydroxy bile salts on rat small intestinal function *in vivo.* Biochim. Biophys. Acta *288:*443–456.

Straub, W., and Triendl, E. (1934): *Naunyn-Schmiedebergs Arch. Pharmacol. 175:*528–535.

Teem, M. V., and Phillips, S. F. (1972): Perfusion of the hamster jejunum with conjugated and unconjugated bile acids: Inhibition of water absorption and effects on morphology. Gastroenterology *62:*261–267.

Tidball, C. S. (1964): Magnesium and calcium as regulators of intestinal permeability. Am. J. Physiol. *206:*243–246.

Tormey, J. M., and Diamond, J. M. (1967): The ultrastructural route of fluid transport in rabbit gall bladder. J. Gen. Physiol. *50:*2031–2060.

Wanitschke, R., and Nell, G. (1974): Transfer of sodium and water through the isolated colonic mucosa as a function of the hydrostatic pressure under the influence of oxyphenisatin. Naunyn-Schmiedebergs Arch. Pharmacol. *282:*Suppl. R 104.

Wanitschke, R., Nell, G., and Rummel, W. (1973): The influence of deoxycholate on the unidirectional sodium fluxes in rat colon *in vitro.* Naunyn-Schmiedebergs Arch. Pharmacol. *277:*Suppl. R 87.

Wanitschke, R., Nell, G., and Rummel, W. (1974): *Manuscript in preparation.*

Wolff, H. P., Henne, G., Krück, F., Roscher, S., Vecsei, P., Brown, J., Düsterdieck, G., Lever, A. F., and Robertson, J. I. S. (1968): Psychosomatische Syndrome mit gastroenteralem und/oder renalem Kalium- und Natriumverlust Hyperreninämie und sekundärem Aldosteronismus. Schweizer Med. Wschr. *98:*1883–1892.

Wolff, H. P., Krück, F., Brown, J. J., Lever, A. F., Vecsei, P., Roscher, S., Düsterdieck, G. O., and Robertson, J. I. S. (1968): Psychiatric disturbance leading to potassium depletion, raised plasma-renin concentration and secondary hyperaldosteronism. Lancet 257–261.

DISCUSSION

DIETSCHY cited work from the literature showing that bile acids in the colon stimulated the secretory phenomena, particularly the secretion of hydrogen and bicarbonate against an electrochemical gradient. This in a sense is contrary to the findings in the present chapter postulating a backflux through the tight junction. RUMMEL referred to the differences in the experimental conditions. If the measurements are made *in vitro,* one can find a net flux only if the hydrostatic pressure which is available *in vivo* is simulated; this is the difference between the quoted experiments and his own.

Intestinal Absorption and Malabsorption,
edited by T. Z. Csáky.
Raven Press, New York © 1975

Intestinal Absorption of Sugars in the Human *In Vivo*

John S. Fordtran

University of Texas, Dallas, Texas 75235

I. REGIONAL CONSIDERATIONS AND COMPARISONS WITH OTHER SOLUTES

Table 1 shows the absorption rates of glucose, xylose, urea, tritiated water, and mannitol from the jejunum and ileum of normal human subjects. Glucose absorption is 1.5 times higher in the jejunum than in the ileum, presumably due to the greater surface area of the proximal small intestine. Absorption rates of xylose, urea, and tritiated water are shown for comparison. These solutes are absorbed in direct proportion to their luminal concentrations (at least within concentration ranges that can be studied before severe hyper-

TABLE 1. *Absorbtion rates in the human small intestine in vivo*

	Jejunum	Ileum	Ratio jejunum/ileum
Glucose 105 mM	1.2[a]	0.82[a]	1.5
Xylose	26.9%	4.5%	6.0
Urea	52.2%	19.7%	2.7
Tritiated water	60.1%	55.7%	1.1
Mannitol	0	0	—

[a] mmole/hr/cm.

tonicity is reached), and the results are expressed as a percent of the perfused solute that was absorbed. The marked variation in the ratio of absorption rates in the jejunum and ileum presumably reflects permeability differences between the proximal and distal small bowel (Fordtran, Rector, Ewton et al., 1965; Fordtran, Rector, Locklear et al., 1967). Mannitol is not absorbed to a measurable extent from either region of the human small intestine.

II. KINETICS OF SUGAR TRANSPORT IN HUMANS

Glucose absorption proceeds avidly against steep concentration gradients, as shown in Fig. 1, and glucose absorption is a saturable process, as shown in Fig. 2 (Saltzman, Rector, and Fordtran, 1972). The apparent K_m and

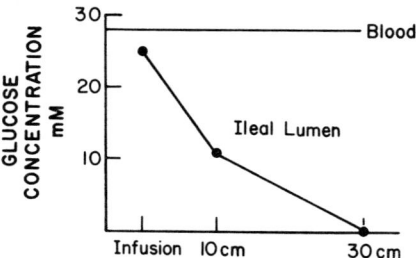

FIG. 1. Ileal absorption of glucose in a subject with diabetes who had marked hyperglycemia. The ileum was perfused with a 25-mM glucose solution. In fluid aspirated 10 and 30 cm distally the glucose concentration was reduced to 10 and 0 mM, due to active glucose absorption against steep concentration gradients.

V_{max} values for ileal absorption of glucose, galactose, 3-O-methyl glucose, and fructose are given in Table 2. Although the K_m is 10 times higher for fructose than for glucose, fructose is absorbed rapidly compared with the other sugars that are not actively transported via the glucose carrier (which

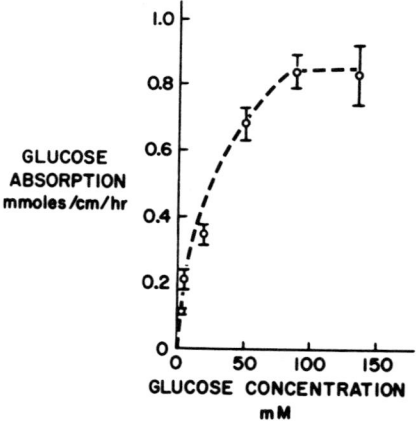

FIG. 2. Rate of human ileal glucose absorption as a function of glucose concentration at the proximal aspiration site of a 3-lumen perfusion tube. From seven to 23 studies were performed at each point. The length of the test segment (between proximal and distal collection sites) varied between 10 and 30 cm, depending on the concentration of sugar infused. Sodium concentration was 50 mEq/l at all glucose concentrations, and mannitol was added to achieve isotonicity with plasma. The test solutions were perfused at a rate of 16 ml/min. Polyethylene glycol was the nonabsorbable volume marker.

TABLE 2. *Apparent kinetic constants for sugar absorption in the human ileum in vivo*

	Km (mM)	V_{max} (mmole/cm/hr)
Glucose	10	0.8
Galactose	71	1.3
3-O-methyl glucose	123	1.4
Fructose	135	1.1

like mannitol are absorbed slowly, if at all). This special mechanism for fructose absorption accounts for the ability of children who lack the glucose-galactose carrier to survive if placed on a fructose diet.

III. EFFECT OF MANNITOL SUBSTITUTION FOR SODIUM

Replacement of sodium by mannitol in the perfusion medium reduces active glucose absorption in the human ileum by approximately 20% (Saltzman et al., 1972). As shown in Fig. 3, even when the sodium concentration rose to only 3 mEq per liter at the end of the test segment, glucose absorption against a concentration gradient occurred almost as rapidly as when luminal sodium concentration was 140 mM.

This limited inhibitory effect of sodium removal was surprising in view of the fact that sugar transport *in vitro* is abolished when sodium is removed completely from the mucosal bathing solution (Schultz, Frizzell, and Nellans, 1974). Moreover, active sugar absorption (or uptake by the mucosal cells)

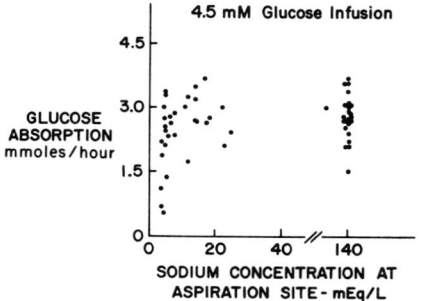

FIG. 3. Rate of human ileal glucose absorption from a 4.5-mM glucose test solution at high and low intraluminal sodium concentrations. The sodium concentration in aspirated ileal fluid is shown. Mannitol replaced sodium in the sodium-free test solutions used to obtain the low intraluminal sodium concentrations.

is reduced eightfold when sodium concentration is reduced from 145 to 24 mEq per liter *in vitro* (Crane, Forstner, and Eicholz, 1965).

IV. EFFECT OF MAGNESIUM SUBSTITUTION FOR SODIUM

It seemed possible that the limited effect of sodium removal on *in vivo* glucose absorption, demonstrated in the previous section, might be related to the fact that mannitol, rather than another cation, was used as a sodium substitute. It is known from the work of others that the mucosal surface of the intestine is negatively charged (Hogben, Tocco, Brodie et al., 1959; Vassar, 1963). These charges might maintain a high intraluminal sodium concentration at the brush border, even when a sodium-free mannitol solution is perfused. The effect of mannitol and magnesium (as substitutes for sodium) on active sugar absorption was therefore compared (Biederdorf, Morawski, and Fordtran, 1974). Mannitol substitution for sodium reduced glucose absorption (4.5 mM) by 23%, whereas when magnesium was the cation, glucose absorption was inhibited by 45%. Kinetic data revealed that magnesium replacement of sodium raised the apparent K_m for glucose transport but had no effect on V_{max}. Magnesium had no effect on the absorption of glucose when 70-mM sodium was present in the perfusate. Results with galactose (10 mM) and 3-O-methyl glucose (10 mM) were somewhat different, in that both mannitol and magnesium substitution for sodium inhibited absorption by about 50%. Fructose absorption (25 mM) was not inhibited by magnesium substitution for sodium.

V. EFFECT OF UNSTIRRED WATER LAYERS

One possible explanation for the limited *in vivo* inhibitory effect of sodium removal on active sugar absorption is that thick unstirred water layers *in vivo* may result in a high concentration of sodium at the brush border, even when luminal sodium concentration is near zero. When sodium is removed from the intestinal lumen, sodium in plasma diffuses into the lumen, either through the intercellular spaces and tight junctions, or across mucosal cell membranes. Thick unstirred water layers might retard sodium diffusion away from the brush border. Therefore, even when sodium-free solutions are perfused into the lumen, sodium concentration at the glucose transport site might be high.

That stirring *in vivo* is relatively poor is supported by the following considerations. The human small bowel cannot be perfused more rapidly than about 30 ml/min without producing severe discomfort, and perfusion rates of this magnitude are unlikely to significantly reduce the unstirred water layer thickness beyond that present at standard perfusion rates of 9 to 16 ml/min. Considering the geometry of the human small bowel lumen, Schultz et al. (1974) have concluded that human perfusion studies have all been done under conditions of very poor stirring, compared to most experiments carried out *in vitro*.

To evaluate this problem, experiments were carried out in the rat ileum *in vivo*, where intestinal loops can be perfused at high rates and where the smaller diameter of the intestine allows greater stirring for any given perfusion rate (Lewis and Fordtran, 1974). Absorption of 4-mM glucose at perfusion rates from 1 to 200 ml/min confirmed an important effect of unstirred water layers on the rate of active glucose absorption. However, even at 200 ml/min perfusion rate, glucose absorption from a magnesium solution occurred at greater than half the rate noted with 140-mM NaCl solutions. There was no evidence that very high perfusion rates, which should thin the unstirred water layer, enhanced the inhibitory effect of sodium removal on glucose absorption. These results confirm our earlier theoretic arguments (Saltzman et al., 1972) against the hypothesis that unstirred water layers can explain that component of active sugar transport that persists during perfusion of sodium-free solutions *in vivo*.

VI. CONCLUSIONS

(a) The greater effect of magnesium than mannitol in depressing glucose absorption in a sodium-free medium is probably due to a greater lowering of sodium concentration at the transport site on the brush border membrane.

(b) The magnesium effect is probably due to displacement of sodium from fixed negative charges on the brush border.

(c) Lowering the sodium concentration at the transport site decreases the apparent affinity of the transport carrier for glucose, galactose, and 3-O-methyl glucose, since sodium removal reduces apparent K_m but not V_{max} for glucose transport.

(d) A modest reduction in sodium concentration at the transport site (mannitol substitution for sodium) results in a near maximum inhibition of absorption of galactose and 3-O-methyl glucose (low-affinity sugars for the glucose transport system); in contrast, absorption of glucose itself (a high-affinity sugar) is minimally inhibited by a modest reduction of sodium.

(e) In the presence of a very low luminal sodium concentration (down to 2 mEq/l) and a very high magnesium concentration (which should effectively displace sodium from fixed negative charges on the brush border), active sugar absorption proceeds at about half the rate noted in the presence of a high luminal sodium concentration.

(f) Although unstirred water layers have a large effect on the rate of ileal active glucose absorption *in vivo*, these layers probably cannot explain the component (approximately half) of active sugar transport which persists during perfusion of sodium-free solutions *in vivo*.

(g) There are at least three possible reasons why active sugar absorption persists *in vivo* but not *in vitro* when luminal sodium concentration is reduced to near zero. First, some unknown mechanism for maintaining a high concentration of sodium at the transport site when luminal sodium concentration is near zero may be operative *in vivo* but not *in vitro*. Second, most *in vitro* experiments have involved sodium removal from the serosal as well as the mucosal side of the intestinal mucosa. Removal of sodium from both surfaces may be needed to completely inhibit active sugar transport. And, third, sodium independent active sugar transport may exist *in vivo* but be lost *in vitro*. There is some precedent for this suggestion; for example, active absorption of chloride is a prominent feature of ileal function *in vivo* but cannot be demonstrated in most *in vitro* preparations of ileal tissue.

REFERENCES

Bieberdorf, F. A., Morawski, S., and Fordtran, J. S. (1974): Effect of sodium, mannitol, and magnesium on glucose, galactose, 3-O-methyl glucose and fructose absorption in the human ileum, submitted for publication.
Crane, R. K., Forstner, G., and Eichholz, A. (1965): Studies on the mechanism of the intestinal absorption of sugars. X. An effect of Na^+ concentration on the apparent Michaelis constants for intestinal sugar transport, *in vitro*. Biochim. Biophys. Acta *109:*467.
Fordtran, J. S., Rector, F. C., Ewton, M. F., et al. (1965): Permeability characteristics of the human small intestine. J. Clin. Invest. *44:*1935.
Fordtran, J. S., Rector, F. C., Locklear, T. W., et al. (1967): Water and solute movement in the small intestine of patients with sprue. J. Clin. Invest. *46:*287.
Hogben, C. A. M., Tocco, D. J., Brodie, B. B., et al. (1959): On the mechanism of intestinal absorption of drugs. J. Pharmacol. Exp. Ther. *125:*275.
Lewis, L. D., and Fordtran, J. S. (1974): Effect of perfusion rate on luminal pressure and on the rate of urea and glucose absorption (with and without NaCl) in the rat ileum *in vivo*. Gastroenterology *66:*A-223 (Abstract).
Saltzman, D. A., Rector, F. C., Jr., and Fordtran, J. S. (1972): The role of intraluminal sodium in glucose absorption *in vivo*. J. Clin. Invest. *51:*876.
Schultz, S. G., Frizzell, R. A., and Nellans, H. N. (1974): Ion transport by mammalian small intestine. Ann. Rev. Physiol. *36:*51.
Vassar, P. S. (1963): The electric charge density of human tumor cell surfaces. Lab. Invest. *12:*1072.

DISCUSSION

FRIZZELL mentioned some of their recent experiments in which sodium was replaced only on the mucosal surface: this abolished the active 3-O-methyl glucose transport into the ileum of the rabbit or rat. FORDTRAN remarked that this would confirm Csáky's finding of several years ago and wondered what would happen if one removed sodium from only the serosal surface. PARSONS stated that in his preparation of the vascularly perfused frog one can replace ions both in the lumen and in the submucosal circulating blood or nutrient medium. He finds that the absence of sodium in the lumen decreases the glucose uptake but does not abolish it. However, when the vascular sodium is also replaced, then the active sugar transport almost completely disappears.

CURRAN wondered if the failure to see a change in the sodium movement in the ileum when glucose is introduced is not due to the fact that the electric potential difference went up to 10 to 15 mV; in *in vitro* preparations one can stop the net sodium absorption by imposing about 10 mV potential difference across the tissue. FORDTRAN agreed and pointed out that Modigliani and Bernier have shown that glucose does not alter net glucose absorption rate in the human ileum but that it increases unidirectional flux rate in both directions across the mucosa (*Biologie et Gastro-Entérologie,* 5:165, 1972). This is strong evidence that glucose enhances active Na absorption in the human ileum but that the PD so generated increases Na backflux so that net Na absorption is not changed.

CSÁKY referred to some of his own experiments in which he found that if sodium is replaced with mannitol only about 50% inhibition was obtained but if the replacing ion was potassium or lithium 80 to 95% inhibition was obtained. He was concerned about sodium leaking out *in vivo* into the unstirred layer, and therefore he repeated the perfusion experiments with a suspension of a special resin which absorbs all the sodium; this decreased further the sugar transport. FORDTRAN wondered what was the difference between their experiments and that of Csáky's as they could never reduce their absorption rate below 50% regardless of whether they replaced sodium with magnesium or with mannitol even at very high perfusion rates that should reduce unstirred water layer thickness.

CURRAN questioned some of Fordtran's experiments in which in some situations there was a substantial stimulation of the fluid reabsorption but not a comparable stimulation of the sodium reabsorption. This would be inconsistent with the hypothesis that the increased fluid flow affects sodium absorption. FORDTRAN replied that much depended on the anion that was present in the lumen. When the passive anion absorption nears zero, one can obtain a lot of water absorption and no stimulation of the sodium transport; consequently, he theorizes that when water flow is generated sodium absorption will be stimulated in either direction depending on the direction of the water flow provided an anion such as chloride, which can move passively across the mucosa, is present with the sodium.

Intestinal Absorption and Malabsorption,
edited by T. Z. Csáky.
Raven Press, New York © 1975

The Role of the Intestinal Flora in Absorption: A Comparative Study Between Germ-free and Conventional Animals

H. A. Gordon

Department of Pharmacology, College of Medicine, University of Kentucky, Lexington, Kentucky 40506

INTRODUCTION

The successful rearing of germ-free animals has permitted the performance of critical studies on the effects of microbial associates in the host animal. Due to the intimate relationship that exists between the intestinal flora and the host, a prime target for research in this area has been the gastrointestinal tract. Actually, the first characteristic observed in germ-free animals around the turn of the century was the marked enlargement and semiliquid contents of the cecum in guinea pigs (1). The lack of effects of the microbial flora in the germ-free gastrointestinal tract becomes evident early and persist throughout life. Essential features in this context are the following: (a) low levels of defensive elements in the intestinal mucosa; (b) altered digestive preparation of nutrients and metabolites in the gut lumen, also affecting electrolyte and water transport; (c) anomalies of intestinal smooth muscle tone; (d) reduction of regional blood flow in the mesenteric area. In spite of these characteristics, germ-free animals grow and mature normally.

The most common animals used in germ-free work are the rat and the mouse. These are descendants of self-reproducing colonies of germ-free parent animals, originally derived by cesarean section and by hand-feeding liquid diets. In gut-oriented germ-free studies, later, other rodents, the chicken, the dog, and the pig have been included. In general, most work in our area attempts to portray the effects of the flora on the host by comparative studies conducted between germ-free and conventional animals. Often antibiotic-treated conventional animals are added to these groups in order to assess the actions of flora neutralization as it may be effected in conventional life. Germ-free animals are housed in isolators and are fed complete diets, fortified for heat sterilization losses. Conventional and antibiotic-treated controls are usually maintained in the open animal colony room and are fed the same sterilized diet as their germ-free counterparts. It is of interest to note that germ-free animals exposed to the conventional environment survive the transition well and within 3 to 4 weeks become indistinguishable from conventional controls. These, and other aspects of germ-free experimentation have recently been reviewed (2).

I. MORPHOLOGIC CONSIDERATIONS

The weight of the wall of the intestinal canal (expressed per unit body weight) has been found significantly reduced in all animal species reared hitherto in the germ-free state (chicken, 3; rat, 4; pig, 5). This is mainly due to a reduction of scattered reticuloendothelial cells, Peyers patches (6, 7), and connective elements (7) in the mucosa and submucosa. The moisture content of the intestinal wall of germ-free animals is often found reduced (3–5), bordering on and sometimes reaching the degree of significance. The counterparts of these characteristics seen in conventional animals (elevated levels of RE cells, connective elements, and of hydration in the gut wall, as well as increased mesenteric blood flow, see Sec. IV) are viewed as a response of the host to the presence of the intestinal flora and have been summed up as representatives of mild "physiologic" inflammation (4). Such changes appear also to have a morphogenic effect on the mucosal contour. In pigs monoassociated with *E. coli* uniformly slender villi have been observed, whereas in conventional controls they appeared club shaped, often stunted, with a tendency to fusion (8). In germ-free rats the greater uniformity of intestinal villi has also been observed. In these animals the total mucosal surface area of the small intestine (mainly in its lower portions) indicated significantly lower values than in conventional controls (9). In the intestinal epithelium of germ-free mice lower renewal rates have been observed (10). The mitosis indices of these cells have been found uniformly low in the duodenum and the ileum of germ-free rats and uniformly high in these gut segments of conventional controls (11). The possibility that the gut flora is directly influencing cell renewal (e.g., by increasing cell attrition) is improbable, because of the great differences in microbial population which exist between the duodenum and ileum of conventional animals. It appears more probable that the proliferative capacity of these cells is uniformly depressed in the germ-free state and elevated in the conventional state (see Secs. III and IV).

II. DIGESTION AND ABSORPTION

Digestive Enzymes

Markedly elevated levels of trypsin and chymotrypsin have been found in intestinal contents (12, 13) and in feces (14) of germ-free animals. Pancreatic trypsinogen and chymotrypsinogen levels, on the other hand, were similar in the opposing animal groups (15). Among releasing enzymes of bioactive peptides, elevated levels of a protease (MAS) tentatively identified as fecal kallikrein have been found in the intestinal contents of germ-free rats and mice (16). The difficulty in differentiating this enzyme from trypsin (17) may in part be resolved by the fact that both glandular kallikrein (18) and MAS (16) show approximately 20 times higher values in rats, in comparison to mice, whereas trypsin levels in the intestinal contents of these two animal species are essentially similar (13). The levels of amylase and lipase in the intestinal contents also seem to be modified in germ-free animals; however the results do not show a uniform trend (12, 15). Thus, at least for proteases in the gut, germ-free life appears to impart an enzyme-sparing effect to the host.

Absorption from the Small Intestine

Relatively little work has been done in this area. In one study (19) in which glucose or 3-methyl glucose was fed by stomach tube to rats enhanced absorption was found in the germ-free group in comparison to conventional controls. This was later corroborated by another study (20), which was conducted in rats using glucose and xylose in an *in vivo* intestinal perfusion-type experiment. The absorption of water from the germ-free small intestine (as indicated by the dry percent of its contents, see Fig. 1) appears to be similar in germ-free and conventional animals. In a recent study (21) increased absorption of glucose and of some vitamins of the B complex has been found from the small intestine of germ-free chickens in comparison to conventional controls. It is speculated that the small intestine of germ-free animals, which

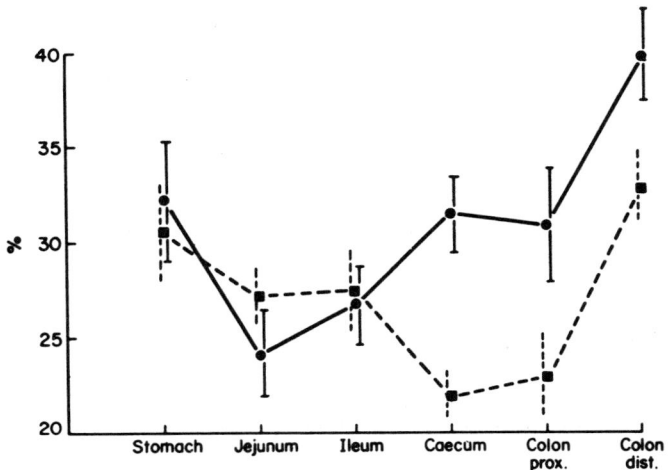

FIG. 1. Percentage of dry matter of the intestinal contents in various segments of the gastrointestinal tract of mice (Swiss-Webster strain, 12 to 13 weeks old, 25 to 30 g females fed sterilized L-462 diet, nine mice per group). Arithmetic means and standard deviations (cross bars). Germ-free, - - -; conventional ———. From ref. 22.

is not burdened by an excess of defensive and connective elements, represents a more effective absorptive membrane than its conventional counterpart. In apparent contradiction to the enhanced absorption of carbohydrates from the germ-free small intestine is the observation, that by the time the germ-free gut content reaches the cecum, its level of free amino acids is markedly elevated (22). This characteristic might be related to the slightly higher food intake of germ-free animals that was observed in some studies (22, 23), to the mentioned increase of digestive enzymes, and to the elevated levels of fecal nitrogen excretion found in germ-free animals (24, 25). The difficulty in assessing the role that the microbial share of nitrogen in the intestinal contents plays in this context (and which is missing in the germ-free group) renders proper evaluation of these results difficult. Yet, as evidenced by their normal growth curves and maturation, no marked difference in nitrogen balance appears to exist between germ-free animals and conventional controls fed complete diets (26).

Solute and Water Absorption from the Lower Bowel

It has previously been mentioned that the contents of the cecum are more liquid in germ-free rodents than in their conventional counterparts (1). This is illustrated for mice in Fig. 1. Recently, these findings could be extended also to the chicken (3), the dog (27), and the pig (5). In addition to the excess of water the contents of the germ-free lower bowel show differences in other components. Thus, elevated levels of mucus (13, 28) and of amino acids that are typical of mucus (22) have been found in cecal contents of germ-free rats and mice. Fecal hexosamine excretion (29) was elevated in germ-free rats. It was indicated (30) that the excess of mucus and of related substances inhibits water absorption and is therefore responsible for the more liquid contents of the germ-free lower bowel. Certain types of mucinases, which are normally present in the intestinal contents of conventional rats, were not found in their germ-free counterparts (31). In addition, it was shown (32) that the Cl^- concentration in the cecal contents of germ-free rats is extremely low and that on feeding chloride-yielding resins to these animals, the cecal enlargement may be reduced. Oral antibiotic treatment of conventional animals, which results in partial neutralization of the intestinal flora appears to cause changes in the lower bowel, which are qualitatively similar to those seen in germ-free animals (33, 34).

In a study (35) aiming at the elucidation of the mechanism of these changes we have harvested contents and prepared supernatants (by spinning at 15,000 g for 10 min) from the cecum of germ-free and conventional rats. An additional group consisted of conventional rats that were receiving over a period of days or weeks streptomycin, bacitracin, and nystatin dissolved in the drinking water (34). Placing the supernatants on a cationic exchange resin column (Biorex 70 in H^+ form), acidic to neutral components were obtained in the initial samples of the effluent ("initial pool"). The characteristics of the initial pool derived from the germ-free cecal supernatant are illustrated on Fig. 2. The presence of mucus and congeners in these samples was shown by coinciding peaks of hexuronic acid content, viscosity, titratable acidity, and colloid osmotic pressure. Despite the H^+ form of the resin used, sizable amounts of Na^+ were found retained in the effluent. Information on the molecular weight of the compounds in the initial pool that were obtained by gel filtration (Sephadex 100) of various supernatants is given in Fig. 3. The effluent of the germ-free initial pool showed a peak of 80,000 MW, containing mucus components, and a second, 20,000 MW peak. Initial pool prepared from conventional rat supernatant showed only the 20,000 MW but not the macromolecular peak. Samples derived from antibiotic-treated conventional rats indicated the presence of a reduced yet

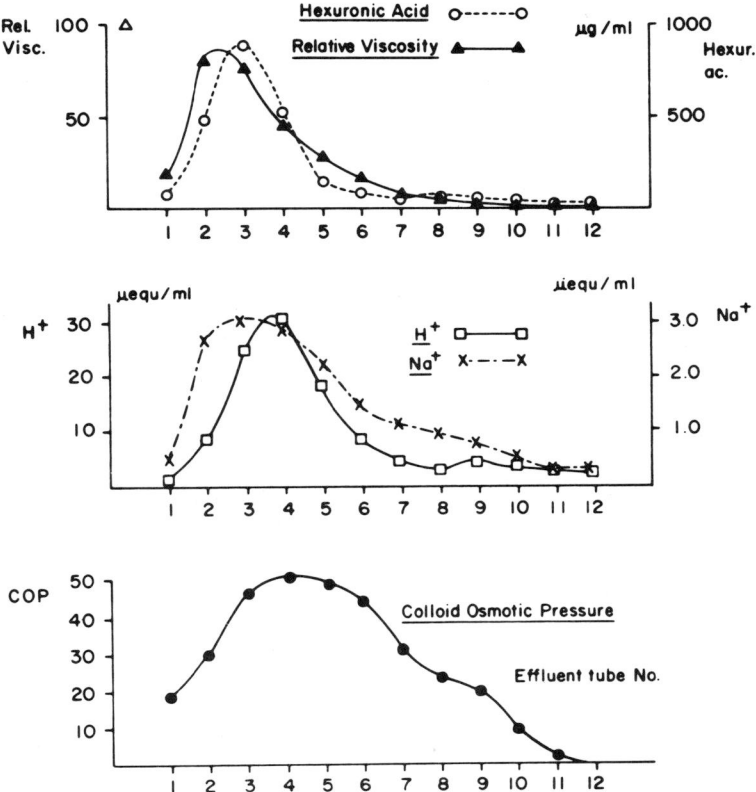

FIG. 2. Characteristics and solutes of effluent (first 12 tubes) from germ-free rat cecal supernatant on cationic exchange resin column (Biorex 70, H^+). Gradient elution: 0.01 to 0.25 N NaOH. "Initial pool." From ref. 34.

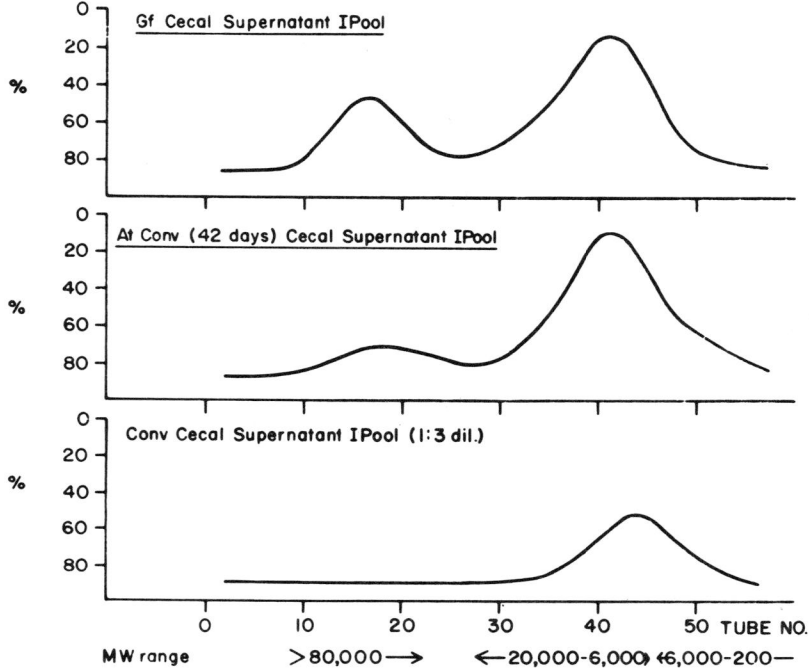

FIG. 3. Gel filtration (Sephadex 100) of effluent (tubes 3–4) from cationic column (Biorex 70, H^+); maximum solute concentration in "initial pool." Transmission at 253 nm. From ref. 35.

sizable quantity of macromolecular substances. Additional observations in the cecal supernatants showed that the total osmolality of the germ-free and of the antibiotic-treated specimens was essentially isosmotic with blood plasma, whereas it was hypertonic in case of the conventional cecal supernatant. Colloid osmotic pressure (in mm Hg), on the other hand, was greatly elevated in the germ-free specimens (107 ± 9) and essentially similar to that of blood plasma in case of the conventional samples (40 ± 8) with the antibiotic-treated specimens showing intermediate values (63 ± 4). An attempt to portray in a simplified form the ionic balance in cecal supernatants of our various animal groups is given in Table 1. Total Na^+ and K^+ were found relatively close in all three groups. Among anions, the germ-free and antibiotic-treated specimens contained little Cl^- or HCO_3^- but held sizable amounts of colloidal anions. In conventional samples Cl^- and HCO_3^- seemed to match the cations, and no colloidal anions were present. Based on these findings, our speculation on the mechanism of the anomalous water absorption in the lower bowel of germ-free and antibiotic-treated conventional animals is illustrated in Fig. 4. Water absorption inhibition (or even water efflux from the tissues into the lumen) under these circumstances might be precipitated by two

TABLE 1. Partial "ionic balance sheet" of cecal supernatants (undiluted)

	Cations		Anions		Muco- polysacch. >80,000	Muco- peptides 20,000–6,000
	Na$^+$	K$^+$	Cl$^-$	HCO$_3^-$		
			μEq/ml			
Germ-free	61	17	0.6	8	+++	+++
At conv (42 days)[a]	77	23	3.5		++	+++
Conventional	58	26	17	30	0	+++

[a] Length of antibiotic treatment.
Reproduced from ref. 35.

additive causes. One of these is the marked luminal colloid water attraction, the other is the trapping of cations by the acidic colloids, "starving" thereby the solute-coupled water absorption system, i.e., the sodium pump. Partial corroboration of this speculation is offered in Fig. 5. Here net water transport is shown from the ligated cecal sac of germ-free rats *in vivo* whose natural content was replaced by various solutions.

In case the luminal liquid was saline (i.e., a plentiful supply of needed ions was present in diffusible form) marked absorption of water and NaCl took place. This was actually the triple value of that seen in conventional controls (see also 36), indicating that there was no inherent defect in the germ-free cecal mucosa. Elevating the colloid osmotic pressure in the lumen to values observed in germ-free cecal supernatant, yet maintaining adequate levels of NaCl (by using a 10% polyvinylpyrrolidone solution in saline), water absorption was reduced but not stopped. Cessation of water absorption could be achieved only by using a germ-free cecal supernatant that showed elevated

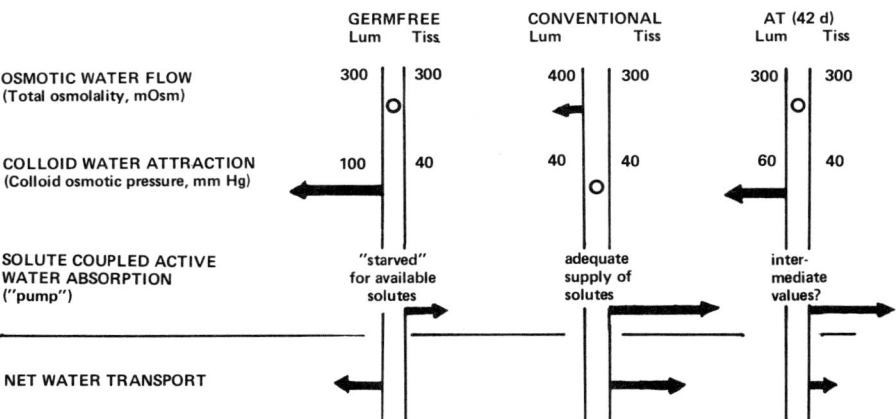

FIG. 4. Water transport across the cecal wall.

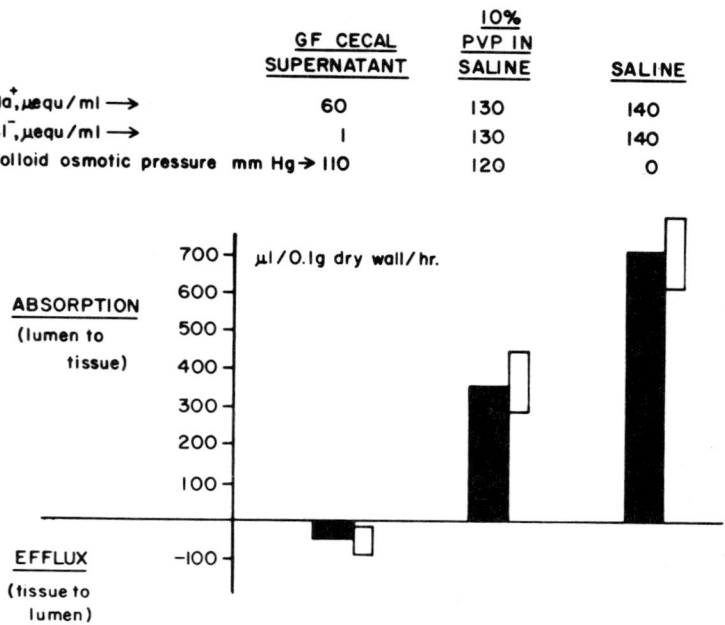

FIG. 5. Net water transport in germ-free rat's ligated cecal sac (3 hr experiment *in vivo*) when natural contents are replaced by similar amounts of GF cecal supernatant, 10% PVP in saline, and saline. From ref. 35.

values of colloid osmotic pressure combined with high levels of (presumably trapped) sodium and low levels of diffusible anions.

The adaptative changes that the germ-free cecal mucosa musters on the constant condition of water absorption inhibition have been indicated also by other observations. Thus, the NaCl threshold levels at which solute-coupled water absorption stops in ligated cecal sacs was found lower in germ-free than in conventional rats (37). Recently, elevated levels of Na^+- and K^+-dependent ATPase were found in the cecal mucosa of germ-free rats (38) which were similar to those that were obtained on inhibiting water absorption via feeding nonabsorbable diet additives (e.g., polyethyleneglycol) in conventional rats (39). By the same token, the intestinal mucosa of germ-free rats was found to utilize more O_2 (in nmoles/min/g scrapings, 516 ± 137) than that of conventional controls (265 ± 116).

III. INTESTINAL MUSCLE TONE AND PERISTALSIS

The considerable distension of the cecum and the reduction of muscle tone of the lower bowel in germ-free rodents are apparent to the observer. Other species (chicken, pig, dog), when reared in the germ-free state either do not show these changes or develop them to a much lesser degree. In germ-free rodents (4) the cecal sac weighs about twice as much as in conventional controls (whereas the weight of the contents amounts to 6 to 20% of the bodyweight in the germ-free group). In the weight-increment of the cecal wall the cytoplasmic component of the muscularis takes the largest share (23). In view of the marked distension all elements of the cecal wall are considerably thinned out. Recently, a detailed study on the ultrastructure of the germ-free rat cecum has been published (40). Lower muscle tone in the germ-free cecal wall has been suggested by observations that showed that on application of epinephrine to quiescent cecal strips *in vitro* the germ-free specimens indicated a significantly lower degree of relaxation than conventional controls (41). Anomalies of the germ-free rat cecal muscle have been shown also by another work (42), which indicated that normal spontaneous contractions could not be shown in germ-free cecal strips and that these preparations were less sensitive to acetylcholine and to epinephrine. Changes in autonomic innervation may also play a role in these phenomena. Thus, structural differences in the primary plexus of Auerbach and a greatly increased size of myenteric neurons have been found in the cecal wall of germ-free rats (43). The passage time of intestinal contents through the entire gastrointestinal tract of germ-free rats has been found to have increased (44).

The cause of the reduced intestinal muscle tone of germ-free rodents is unclear. The nature of the diet appears to modify it. It is common experience that feeding purified diets to germ-free rodents will result in smaller ceca, while high bulk-type diets will have opposite effects. Attempts have been made to correlate the presence of certain metabolites that accumulate in the lower bowel contents of germ-free rodents to the reduced intestinal muscle tone. Among these is the substance tentatively identified as a direct-acting fecal kallikrein (16). Recently, it was indicated that the elevated levels of free amino acids that were found in the lower bowel contents of germ-free rodents (22) might also be implicated in this phenomenon (45, 46). Thus a chromatographic fraction rich in free amino acids prepared from germ-free cecal supernatant or individual implicated amino acids proved strongly inhibitory to the spontaneous rhythmic contractions of intestinal villi in dogs. The possibility that free amino acids are involved in germ-free rodents' reduced intestinal smooth muscle tone is indicated also by preliminary observations that suggest that animal species that do not show elevated levels of free amino acids in their lower bowel contents (dog, pig) do not develop pronounced signs of intestinal muscle anomalies.

IV. CIRCULATORY EFFECTS

In germ-free rats (the only germ-free animal whose circulation has been studied to date) regional blood flow was found to be depressed. The reduction was most conspicuous in areas that in normal life are intimately associated with the microbial flora, i.e., in all elements of the gastrointestinal tract, the airways, and the integument (23). Cardiac output (47) and metabolic rate (O_2 consumption, 48) were also reduced. Probing vascular responsiveness to various smooth muscle agonists, mesenteric microvessels (precapillary arterioles) in germ-free rats were found highly refractory to epinephrine, vasopressin, and angiotensin (49, 50). On surgical removal of the enlarged cecum early in life and maintaining the germ status of these animals, the listed elements of circulatory and metabolic depression were found to wane (48 and Table 2). This has concentrated our search on substances in the intestinal contents of germ-free animals which on uptake into the enterohepatic circulation might be responsible for the state of depression.

By ion exchange chromatography and gel filtration, a pigment (named alpha pigment) was found (51) in the effluent from the germ-free rat cecal supernatant, which on intravenous injection reduced the hypertensive effect of epinephrine in conventional rats. On topical application onto the exteriorized jejunal mucosa of dogs the alpha pigment increased the spontaneous rhythmic contractions of intestinal villi (a sign that follows the application of epinephrine inhibitory substances). Considering various agents that are known to impart epinephrine refractoriness to smooth muscle, the effects of the alpha pigment were compared to those of ferritin, whose VDM-type actions ("vasodepressor material") have previously been described (52).

TABLE 2. Cardiac output,[a] epinephrine threshold, vascular smooth muscle[b] regional blood flow[c] in unoperated and cecectomized germ-free and conventional rats

	Germ-free[i]	Conventional[i]
I. Unoperated		
Cardiac output[d]	137 ± 7	203 ± 11
Epinephrine threshold[e]		
Vascular sm. muscle	13.7 ± 3.2	0.4 ± 0.1
Regional blood flow[f]		
Small intestine	11.8 ± 2.6	25.6 ± 4.7
Cecum	2.6 ± 0.4	3.3 ± 1.1
Large intestine	2.3 ± 0.6	4.0 ± 0.8
Liver (arterial)	7.4 ± 1.5	14.5 ± 0.8
Liver (portal)	17.7 ± 2.9	32.6 ± 5.1
II. Cecectomized		
Cardiac output[g]	201 ± 11	218 ± 5
Epinephrine threshold[h]	1.8 ± 0.80	0.8 ± 0.1

[a] ml/min/kg bwt.
[b] Dose of norepinephrine (μg/ml) which on topical application causes 40 to 50% constriction in exteriorized precapillary arterioles.
[c] Whole organ, ml/min/kg bwt.
[d] From ref. 47.
[e] From ref. 49.
[f] From ref. 23.
[g] From ref. 48.
[h] From ref. 50.
[i] Means ± SD.

On successive bioassay on the dog villus model, using a variety of specific activator and blocking substances, the effects of the germ-free alpha pigment aligned closely to that of ferritin (51). We speculate that the alpha pigment in the intestinal contents originates from ferritin which on desquamation of the epithelial cells is known to reach the lumen in sizable quantities. Here digestive enzymes break up the large ferritin molecule to smaller fractions (MW of the alpha pigment averages around 4,000, but smaller fractions capable of absorption appear to exist) that in germ-free conditions retain their VDM effect. Partial evidence of absorption of the alpha pigment (in addition to epinephrine refractoriness found in germ-free rat mesenteric microvessels, 49) was supplied by observations that indicated that the portal blood of germ-free rats, on topical application, enhances villus motility, whereas this effect was essentially absent when conventional portal blood is used (53). In addition, samples rich in the alpha pigment, prepared from the germ-free rat cecal supernatant, when topically applied onto the mesocecum of conventional rats was found to impart epinephrine refractoriness to precapillary arterioles in a reversible fashion (54). In conventional animals, on action of the intestinal flora, the quantity and effectiveness of the alpha pigment is greatly reduced. The mechanism whereby the flora inactivates the alpha pigment is unknown. The refractoriness to vasopressin and angiotensin found in vascular smooth muscle of germ-free rats also awaits elucidation.

No studies have been conducted to date on the correlation between intestinal absorption and mesenteric blood flow in germ-free animals. Considering the marked reduction of mesenteric blood flow, along with the evidence of intact nutrient supply of these animals, the absorptive function of the germ-free intestinal mucosa (chiefly of the small intestine) must be considered fairly efficient. Perhaps the reduction of the germ-free mucosa to its "absorptive essentials" (by reduced participation of defensive and connective elements) contributes to this picture.

V. SUMMARY AND COMMENT

It appears that in normal life the flora affects intestinal function by imparting elements of mild inflammation to the gut wall, and by neutralizing bioactive metabolites of the host in the lower bowel, which when left unchecked, will depress water absorption, intestinal muscle tone, and blood circulation. These effects of the flora have been observed in all hitherto examined animal species, except the action on intestinal muscle tone, which is evident only in rodents. The identity of flora elements which by eliminating the anomalies of intestinal absorption in germ-free animals exert a clearly synergistic, needed effect on the host is essentially unknown.

In absorption from the upper reaches of the intestine an obstructive action of the flora has been observed, which might be caused by the mild inflammatory response elicited in the mucosa. This effect, however, is probably slight and compensated for by the flora-induced, increased mesenteric blood circulation.

In the lower portions of the bowel, starting with a fairly sharp demarcation line at the ileocecal valve, the presence of the flora is indispensable for maintaining the integrity of intestinal function. Here the host appears to rely on the flora for the enzymatic degradation of the "colloid pool" that results in the lumen from partly digested glandular secretions and epithelial desquamation. In the case of the absence of the flora, or when the implicated flora elements are neutralized by antibiotics, the accumulation of nonabsorbable, acidic colloids will retain water in the lumen and trap cations, which are needed for the maintenance of solute-coupled water absorption. Through these, chronically loose stools or even diarrhea will ensue. These changes by themselves do not appear to be particularly detrimental to the animal's health, although, e.g., on discontinuation of antibiotics, it may be difficult to establish a balanced flora that is capable of normal mucus degradation.

It is speculated that germ-free-type anomalies of the intestinal muscle tone, which develop mainly in rodents, are based on the accumulation of directly or indirectly acting depressant metabolites in the gut lumen, whose effect will reach the intestinal muscle. In this context, free amino acids and kallikrein, a releasing enzyme of hypotensive peptides, have been implicated. Among the anomalies of germ-free animals, this is the one that leads to life-threatening situations, indicating therefore the importance of the microbial associates which are engaged in redressing it. This is illustrated by the fact that in colonies of aging germ-free mice (55) the prevalent lesions observed at natural death were extreme distension of the lower bowel, cessation of peristaltic movement, and generally the development of conditions that resemble the paralytic ileum. In addition, considerable dilatation of the gall bladder and, paradoxically, obstructing intestinal volvuli have been observed in these animals.

Another class of bioactive metabolites that await neutralization by the flora in the gut lumen are depressant substances that on absorption impart contractile refractoriness to vascular smooth muscle. The variety of agonists (epinephrine, vasopressin, angiotensin) to which such refractoriness develops in the absence of the flora indicates that several types of depressors in the gut are involved here. Ferritin components derived from the desquamation of epithelial cells, with their epinephrine inhibitory VDM effects, appear to form one group of them. The importance of this class of substances is also indicated by the fact that in the absence of the flora, from young age on, they seem to be implicated not only in the reduction of mesenteric blood flow, but also in generalized circulatory effects, such as the depression of cardiac output. It might even be conceivable that the flora, by neutralization of these absorbable epinephrine inhibitory agents in the gut, indirectly support the calorigenic action of endogenous epinephrine, thereby raising the overall metabolic rate. This may be reflected by the reduced oxygen consumption observed in germ-free animals and by the waning of the reduced cardiac output and oxygen consumption in these hosts after surgical removal of their large cecal pool of depressant substances. The state of vascular hyporesponsiveness of germ-free animals does not appear to have adverse effects on their health.

These observations indicate that in studies on intestinal absorption, the "physiologic" effects of the flora must be considered in a variety of details, and that gnotobiotic methodology, which is readily available today, represents a critical tool in their evaluation.

ACKNOWLEDGMENTS

This work was supported by U.S. Public Health Service grant AM 14621 from the National Institute of Arthritis, Metabolism, and Digestive Diseases, for which the author expresses his sincere gratitude. He also thanks Academic Press, Inc., New York, for kindly permitting reproduction of article, Table 1 and Figs. 1–3 and 5 that have appeared in two of their publications (refs. 23 and 35, respectively).

REFERENCES

1. Nuttal, G. H. F., and Thierfelder, H. (1896–1897): Thierisches Leben ohne Bakterien im Verdauungskanal. II. Mitt. Hoppe Seyler's Z. Physiol. Chem. 22:62–73.
2. Gordon, H. A., and Pesti, L. (1971): The gnotobiotic animal as a tool in the study of host microbial relationships. Bact. Rev. 35:390–429.
3. Reyniers, J. A., Wagner, M., Luckey, T. D., and Gordon, H. A. (1960): Survey of germfree animals: The white Wyandotte Bantam and white Leghorn chicken. In: *Lobund Reports* No. 3, edited by J. A. Reyniers, University of Notre Dame Press, Notre Dame, Indiana, pp. 7–159.
4. Gordon, H. A., Bruckner-Kardoss, E., Staley, T. E., Wagner, M., and Wostmann, B. S. (1966): Characteristics of the germfree rat. Acta. Anat. 64:367–389.
5. Miniats, O. P., and Valli, V. E. (1973): The gastrointestinal tract of gnotobiotic pigs. In: *Germfree Research,* edited by J. B. Heneghan. Academic Press, New York, p. 575.
6. Bauer, H., Horowitz, R. E., Levenson, S. M., and Popper, H. (1963): The response of the lymphatic tissue to the microbial flora. Studies on germfree mice. Amer. J. Pathol. 42:471–483.
7. Gordon, H. A., and Bruckner-Kardoss, E. (1961): Effects of the normal flora on various tissue elements of the small intestine. Acta Anat. 44:210–225.
8. Keworthy, R., and Allen, W. D. (1966): Influence of diet and bacteria on small intestinal morphology, with special reference to early weaning and *Escherichia coli.* J. Comp. Pathol. 76:291–296.
9. Gordon, H. A., and Bruckner-Kardoss, E. (1961): Effect of normal microbial flora on intestinal surface area. Amer. J. Physiol. 201:175–178.
10. Abrams, G. D., Bauer, H., and Sprinz, H. (1963): Influence of the normal flora on mucosal morphology and cellular renewal in the ileum. A comparison of germfree and conventional mice. Lab. Invest. 12:355–364.
11. Guenet, J. L., Sacquet, E., Gueneau, G., and Meslin, J. C. (1970): Action de la

microflore total du rat sur l'activité mitotique des cryptes de Lieberkühn. C.R. Acad. Sci. Paris *270:*3087–3090.
12. Lepkovsky, S., Furuta, F., Ozone, K., Koike, T., and Wagner, M. (1966): The proteases, amylase and lipase of the pancreas and intestinal contents of germfree and conventional rats. Brit. J. Nutr. *20:*257–261.
13. Loesche, W. J. (1968): Protein and carbohydrate composition of cecal contents of gnotobiotic rats and mice. Proc. Soc. Exp. Biol. Med. *128:*195–199.
14. Borgström, B., Dahlqvist, A., Gustafsson, B. E., Lundh, G., and Malmquist, J. (1959): Trypsin, invertase and amylase content of feces of germfree rats. Proc. Soc. Exp. Biol. Med. *102:*154–155.
15. Reddy, B. S., Pleasants, J. R., and Wostmann, B. S. (1969): Pancreatic enzymes in germfree and conventional rats fed chemically defined, water-soluble diet free from natural substrates. J. Nutr. *97:*327–334.
16. Gordon, H. A. (1967): A substance acting on smooth muscle in intestinal contents of germfree animals. Ann. N.Y. Acad. Sci. *147:*83–106.
17. Back, N., Steger, R., and Mirand, E. A. (1969): Kinin forming activity in cecal contents of germfree and conventional mice. In: *Germfree Biology,* edited by E. A. Mirand and N. Back, Plenum Press, New York, p. 173–177.
18. Werle, E. (1960): Kallikrein, kallidin and related substances. In: *Polypeptides that Affect Smooth Muscles and Blood Vessels,* edited by M. Schachter, Pergamon Press, Oxford, p. 199.
19. Csáky, T. Z.: *personal communication.*
20. Heneghan, J. B. (1963): Influence of microbial flora on xylose absorption in rats and mice. Amer. J. Physiol. *205:*417–420.
21. Ford, D. J., and Coates, M. E. (1971): Absorption of glucose and vitamins of the B complex by germfree and conventional chicks. Proc. Nutr. Soc. *30:*10–11A.
22. Combe, E., Penot, E., Charlier, H., and Sacquet, E. (1965): Métabolisme du rat "germfree." Teneurs des contenus digestifs en certains composés azotés, en sodium et en potassium. Teneurs de quelques tissus en acides nucléiques. Ann. Biol. Anim. Biochim. Biophys. *5:*189–206.
23. Gordon, H. A. (1968): Is the germfree animal normal? In: *The Germfree Animal in Research,* edited by M. E. Coates, Academic Press, New York, pp. 127–150.
24. Levenson, S. M., and Tennant, B. (1963): Contributions of intestinal microflora to the nutrition of th host animal. Some metabolic and nutritional studies with germfree animals. Fed. Proc. *22:*109–119.
25. Evrard, E., Hoet, P. P., Eyssen, H., Charlier, H., and Sacquet, E. (1964): Fecal lipids in germfree and conventional rats. Brit. J. Exp. Pathol. *45:*409–414.
26. Pleasants, J. R. (1968): Characteristics of the germfree animal. In: *The Germfree Animal in Research,* edited by M. E. Coates, Academic Press, New York, pp. 113–125.
27. Heneghan, J. B.: *personal communication.*
28. Loesche, W. J. (1968): Accumulation of endogenous protein in the cecum of the germfree rat. Proc. Soc. Exp. Biol. Med. *129:*380–384.
29. Lindstedt, G., Lindstedt, S., and Gustafsson, B. E. (1965): Mucus in intestinal contents of germfree rats. J. Exp. Med. *121:*201–213.
30. Csáky, T. Z. (1968): Intestinal water permeability regulation involving the microbial flora. In: *The Germfree Animal in Research,* edited by M. E. Coates, Academic Press, New York, pp. 151–159.
31. Hoskins, L. C. (1968): Bacterial degradation of gastrointestinal mucins. II. Bacterial origin of fecal ABH(O) blood group antigen-destroying enzymes. Gastroenterology *54:*218–224.
32. Asano, T. (1969): Modification of cecal size in germfree rats by long-term feeding of anion exchange resins. Amer. J. Physiol. *217:*911–918.
33. Wostmann, B. S., Reddy, B. S., Bruckner-Kardoss, E., Gordon, H. A., and Singh, B. (1973): In: *Germfree Research: Biological Effect of Gnotobiotic Environments,* edited by J. B. Heneghan. Academic Press. New York, p. 261–270.
34. Wiseman, R. F. and Gordon, H. A. (1971): Neutralization of the intestinal flora

and development of germfree-like characteristics in antibiotic treated rats. J. Lab. Clin. Med. 78:834.
35. Gordon, H. A., and Wostmann, B. S. (1973): Chronic mild diarrhea in germfree rodents: A model portraying host-flora synergism. In: *Germfree Research,* edited by J. B. Heneghan. Academic Press. New York, p. 261–270.
36. Loeschke, K., and Gordon, H. A. (1970): Water movement across the cecal wall of the germfree rat. Proc. Soc. Exp. Biol. Med. 133:1217–1222.
37. Nakamura, S., and Gordon, H. A. (1973): Threshold levels of NaCl upholding solute-coupled water transport in the cecum of gremfree and conventional rats. Proc. Soc. Exp. Biol. Med. 142:1336–1340.
38. Simonetta, M., Faelli, A., and Cremaschi, D.: *personal communication.*
39. Loeschke, K., and Uhlich, E. (1974): Stimulation of sodium transport and Na^+-K^+-ATPase activity in the hypertrophying rat cecum. Pflügers Arch. 346:233–249.
40. Gustafsson, B. E., and Maunsbach, A. B. (1971): Ultrastructure of the enlarged cecum in germfree rats. Z. Zellforsch 120:555–578.
41. Staley, T. E., quoted by H. A. Gordon. (1968): Is the germfree animal normal? In: *The Germfree Animal in Research,* edited by M. E. Coates. Academic Press, New York, p. 131–132.
42. Strandberg, K., Sedval, G., Midtvedt, T., and Gustafsson, B. E. (1966): Effect of some biological active amines on the cecum wall of germfree rats. Proc. Soc. Exp. Biol. Med. 121:699–702.
43. Dupont, J. R., Jervis, H. R., and Sprinz, H. (1965): Auerbach's plexus of the rat cecum in relation to the germfree state. J. Comp. Neurol. 125:11–18.
44. Abrams, G. D., and Bishop, J. E. (1967): Effect of the normal flora on gastrointestinal motility. Proc. Soc. Exp. Biol. Med. 126:301–304.
45. Gordon, H. A., and Bruckner, G. (1974): Depressant smooth muscle effect of fractions containing acidic amino acids prepared from cecal supernatant of germfree rats. Fed. Proc. 33, No. 3, Part I.
46. Kokas, E., and Valentine, R. (1974): Effects of free amino acids in intestinal contents on the rhythmic contraction of villi in dogs. Fed. Proc. 33, No. 3, Part I.
47. Gordon, H. A., Wostmann, B. S., and Bruckner-Kardoss, E. (1963): Effects of microbial flora on cardiac output and other elements of blood circulation. Proc. Soc. Exp. Biol. Med. 114:301–304.
48. Wostmann, B. S., Bruckner-Kardoss, E., and Knight, P. L., Jr. (1968): Cecal enlargement, cardiac output and oxygen consumption in germfree rats. Proc. Soc. Exp. Biol. Med. 128:137–141.
49. Baez, S., and Gordon, H. A. (1971): Tone and reactivity of vascular smooth muscle in germfree rat mesentery. J. Exp. Med. 134:846–856.
50. Baez, S., Bruckner, G., and Gordon, H. A. (1973): Responsiveness of jejunal-ileal mesentery microvessels in unoperated and cecectomized germfree rats to some smooth muscle agonists. In: *Germfree Research,* edited by J. B. Heneghan, Academic Press, New York, p. 527–533.
51. Gordon, H. A., and Kokas, E. (1968): A bioactive pigment ("alpha pigment") in cecal contents of germfree animals. Biochem. Pharmacol. 17:2333–2347.
52. Mazur, A., and Shorr, E. (1948): Hepatorenal factors in circulatory homeostasis. IX. The identification of the hepatic vasodepressor substance, VDM, with ferritin. J. Biol. Chem. 176:771–787.
53. Kokas, E.: *personal communication.*
54. Bruckner, G. (1973): Epinephrine inhibitory substance in intestinal contents of germfree rats. In: *Germfree Research,* edited by J. B. Heneghan, Academic Press, New York, p. 535–540.
55. Gordon, H. A., Bruckner-Kardoss, E., and Wostmann, B. S. (1966): Aging in germfree mice: Life tables and lesions observed at natural death. J. Gerontol. 21:380–387.

Intestinal Absorption and Malabsorption,
edited by T. Z. Csáky.
Raven Press, New York © 1975

Cholera Toxin and Intestinal Transport

Thomas R. Hendrix

Johns Hopkins University, Baltimore, Maryland 21205

INTRODUCTION

Interest in the past has focused primarily on the absorptive functions of the intestine. Recent studies of the pathogenesis of cholera, however, have created an awareness of the large volumes of fluid that can move into the intestine. To understand the mechanisms involved in producing this reversal of the normal direction of fluid movement is one of the most challenging questions in pathophysiology (Hendrix and Bayless, 1970).

I. CHOLERA AND CHOLERA ENTEROTOXIN

A. The Disease

Cholera is caused by the transient colonization of the intestine by large numbers of cholera organisms, *Vibrio cholerae* (Gorbach, Banwell, Jacobs, Chatterjee, Mitra, Brigham, and Neogy, 1970; Hornick, Music, Wenzel, Cash, Lebonati, Snyder, and Woodward, 1971. It has been demonstrated that the cholera vibrios do not invade the mucosa but rather elaborate an enterotoxin which reacts with the mucosa to provoke massive outpouring of fluid with daily fecal fluid losses as great as 17 liters or more per day (Watten, Morgan, Songkhla, Vanikiati, and Phillips, 1959. This massive fluid and electrolyte loss can be duplicated in man and experimental animals by placing the bacteria-free filtrate of *V. cholerae* cultures into the intestine. Indeed, the clinical manifestations of cholera are solely the consequence of the massive fluid and electrolyte losses induced by the enterotoxin (Hendrix, 1971; Banwell and Sherr, 1973).

B. The Toxin

Cholera enterotoxin is a heat-labile, neutral protein with molecular weight (MW) of 84,000 (Finkelstein and Lo Spalluto, 1970; Pierce, Greenough, and Carpenter, 1971). The toxin appears to be composed of one heavy component, MW 28,000, and seven light components with MW of 8,000 each. In the preparation of purified toxin (choleragen), a nontoxic "toxoid" (choleragenoid) is also isolated. This latter material binds to the intestinal mucosa and blocks the secretory effect of toxin administered subsequently. Since choleragenoid lacks the heavy component, it has been suggested that the light components are responsible for the binding of the toxin to the mucosa and the heavy component initiates the train of events leading to secretion (Lönnroth and Holmgren, 1973).

C. Toxin-Epithelial Cell Interaction

Binding of toxin to the mucosa is rapid and not reversible. A 5-min exposure of the mucosa to toxin is as effective in eliciting maximum intestinal secretion as is continuous exposure (Goodgame, Banwell, and Hendrix, 1973). The toxin appears to bind to the brush border (microvilli) of the intestinal epithelium, crypts, and villi alike (Peterson, Lo Spalluto, and Finkelstein, 1972), and this binding appears to be due to specific affinity of the toxin for a specific membrane ganglioside, G_{M1}. The cholera organism has a sialidase which although inactive against G_{M1} ganglioside can convert a variety of other gangliosides to G_{M1}. It, thus, appears possible that the infecting organism itself can increase the number of binding sites on the epithelium and thus magnify the secretory effect (Holmgren, Lönnroth, and Svennerholm, 1973).

Following binding of cholera toxin to the intestinal cell, adenylate cyclase is activated (Kimberg, Field, Johnson, Henderson, and Gershon, 1971), and cellular levels of cyclic 3′,5′-adenosine monophosphate (cAMP) rise (Shafer, Lust, Sircar, and Goldberg, 1970). This phenomenon of binding of cholera toxin to the cell membrane with activation of adenylate cyclase and consequent elevation of cellular cAMP is not unique to the intestinal epithelium but is seen in a host of cell types, hepatocytes, fat cells, lymphocytes, platelets, adrenal cortical cells, etc. (Pierce et al., 1971). It is unclear at present whether or not this entire series of events takes place in the brush border and, if so, in which of the cell types that make up the intestinal epithelium. It has been suggested that the toxin or an active fragment is taken into the cell where adenylate cyclase is activated with subsequent stimulation of secretion. This suggestion was based on the report that the activity of adenylate cyclase was much greater in isolated lateral-basal membranes than in microvillous membranes (brush borders) (Parkinson, Ebel, DiBona, and Sharp, 1972).

A great deal has been made of the delay between time of exposure and the onset of intestinal secretion, but it is not as long as is frequently stated. Statistically significant differences between control and toxin-exposed animals occur as early as 10 min in the rabbit and 45 min in the dog, although maximal rate of secretion is not reached until the second hour (McGonagle, Serebro, Iber, Bayless, and Hendrix, 1969; Goodgame et al., 1973).

A striking feature of cholera toxin action on cells is its prolonged effect after a brief exposure. Intestinal secretion may persist as long as 36 hr. It has been suggested that the effect is limited by the lifespan of the cell. Other agents that produce their effects through elevation of cAMP are characterized by very rapid onset and prompt return to normal when the stimulant is removed (Pierce et al., 1971).

II. ORIGIN AND COMPOSITION OF CHOLERA TOXIN-INDUCED INTESTINAL FLUID

A. Site of Fluid Production

Although the cholera organisms and toxin are found throughout the alimentary canal in cholera, massive outpouring of fluid occurs solely in the small intestine. The volume secreted per unit length of intestine is greatest in the duodenum and least in the ileum (Carpenter, Sack, Feeley, and Steinberg, 1968; Carpenter and Greenough, 1968). There is no evidence that the absorptive function of the colon is altered during cholera.

B. Composition of Cholera Fluid

The electrolyte compositions of jejunal and ileal fluids are characteristic. In general, bicarbonate is lower and chloride is higher than plasma in jejunal

TABLE 1. Composition of intestinal fluid (mEq/l)

	Na	K	Cl	HCO_3
Jejunum (cholera and normal)	148	5.6	138	15
Ileum (cholera and normal)	146	5.7	121	42
Cholera stool	140	10	110	48
Normal stool	30	100	15[a]	32[a]

[a] In normal stool, organic anion account for the discrepancy between cations (Na + K) and anions (Cl + HCO_3). The great volume of choleraic stool purges the colon of organic anion which are normally derived from unabsorbed foodstuff and shed cells.

fluid, whereas the opposite is found in the ileum. These differences are maintained during cholera-induced secretion. On the other hand, the electrolyte composition of the stool changes, as the volume of fluid delivered from the small intestine to the colon increases. The colon's limited ability to absorb fluid and conserve sodium and other electrolytes is overwhelmed, hence the electrolyte composition of stool approaches that of the ileal fluid (Table 1). The intestinal fluid is approximate isomotic with plasma and contains very little protein, 85 mg/100 ml (Hendrix, 1971).

III. MECHANISMS OF FLUID PRODUCTION

Over the years several hypotheses have been proposed to explain the striking intestinal fluid loss that characterizes cholera: (a) increased exudation; (b) increased filtration; (c) decreased absorption; and (d) increased secretion.

A. Exudation

The hypothesis enjoying the longest popularity with the least evidence for its support was presented by Virchow and Koch. They believed that the cholera infection lead to extensive sloughing of the intestinal epithelium. The process can be likened to an extensive burn. Cohnheim pointed out as early as 1882 that this could not possibly be the explanation of cholera diarrhea since, among other considerations, the protein content of cholera stool was very low (Pierce et al., 1971). Nevertheless, exudation hypothesis was not put to rest until Gangarosa, Beisel, Benyajati, Sprinz, and Piyaratn (1960) found normal intestinal mucosa by peroral intestinal biopsy during the course of cholera. These studies have been amplified by morphologic studies of cholera in animals in which mucosa can be biopsied repeatedly from the first contact of the mucosa with the cholera organism or cholera enterotoxin through to recovery (Norris and Majno, 1968; Elliott, Carpenter, Sack, and Yardley, 1970). Except for discharge of mucus from the goblet cells, no morphologic alterations are detected by light or electronmicroscopy (Yardley, Bayless, Leubbers, Halsted, and Hendrix, 1972). Although the mucosal capillary bed is more dilated in choleraic animals, no new or abnormal pathways through the walls of the capillaries were detected (Yardley and Brown, 1973). These experimental studies in animals as well as studies in man indicate that the intestinal fluid losses in cholera are brought about by a functional rather than a morphologic alteration of the intestine.

B. Increased Filtration

Although the low protein content of choleraic intestinal fluid is consistent with the hypothesis that the fluid is produced by filtration, there are several other conditions to be met.

Increased filtration through the epithelium requires an increase in the driving force across the epithelium or an increase in epithelial permeability or both. The sources of the driving forces across the epithelium are osmotic and hydrostatic. The osmotic force in cholera is oriented in the wrong direction. As the diarrhea increases in severity, the cholera patient becomes very hemoconcentrated with plasma protein concentration as high as 13.4 g/100 ml (Watten et al., 1959). From clinical and experimental observations there is no evidence that hydrostatic pressure across the capillary bed is increased. In clinical cholera the patient continues to pour fluid into his intestine even though his blood pressure has fallen so low that the pulse is undetectable. In experimental cholera, flow through the mesenteric artery was reduced to 30% of normal without altering the rate of cholera-induced fluid production (Carpenter, Greenough, and Sack, 1969).

Finally, acute volume expansion in experimental animals reverses net intestinal movement from absorption to net secretion, presumably through the mechanism of increased hydrostatic pressure in the mucosal capillaries of the intestine. Morphologic studies show the appearance of the epithelium in this secretory state to be completely different from those seen with enterotoxin-induced intestinal secretion (Di Bona, Chen, and Sharp, 1974).

It has been suggested that cholera toxin leads to intestinal fluid production by increasing the permeability of the intestinal epithelium (Love, 1969a,b). If increased permeability was indeed an important factor, the electrolyte composition of jejunal and ileal fluids should approach the composition of

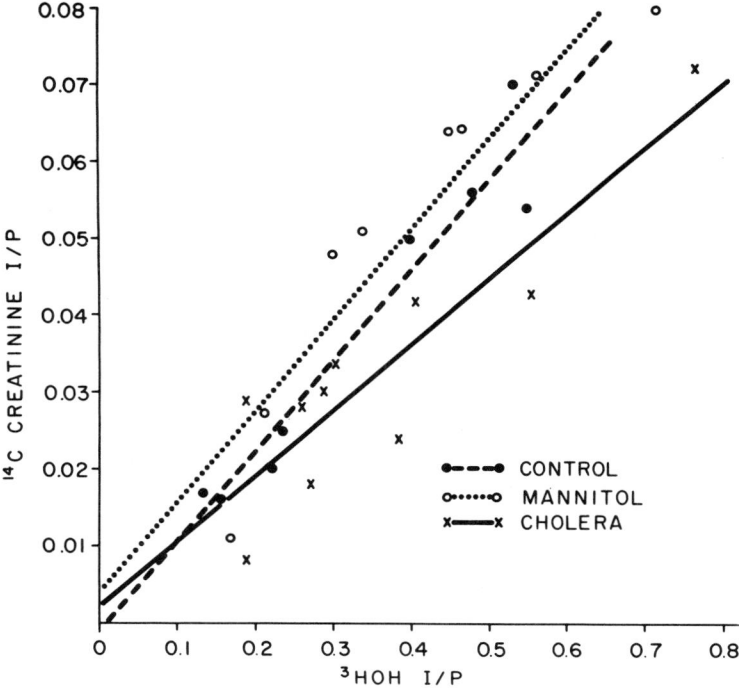

FIG. 1. A plot of the intestinal:plasma ratios of labeled creatinine and water after intravenous injection of the isotopically labeled compounds indicates that there is no increase above control values in intestinal permeability when intestinal secretion is stimulated by cholera enterotoxin or hypertonic mannitol (450 mOsm/l). In all studies the permeability of the cholera toxin-exposed mucosa was less than the other two groups. (As the mucosa becomes more permeable, it offers less resistance to the passage of the larger molecule of the isotope pair and the slope of the line becomes steeper.)

plasma. Since they do not, but rather maintain normal composition with jejunal fluid electrolyte composition differing significantly from ileal fluid and both differing from plasma, there is strong evidence against a permeability change being induced by cholera toxin.

More direct evidence against a cholera toxin induced permeability change has been obtained in clinical and experimental cholera. When isotopically labeled mannitol was injected intravenously and the radioactivity of stools was measured, no difference was found between cholera and control patients (Gordon, Gardner, and Kinzie, 1972).

To assess more directly whether or not cholera toxin increased the permeability of the mucosa, the ratio of intestinal to plasma radioactivity was measured after pairs of isotopically labeled molecules of varying sizes were injected intravenously (^{3}HOH and ^{14}C urea, ^{3}HOH and ^{14}C creatinine, and ^{3}HOH and ^{14}C lactose). The data obtained were compared with ratios measured in control animals and animals in which an equal net fluid secretion was produced by infusing the lumen with a hypertonic mannitol solution. With each of the three isotope pairs, there was no difference in intestinal:plasma ratios among the three groups of animals, controls, osmotic-induced secretion, and cholera-induced secretion (Rohde and Chen, 1972; Scherer, Harper, Banwell, and Hendrix, 1974) (Fig. 1).

IV. IMPAIRED ABSORPTION

The bidirectional fluxes of water and electrolytes across the intestinal epithelium are large compared to the net flux (Visscher, Fetcher, Carr, Gregor, Bushey, and Barker, 1944a; Visscher, Varco, Carr, Dean, and Erickson, 1944b). The magnitude and direction of the net fluxes are an algebraic sum of the unidirectional diffusive, connective, and transport fluxes, which in turn are determined by electrochemical gradients, osmotic and hydrostatic pressure gradients, epithelial permeability, and "transport mechanisms."

A. Sodium Absorption

Since in the past active transport of sodium has been extensively studied, it is not surprising that impaired sodium absorption was suggested as the cause of the fluid losses in cholera. Watten et al. (1959), using Visscher's et al. (1944a,b) figure of 83 min for clearance of sodium from the plasma, and assuming plasma volume to be 5% of body weight calculated that the intestine of a 55-kg man would receive 48 l of isotonic fluid per 24 hr. They suggested that if there was a 35% impairment of intestinal reabsorption a 24 hr fecal volume in excess of 17 l would result, a defect sufficient to account fecal fluid losses seen in cholera. Apparent support for this notion was provided by the observation that crude cholera toxin inhibited active sodium transport by frog skin (Fuhrman and Fuhrman, 1960).

In vivo perfusion studies in human and experimental cholera have given contradictory results, some report no change $J_{m\text{-}s}^{Na}$ (unidirectional sodium flux lumen to blood) (Banwell, Pierce, Mitra, Caranosos, Keimowitz, Mondal, and Manji, 1968; Iber, McGonagle, Serebro, Leubbers, Bayless, and Hendrix, 1969; Love, 1969b); whereas, others have suggested that it is decreased and contributes to the fluid loss (Phillips, 1968; Swallow, Code, and Freter, 1968).

In vitro studies of stripped ileal mucosa short circuited in an Ussing-type chamber demonstrated absorption of sodium against an electrochemical gradient. Addition of cholera toxin in vivo or in vitro abolishes this active transport of sodium (Field, 1971a,b; Field, Fromm, All-Awaqati, and Greenough, 1972). There are many possible explanations for these discrepant results, e.g., in vivo versus in vitro, bolus versus steady-state method, jejunum versus ileum, composition of luminal fluid, animal species differences.

B. Glucose-Associated Sodium Absorption

Regardless of whether or not sodium absorption is normal or depressed in cholera, all agree that glucose absorption and glucose-enhanced sodium absorption are normal in spite of a striking reversal of the direction net intestinal fluid movement (Hirschhorn, Kinzie, Sachar, Northrup, Taylor, Ahmad, and Phillips, 1968; Pierce, Banwell, Mitra, Caranosos, Keimowitz, Mondal, and Manji, 1968; Serebro, Bayless, Hendrix, Iber, and McGonagle, 1968; Iber et al., 1969; Nalin, Cash, Rahman, and Yunus, 1970; Rohde and Cash, 1973). Indeed, the capacity of these active transport mechanisms for glucose and amino acids to entrain sodium and other electrolytes and water along with the actively transported solute is so great that they can be employed to replace the fecal water and electrolyte losses.

V. INTESTINAL SECRETION

The observations that cholera toxin causes a reversal of the normal direction of water and electrolyte movement on one hand, while on the other, the provision that an actively transported solute such as glucose can carry sufficient water and electrolytes in the opposite direction to compensate for the losses present a paradox. A solution for this paradox may be provided if we consider the sites for absorption and secretion to be separate.

A. Site of Intestinal Secretion

It is generally accepted that the site of absorption is at the crests of the villi (Kinter and Wilson, 1965), and there are a number of observations compatible with the notion that cholera toxin-induced secretion originates in the crypt as a specific process. This latter notion is not new for in the nineteenth century Cohnheim concluded that "the process of cholera may be . . . an extra-ordinary profuse secretion from the glands of the small intestine," (Hendrix, 1971).

First, the lumina of the crypts of Lieberkühn are dilated and the crypt epithelium flattened in experimental canine cholera (Elliott et al., 1970). Second, selective damage to the villus crests while interfering with glucose

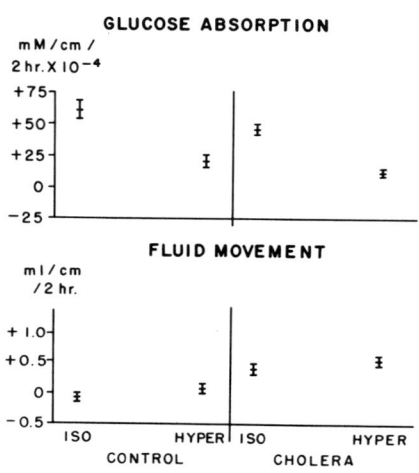

FIG. 2. To test Cohnheim's hypothesis that cholera-induced intestinal secretion originates in the crypts of Lieberkühn, the effect of damaging the epithelium of the villus crests or of the crypts on glucose absorption (a villus crest function) and on cholera enterotoxin-induced intestinal secretion was studied. In both control and cholera groups damage to the villus crests by exposure to hypertonic Na_2SO_4 decreased glucose absorption (upper graph). On the other hand, net fluid movement was not altered by damage to the villus crests in either the control or cholera groups (lower graph).

absorption did not alter toxin-induced intestinal secretion (Roggin, Banwell, Yardley, and Hendrix, 1972). On the other hand, selective damage to the crypts induced by cycloheximide, a reversible inhibitor of protein synthesis blocked cholera-induced secretion without altering glucose absorption (Serebro, Iber, Yardley, and Hendrix, 1969) (Figs. 2 and 3).

Third, Hirschhorn and Frazier (1973) found that theophylline, which also produces net electrolyte transport from serosa to mucosa *in vivo* resulted in a decrease in intracellular electrical potential of the intravillus cells (cells adjacent to the crypts), whereas the villus cells are unaffected.

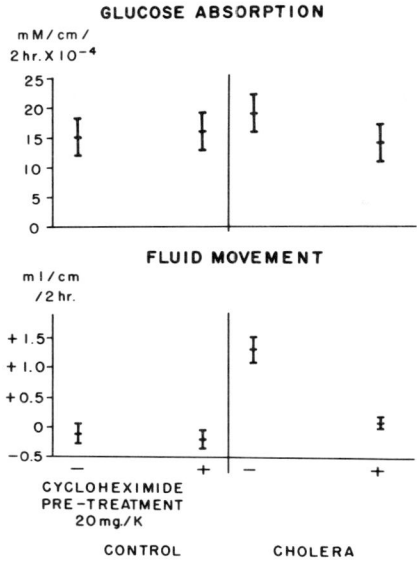

FIG. 3. Cycloheximide 20 mg/kg suppresses mitosis without producing histologic damage in the crypts (40 mg/kg produces selective histologic damage in crypts). No significant alteration in glucose absorption was found in the groups exposed to cycloheximide. However, cholera-induced secretion was strikingly inhibited.

B. Evidence for Active Secretion

The observations that jejunal and ileal fluids maintain their characteristic anion compositions during cholera-induced secretion suggests that there is an active component to the process. Much more direct evidence, however, is provided by *in vitro* studies employing Ussing chambers. In this preparation electrochemical gradients across the mucosa can be eliminated, and the net and unidirectional fluxes measured by observing the transfer of isotopically labeled ions. From this model, Field, Fromm, and McColl (1971) concluded that there was an active absorptive mechanism for both sodium and chloride ions and that there was an active secretory process for bicarbonate or an equivalent process, such as active absorption of hydrogen ions, causing alkalinization of the luminal fluid.

Pretreatment of rabbit ileal mucosa or addition of purified toxin to the mucosa side of the chamber leads to an increase in the transepithelial potential difference (PD) and the short-circuited current (SCC). The net absorptive flux of Na seen in control tissue was reduced to zero, whereas the net Cl flux was reversed from absorption to secretion, and the secretory bicarbonate flux was unchanged. The addition of glucose to the mucosal chamber produces net sodium absorption without altering the cholera toxin-induced secretory fluxes (Field, Fromm, Al-Awqati, and Greenough, 1972). Using a similar technique, Powell, Binder, and Curran (1973) came to a somewhat different interpretation, namely that cholera toxin stimulated an electrically neutral active transport of NaCl and/or $NaHCO_3$ from serosa to mucosa. In this model, active sodium absorption is unaffected but net sodium absorption is reduced to zero because of the toxin-induced sodium flux in the opposite direction. The major difference is that Field et al. (1972) attribute the increase in short-circuit current to electrogenic anion secretion and inhibition of active electrogenic sodium absorption, whereas Powell et al. (1973) attribute the short circuit current to an unaffected active electrogenic sodium absorption and the change in net electrolyte movement to a neutral NaCl and/or $NaHCO_3$ secretory mechanism. *In vivo* studies of ion transport in the cholera-exposed canine ileum indicate that both HCO_3 and Cl enter the lumen against their electrochemical gradients. In addition, it was found that the sodium in the ileal fluid could be accounted for by passive movement down its electrochemical gradient, whereas more K was present than could be accounted for by passive movement (Moore, Bieberdorf, Morawaski, Finkelstein, and Fordtran, 1971).

One point is clearly established by all of these studies—cholera toxin stimulates the transport of anions into the lumen against an electrochemical gradient and the steepest gradient is for bicarbonate.

C. Role of cAMP

Cyclic AMP has been shown to influence transport in several epithelia, frog skin, toad urinary bladder, and renal collecting tubule. It also alters transport characteristics of the ileal mucosa *in vivo* in a manner similar to cholera toxin (Field, 1971a,b). In addition, intestinal adenylate cyclase activity and cAMP have been found to be elevated in clinical and experimental cholera suggesting the possibility that cholera toxin exerts its effect through the activation of adenylate cyclase and subsequent elevation of epithelial cAMP (Kimberg et al. 1971; Sharp and Hynie, 1971; Chen, Rohde, and Sharp, 1972; Field et al., 1972). This possibility is strengthened by the observation that the level of jejunal mucosal adenylate cyclase activity parallels the secretory rate over the 48 hr after exposure to cholera toxin (Guerrant, Chen, and Sharp, 1972). The changes in *in vitro* ion transport induced by cAMP directly or by increasing cAMP production by stimulating adenylate cyclase with prostaglandin E_1 or preventing its breakdown by inhibiting phosphodiesterase with theophylline are rapid in onset, peak SCC (short-circuit current) reached in 1 to 2 min and subsides to 50% in 20 min and base line in 1 hr. The changes induced by cholera toxin, on the other hand, are slower in onset requiring 1 to 2 hr to reach a plateau, which is then maintained for hours (Field, 1971a; Field et al., 1972). In spite of these differences it appears that cholera toxin is producing its effect on *in vitro* SCC by increasing mucosa cAMP since the effects of cholera toxin and cAMP (induced by theophylline) are not additive (Fig. 4).

What then is the explanation of the difference between the effect of cholera toxin and direct application of cAMP? Several possibilities have been considered but none substantiated: (a) Cholera toxin might lead to synthesis of adenylate cyclase and the time required for synthesis accounts for the delay.

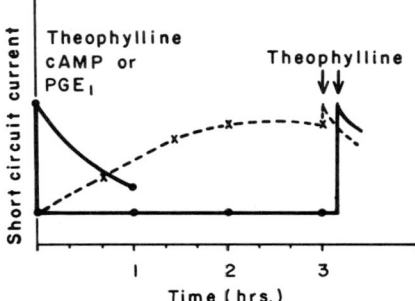

FIG. 4. Raising mucosal AMP by theophylline, PGE, or cAMP itself causes a prompt increase in short-circuit current (SCC) across the mucosa mounted in an Ussing chamber. This response is contrasted to the gradual increase SCC produced by cholera enterotoxin exposure (x__x). It is suggested that the two processes involve the same final common pathway since addition of theophylline at the peak SCC response to cholera toxin is not additive. The tissue maintains its responsiveness to theophylline as indicated by response in control mucosa (●——●).

This is unlikely since Kimberg et al. (1971) showed that NaF-stimulated adenylate cyclase activity is no greater after exposure of the mucosa to active than inactive toxin. (b) The toxin that is bound to the surface must be taken into the cell to reach the active sites. Support for this notion was provided by the report that the majority of the epithelial cell cyclase activity is to be found in the lateral and basal membranes of the cell rather than in the brush border (Parkinson et al., 1972). On the other hand, cholera toxin is a large molecule (MW 84,000), so the amounts taken into the cell must be small. To date, no direct evidence is available indicating uptake of the toxin or toxin fragments. (c) Cholera toxin produces stimulation of adenylate cyclase through an intermediate, prostaglandin, for instance. That a mediator may be involved is suggested by the studies of Serebro, McGonagle, Iber, Royall, and Hendrix (1968) and Vaughan-Williams and Dohadwalla (1969), which show a secretory response in intestinal segments not exposed to toxin but perfused with blood from a loop containing toxin. The effect is not due to absorbed toxin since parenterally administered toxin has no secretory effect on the intestine (Pierce, Graybill, Kaplan, and Bouwman, 1972).

Prostaglandins have been suggested as a possible intermediate between toxin and cAMP-mediated intestinal secretion (Pierce, Carpenter, Elliott, and Greenough, 1971). This possibility is strengthened by the observation that cholera-induced secretion is inhibited by aspirin and indomethacin (Finch and Katz, 1972; Jacoby and Marshall, 1972), agents shown to inhibit the synthesis of prostaglandins (Vane, 1971). Bourne (1973), on the other hand, was unable to detect any inhibition of cholera toxin-induced elevation of leucocyte cAMP by these agents. Furthermore, the effects of prostaglandin E_1 on the intestinal mucosa maximally stimulated by cholera toxin was found to be additive suggesting that they elevate cAMP by different pathways (Kimberg, Field, Gershon, and Henderson, 1974). Alterations in activity of cyclic nucleotide phosphodiesterase, the enzyme which inactivates cAMP, are not produced by cholera toxin, hence can play no role in toxin-induced secretion (Kimberg et al., 1974).

Cholera toxin and cAMP have been found to increase the electrical resistance and decrease the conductance of the intestinal mucosa (Field et al., 1972; Powell et al., 1973).

At the present time, the mechanism by which cholera toxin stimulates adenylate cyclase is not known, nor is the explanation of its long action, perhaps extending for the functional life of the affected cell.

VI. INHIBITORS OF CHOLERA-INDUCED SECRETION

Cholera enterotoxin-induced secretion can be blocked at several steps. Defining the nature of the inhibition may provide insight into the mechanisms involved in intestinal secretion.

Complexing cholera toxin with specific antitoxin or ganglioside prevents its binding to the mucosa and subsequent stimulation of intestinal secretion (Greenough, Carpenter, Bayless, and Hendrix, 1970). On the other hand, these agents are ineffectual if added after the toxin has come in contact with the mucosa (Fig. 5).

Polymixin, an antibiotic which binds to phospholipids (Kunin, 1971), was used in an attempt to prevent binding of the toxin to the mucosa. It was shown that it did not block binding of the toxin but rather prevented secretion by blocking the activation of adenylate cyclase possibly by binding to the phospholipid necessary for the coupling of the receptor and catalytic sites of the enzyme (Maimon, Banwell, and Hendrix, 1972).

Cycloheximide, a reversible inhibitor of protein synthesis, will prevent cholera-toxin-induced intestinal secretion but does not prevent activation of adenylate cyclase and elevation of cAMP (Serebro et al., 1969; Kimberg,

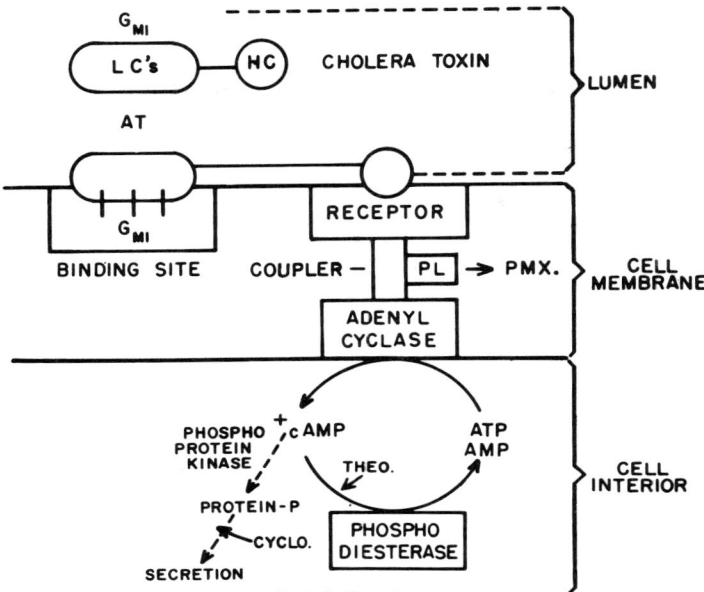

FIG. 5. Schematic representation postulated sites of action of several inhibitors of cholera enterotoxin-induced secretion. From these considerations hypotheses can be developed and tested to explain intestinal secretion. In the lumen ganglioside (G_{MI}) or specific antitoxin (AT) bind to the light components (LCs) of cholera toxin and make it impossible to bind to the mucosa with subsequent stimulation of secretion. The light components of cholera toxin are believed to be bound to the surface of the epithelial cells by a specific ganglioside (G_{MI}), but this is not the step that initiates secretion. The heavy component (HC) appears to be responsible for initiating secretion through the activation of adenylate cyclase. The line connecting LCs and HC is made of different lengths to indicate that there may be intermediate steps between binding and enzyme activation. Polymixin (PMX) an antibiotic that binds to phospholipids of cell membranes does not block binding of the toxin to the epithelium but does block secretion probably by interfering with phospholipid (PL) coupling of the receptor and catalytic components of adenylate cyclase. Elevation of intestinal epithelial cAMP is associated with intestinal secretion regardless of how induced, by stimulating adenylate cyclase by cholera toxin, prostaglandins, or intestinal hormones such as vasoactive intestinal peptide (VIP), or by blocking phosphodiesterase activity with theophylline (Theo). Cycloheximide (cyclo) presumably acts by inhibiting a protein synthetic step essential for the secretory process.

Field, Gershon, Schooley, and Henderson, 1973). If cycloheximide is given after cholera-induced secretion is established, fluid production persists for 2.5 to 3 hr before being inhibited (Harper, Yardley, and Hendrix, 1970). If the animal is pretreated with cycloheximide and challenged with toxin after varying intervals, no secretion is induced until there is a return of protein synthesis as manifest by reappearance of mitotic figures in the crypts, 8 to 12 hr after administration of the drug (Banwell and Hendrix, *unpublished observations*). These findings suggest that there is a protein synthetic step involved in cholera-induced secretion and one of the proteins has a functional existence of 2.5 to 3 hr.

Ethacrynic acid inhibits cholera toxin-induced secretion but the mechanism remains to be defined. It is not a property of all diuretics since furosimide was without effect (Carpenter, Curlin, and Greenough, 1969).

The effect of the carbonic anhydrase inhibitor, acetazoleamide, has been reported to block cholera secretion (Norris, Curran, and Schultz, 1969), whereas Carpenter et al. (1969) found no effect.

Ouabain, an inhibitor of Na-K ATPase, was also found to be without effect. Finally, the anti-inflammatory drugs that inhibit the synthesis of prostaglandins have been reported to prevent cholera toxin-induced secretion (Finch and Katz, 1972; Jacoby and Marshall, 1972).

VII. SPECULATION

Is cholera-induced intestinal secretion a specific pathologic response to a noxious agent, the enterotoxin of the cholera organism, or is it rather a morbid exaggeration of a normal physiologic response? I wish to suggest that it is an exaggeration of the process that Florey, Wright, and Jennings (1941) suggested was turned on with each meal: "It may be necessary for a constant secretion of fluid to take place from the crypts of Lieberkühn . . . and as the products of digestion are absorbed water and salt go with them. One may envisage a circulation of fluid during active digestion, the secretion passing out from the crypts of Lieberkühn and back into the villi" (Fig. 6). Studies

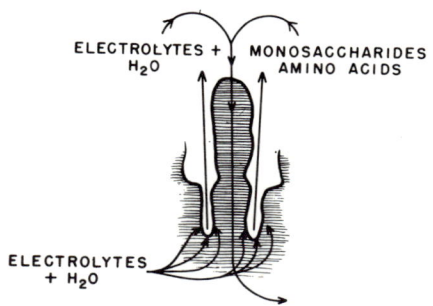

FIG. 6. It has been suggested that intestinal secretion is an integral part of the absorptive process, water and electrolytes entering the lumen by secretion from the crypts to prevent the oncotic pressure of the luminal contents from rising as hydrolysis of carbohydrates and proteins occur in the lumen. It is a reasonable hypothesis that this process is mediated by intestinal hormones such as vasoactive intestinal peptide (VIP). The secretion initiated by hormones is probably rapid in onset and responsive to negative feedback inhibition. Cholera enterotoxin may act by locking the secretory mechanism in the "full on position."

on the pathogenesis of cholera may be interpreted as suggesting that the process is mediated by cAMP in two ways: First, stimulation of electrolyte and water secretion by the crypts, and second facilitate absorption by decreasing conductance over the inter epithelial cell shunt pathway. Since cAMP decreases the mucosal conductance, this would serve to increase the efficiency of absorption, since the osmotic gradient developed in the lateral spaces between columnar cells would not tend to be dissipated back into the lumen through the tight junction.

REFERENCES

Banwell, J. G., Pierce, N. F., Mitra, R., Caranosos, G. J., Kermowitz, R. I., Mondal, A., and Manji, P. M. (1968): Preliminary results of a study of small intestinal water and solute movement in acute and convalescent human cholera. Ind. J. Med. Res. 56:633–639.

Banwell, J. G., and Sherr, H. (1973): Effect of bacterial enterotoxins on the gastrointestinal tract. Gastroenterology 65:467–497.

Bourne, H. R. (1973): Failure of anti-inflammatory drugs to prevent cyclic AMP accumulation. Nature 241:339.

Carpenter, C. C. J., Curlin, G. T., and Greenough, W. B. (1969): Response of canine Thirty-Vella jejunal loop to cholera exotoxin and its modification by ethacrynic acid. J. Infect. Dis. 120:332–338.

Carpenter, C. C. J., and Greenough, W. B. (1968): Response of canine duodenum to intraluminal challenge with cholera exotoxin. J. Clin. Invest. 47:2600–2607.

Carpenter, C. C. J., Greenough, W. B., and Sack, R. B. (1969): The relationship of superior mesenteric blood flow to gut electrolyte loss in experimental cholera. J. Infect. Dis. 119:182–193.

Carpenter, C. C. J., Sack, R. B., Feeley, J. C., and Steinberg, R. W. (1968): Site and characteristic of electrolyte loss and effect of intraluminal glucose in experimental canine cholera. J. Clin. Invest. 47:1210–1220.

Chen, L. C., Rohde, J. E., and Sharp, G. W. G. (1971): Intestinal adenyl-cyclase activity in human cholera. Lancet 1:939–941.

Chen, L. C., Rohde, J. E., and Sharp, G. W. G. (1972): Properties of adenyl-cyclase from human jejunal mucosa during naturally acquired cholera and convalescence. J. Clin. Invest. 51:731–740.

Di Bona, D. R., Chen, L. C., and Sharp, G. W. G. (1974): A study of intercellular spaces in the rabbit jejunum during acute volume expansion and after treatment with cholera toxin. J. Clin. Invest. 53:1300–1307.

Elliott, H. L., Carpenter, C. C. J., Sack, R. B., and Yardley, J. H. (1970): Small bowel morphology in experimental canine cholera. A light and electron microscopy study. Lab. Invest. 22:112–120.

Field, M. (1971a): Intestinal secretion: Effect of cyclic AMP and its role in cholera. New Engl. J. Med. 284:1137–1144.

Field, M. (1971b): Ion transport in rabbit ileal mucosa. II. Effects of cyclic 3′,5′-AMP. Amer. J. Physiol. 221:992–997.

Field, M., Fromm, D., Al-Awqati, Q., and Greenough, W. B., III. (1972): Effect of cholera enterotoxin on ion transport across isolated ileal mucosa. J. Clin. Invest. 51:796–804.

Field, M., Fromm, D., and McColl, I. (1971): Ion transport in rabbit ileal mucosa. I. Na and Cl fluxes and short circuit current. Amer. J. Physiol. 220:1388–1396.

Finch, A. D., and Katz, R. L. (1972): Prevention of cholera-induced intestinal secretion by aspirin. Nature 238:273–274.

Finkelstein, R. A., and Lo Spalluto, J. J. (1970): Production of highly purified choleragen and choleragenoid. J. Infect. Dis. 121:63–72.

Fuhrman, G. J., and Fuhrman, F. A. (1960): Inhibition of active sodium transport by cholera toxin. Nature *188:*71–72.
Florey, H. W., Wright, R. D., and Jennings, M. A. (1941): The secretions of the intestine. Physiol. Rev. *21:*36–69.
Gangarosa, E. J., Beisel, W. R., Benyajati, C., Sprinz, H., and Piyaratn, P. (1960): The nature of the gastrointestinal lesion in Asiatic cholera and its relation to pathogenesis: A biopsy study. Amer. J. Trop. Med. Hyg. *9:*125–135.
Goodgame, J. T., Banwell, J. G., and Hendrix, T. R. (1973): The relationship between duration of exposure to cholera toxin and the secretory response of rabbit jejunal mucosa. Johns Hopkins Med. J. *132:*117–126.
Gorbach, S. L., Banwell, J. G., Jacobs, B., Chatterjee, B. D., Mitra, R., Brigham, K. L., and Neogy, K. N. (1970): Intestinal flora in Asiatic cholera. II. The small bowel. J. Infect. Dis. *21:*38–45.
Gordon, R. S., Jr., Gardner, J. D., and Kinzie, J. L. (1972): Low mannitol clearance into cholera stool as evidence against filtration as the source of stool fluid. Gastroenterology *63:*407–412.
Greenough, W. B., Carpenter, C. C. J., Bayless, T. M., and Hendrix, T. R. (1970): The role of cholera exotoxin in the study of intestinal water and electrolyte transport. *In: Progress in Gastroenterology II,* edited by G. B. Jerzy Glass, Grune and Stratton, New York.
Guerrant, R. L., Chen, L. C., and Sharp, G. W. G. (1972): Intestinal adenyl-cyclase activity in canine cholera: Correlation with fluid accumulation. J. Infect. Dis. *125:*377–381.
Harper, D. T., Jr., Yardley, J. H., and Hendrix, T. R. (1970): Reversal of cholera exotoxin-induced jejunal secretion by cycloheximide. Johns Hopkins Med. J. *126:*258–266.
Hendrix, T. R. (1971): The pathophysiology of cholera. Bull. N.Y. Acad. Med. *47:*1169–1180.
Hendrix, T. R., and Bayless, T. M. (1970): Intestinal secretion. Ann. Rev. Physiol. *32:*139–164.
Hirschhorn, N., and Frazier, H. S. (1973): The electrical profile of stripped, isolated rabbit ileum. Johns Hopkins Med. J. *132:*271–281.
Hirschhorn, N., Kinzie, J. L., Sachar, D. B., Northup, R. S., Taylor, J. O., Ahmad, Z., and Phillips, R. A. (1968): Decrease in net stool output in cholera during intestinal perfusion with glucose-containing solutions. New Engl. J. Med. *279:*176–181.
Holmgren, J., Lönnroth, I., and Svennerholm, L. (1973): Tissue receptor for cholera exotoxin: Postulated structure from studies with G_{M1} ganglioside and related glycolipids. Infect. Immunity *8:*208–214.
Hornick, R. B., Music, S. I., Wenzel, R., Cash, R., Libonati, J. P., Snyder, J. M., and Woodward, T. E. (1971): The Broad Street pump revisited: Response of volunteers to ingested cholera vibrios. Bull. N.Y. Acad. Med. *47:*1181–1191.
Iber, F. L., McGonagle, T. J., Serebro, H. A., Luebbers, E. H., Bayless, T. M., and Hendrix, T. R. (1969): Unidirectional sodium flux in small intestine in experimental canine cholera. Amer. J. Med. Sci. *258:*340.
Jacoby, H. I., and Marshall, C. H. (1972): Antagonism of cholera enterotoxin by anti-inflammatory agents in the rat. Nature *235:*163–165.
Kimberg, D. V., Field, M., Gershon, E., Schooley, R. T., and Henderson, A. (1973): Effects of cycloheximide on the response of intestinal mucosa to cholera enterotoxin. J. Clin. Invest. *52:*1376–1383.
Kimberg, D. V., Field, M., Gershon, E., and Henderson, A. (1974): Effects of prostaglandins and cholera enterotoxin on intestinal mucosal cyclic AMP accumulation. Evidence against an essential role for prostaglandins in the action of toxin. J. Clin. Invest. *53:*941–949.
Kimberg, D. V., Field, M., Johnson, J., Henderson, A., and Gershon, E. (1971): Stimulation of intestinal mucosal adenyl cyclase by cholera enterotoxin and prostaglandins. J. Clin. Invest. *50:*1218–1230.
Kinter, W. G., and Wilson, T. H. (1965): Autoradiographic studies of sugar and amino acid absorption by everted sacs of hamster intestine. J. Cell. Biol. *25:*19–40.

Kunin, C. M. (1971) Binding of polymixin antibiotics to tissues: The major determinant of distribution and persistence in the body. J. Infect. Dis. *124:*394–400.
Lönnroth, I., and Holmgren, J. (1973): Subunit structure of cholera toxin. J. Gen. Microbiol. *76:*417–427.
Love, A. H. G. (1969a): Permeability characteristics of the cholera infected small intestine. Gut *10:*105–107.
Love, A. H. G. (1969b): Water and sodium absorption by the intestine in cholera. Gut *10:*63–67.
Maimon, H. N., Banwell, J. G., and Hendrix, T. R. (1972): Inhibition of cholera toxin induced secretion. Clin. Res. *20:*459.
McGonagle, T. J., Serebro, H. A., Iber, F. L., Bayless, T. M., and Hendrix, T. R. (1969): Time of onset of action of cholera toxin in dog and rabbit. Gastroenterology *57:*5–8.
Moore, W. L., Bieberdorf, F. A., Morawski, S. G., Finkelstein, R. A., and Fordtran, J. S. (1971) Ion transport during cholera-induced ileal secretion in the dog. J. Clin. Invest. *50:*312–318.
Nalin, D. R., Cash, R. A., Rahman, M., and Yunus, M. (1970): Effect of glycine and glucose on sodium and water absorption in patients with cholera. Gut *11:*768–772.
Norris, H. T., Curran, P. F., and Schultz, S. G. (1969): Modification of intestinal secretion in experimental cholera. J. Infect. Dis. *119:*117–125.
Norris, H. T., and Majno, G. (1968): On the role of the ileal epithelium in the pathogenesis of experimental cholera. Am. J. Path. *53:*268–279.
Parkinson, D., Ebel, H., Di Bona, D. R., and Sharp, G. W. G. (1972): Localization of the action of cholera toxin on adenyl cyclase in mucosal epithelial cells of rabbit intestine. J. Clin. Invest. *51:*2292–2298.
Peterson, J. W., Lo Spalluto, J. J., and Finkelstein, R. A. (1972): Localization of cholera toxin *in vivo.* J. Infect. Dis. *126:*617–628.
Phillips, R. A. (1968): Asiatic cholera (with emphasis on pathophysiological effects of the disease). Ann. Rev. Med. *19:*69–80.
Pierce, N. F., Banwell, J. G., Mitra, R. C., Caranosos, G. J., Keimowitz, R. I., Mondal, A., and Manji, P. M. (1968): Effect of intra gastric glucose-electrolyte infusion upon water and electrolyte balance in Asiatic cholera. Gastroenterology *55:*333–343.
Pierce, N. F., Carpenter, C. C. J., Elliott, H. L., and Greenough, W. B., III. (1971): Effects of prostaglandins, theophylline and cholera exotoxin upon transmucosal water and electrolyte movement in canine jejunum. Gastroenterology *60:*22–32.
Pierce, N. F., Graybill, J. R., Kaplan, M. M., and Bouwman, D. L. (1972): Systemic effects of parenteral cholera enterotoxin in dogs. J. Lab. Clin. Med. *79:*145–156.
Pierce, N. F., Greenough, W. B., and Carpenter, C. C. J. (1971): *Vibrio cholerae* enterotoxin and its mode of action. Bact. Rev. *35:*1–13.
Powell, D. W., Binder, J. H., and Curran, P. F. (1973): Active electrolyte secretion stimulated by choleragen in rabbit ileum *in vitro.* Amer. J. Physiol. *225:*781–787.
Rohde, J. E., and Cash, R. A. (1973): Transport of glucose and amino acids in human jejunum during Asiatic cholera. J. Infect. Dis. *127:*190–192.
Rohde, J. E., and Chen, L. C. (1972): Permeability and selectivity of canine and human jejunum during cholera. Gut *13:*191–196.
Roggin, G. M., Banwell, J. G., Yardley, J. H., and Hendrix, T. R. (1972): Unimpaired response of rabbit jejunum to cholera toxin after selective damage to villus epithelium Gastroenterology *63:*981–989.
Serebro, H. A., Bayless, T. M., Hendrix, T. R., Iber, F. L., and McGonagle, T. (1968): Absorption of *d*-glucose by rabbit jejunum during cholera toxin-induced diarrhea. Nature *217:*1272–1273.
Serebro, H. A., Iber, F. L., Yardley, J. H., and Hendrix, T. R. (1969): Inhibition of cholera toxin action in the rabbit by cycloheximide. Gastroenterology *56:*506–511.
Serebro, H. A., and McGonagle, T., Iber, F. L., Royall R. and Hendrix, T. R. (1968): An effect of cholera toxin on the small intestine without mucosal contact. Johns Hopkins Med. J. *123:*229–232.
Shafer, D. E., Lust, W. D., Sircar, B., and Goldberg, N. D. (1970): Elevation of

adenosine 3′,5′ cyclic monophosphate concentration in intestinal mucosa after treatment with cholera toxin. Proc. Nat. Acad. Sci. *67*:851–856.

Sharp, G. W. G., and Hynie (1971): Stimulation of intestinal adenyl cyclase by cholera toxin. Nature *229*:266–269.

Scherer, R. W., Harper, D. T., Banwell, J. G., and Hendrix, T. R. (1974): Absence of concurrent permeability changes in intestinal mucosa with secretion. Johns Hopkins Med. J. *134*:156–167.

Swallow, J. H., Code, C. F., and Freter, R. (1968): Effect of cholera toxin on water and ion fluxes in the canine bowel. Gastroenterology *54*:35–40.

Vane, J. R. (1971): Inhibition of prostaglandin synthesis as a mechanism of action of aspirin-like drugs. Nature (New Biol.) *231*:232–235.

Vaughan-Williams, E. M., and Dohadwalla, A. N. (1969): The appearance of a choleragenic agent in the blood of infant rabbits infected intestinally with *Vibrio cholerae*, demonstrated by cross-circulation. J. Infect. Dis. *120*:658–663.

Visscher, M. B., Fetcher, E. S., Jr., Carr, C. W., Gregor, H. P., Bushey, M. S., and Barker, D. E. (1944a): Isotopic tracer studies on the movement of water and ions between intestinal lumen and blood. Amer. J. Physiol. *142*:550–575.

Visscher, M. B., Varco, R. H., Carr, C. W., Dean, R. B., and Erickson, D. (1944b): Sodium ion movement between intestinal lumen and blood. Amer. J. Physiol. *141*:488–505.

Watten, R. H., Morgan, F. M., Songkhla, Y. N., Vanikiati, B., and Phillips, R. A. (1959): Water and electrolyte studies in cholera. J. Clin. Invest. *38*:1879–1889.

Yardley, J. H., Bayless, T. M., Luebbers, E. H., Halsted, C. H., and Hendrix, T. R. (1972): Goblet cell mucus in the small intestine. Findings after net fluid production due to cholera toxin and hypertonic solutions. Johns Hopkins Med. J. *131*:1–10

Yardley, J. H., and Brown, G. D. (1973): Horseradish peroxidase tracer studies in the intestine in experimental cholera. Lab. Invest. *28*:482–493.

DISCUSSION

CSÁKY remarked that, if cholera is a disease of the crypts caused by the binding of the toxin to the ganglioside and a few seconds of exposure seem to be sufficient to produce the effect, the toxin must reach a receptor very rapidly and bind with it. How does this appraisal stand up in view of the theory of the unstirred layer particularly as far as the crypts are concerned. HENDRIX called attention to the fact that on the photomicrographs one can actually see the bacteria that produce the toxin sitting on the microvilli so that the unstirred layer between the bacteria and the site of the receptor must be very small. It is not known where the receptor is exactly localized but it is suspected that the toxin activates adenosine cyclase in all the intestinal cells. What happens in response to the elevated level of cyclic AMP depends on the individual cell. It is conceivable that the crypt cells and the villus cells behave differently when their intracellular level of cyclic AMP is raised.

DIETSCHY raised the question of whether cholera toxin acts on a variety of cells, consequently the cholera receptors must not be unique in the intestinal cell. HENDRIX answered that cyclic AMP of course is produced in many other cells in response to cholera toxin. The intestinal secretion due to cholera is associated with elevated cyclic AMP but a causal relationship between the two is not absolutely proven. Presently no evidence is available to suggest that in cholera the toxin acts on any cells other than the epithelial cells of the intestine. The interesting thing is that once the cholera toxin is bound it cannot be washed off and its effect will continue for 25 to 36 hours.

RUMMEL asked about the time relationship between the onset of the clinical cholera and the increase of the intracellular AMP content. It appears that the AMP is produced much slower than the clinical effect. HENDRIX admitted that indeed this is one of the discrepancies which still raises the question of whether or not the production of cyclic AMP is causally involved in the typical *in vivo* clinical cholera since its elevation occurs later than the onset of cholera toxin induced secretion *in vivo*.

POWELL called attention to mounting evidence that both sodium and anion are being secreted under the influence of cholera toxin. He showed recently that there is an increase in the resistance of the gut after cholera toxin or after cyclic AMP. This suggests further that instead of an increase in permeability there may be a decrease of the passive permeability.

Intestinal Absorption and Malabsorption,
edited by T. Z. Csáky.
Raven Press, New York © 1975

The Influence of *Escherichia coli* and Other Bacterial Enterotoxins on Intestinal Fluid Transport

John G. Banwell

University of Kentucky Medical Center, Department of Medicine, Division of Gastroenterology, Lexington, Kentucky 40506

INTRODUCTION

Several bacteria, in addition to *V. cholerae,* are known to elaborate exoenterotoxins. *Escherichia coli, Shigella dysenteriae, Staphylococcus aureus, Clostridium perfringens,* and *Pseudomonas aeroginosa* have all been shown to have this capacity (Banwell and Sherr, 1973). These toxins, in contradistinction to cholera toxin, are only available at present in a crude or impure form and their structural characteristics have yet to be defined. Nevertheless, they fulfill the usually accepted criteria for classification as exoenterotoxins.

In this chapter major interest will be directed to an analysis of the effects of *E. coli* enterotoxin on the mucosa for three major reasons. (a) The significance of *E. coli* enterotoxin induced diarrheal disease in relation to health and the economy is considerable and its pathogenetic role in human (childhood and traveler's diarrhea) (Rowe, Taylor, and Bettelheim, 1970; South, 1971), as well as in animal illness (infantile gastroenteritis of pigs and calves) (Tennant, 1971), is now well defined. (b) Although presently available preparations of *E. coli* enterotoxin are impure, several interesting similarities and differences are already apparent in the mode of action of this toxin in comparison with cholera enterotoxin. (c) Two distinct forms of *E. coli* enterotoxin are known, a heat labile (LT) and a heat stable (ST) form (Gyles and Barnum, 1969; Smith and Gyles, 1969), which may cause intestinal fluid secretion by different pathogenetic mechanisms.

I. ESCHERICHIA COLI ENTEROTOXINS

It can be demonstrated by a variety of techniques that enterotoxin producing strains of *E. coli* do not invade the mucosal surface or cause intestinal mucosal injury; broth culture filtrates of *E. coli* containing the enterotoxin do not cause inflammatory changes in the mucosa when examined by light or electron microscopy (Dupont, Formal, Hornick, Snyder, Libonati, Sheahan, LaBrec, and Kalas, 1971; Moon, Whipp, and Baetz, 1971).

Both ST and LT enterotoxins are elaborated and released into broth culture filtrates during the log phase of cell growth in a manner similar to cholera toxin (Evans, Evans, and Gorbach, 1973) and into intestinal fluid during small intestinal colonization of experimental animals (Guerrant, Ganguly, Casper, Moore, Pierce, and Carpenter, 1973) as well. A variety of factors may determine whether the organism can colonize the small intestine successfully (Table 1). In the pig the presence of the K88 plasmid transmitted fimbrial antigen is involved in the ability of enterotoxigenic organism to colonize the upper intestine, perhaps by favoring adherence of the bacteria to the mucosal surface (Jones and Rutter, 1972). Bertschinger, Moon, and Whipp (1972a) have shown that enteropathogenic strains of *E. coli* are as-

TABLE 1. *Some factors that may influence the enteropathogenicity of E. coli*

1. Intestinal motility—gross—flow of contents and muscular activity
   —fine —villikinin

2. Bacterial fimbriae (pili) —K88 antigen

3. Association between bacteria and intestinal microvillus membrane
   —special receptors, steric configuration
   —physical factors

4. Antibacterial or antitoxic antibodies

5. Mucosal cell turnover

sociated with porcine intestinal epithelium, being characteristically distributed along the villi from the tip to base, contiguous to the brush border membrane. In contrast, nonenteropathogenic strains remained near the central lumen and tips of the villi and were only occasionally close to the brush border. Although in another study (Bertschinger, Moon, and Whipp 1972b) no close correlation was demonstrated between the degree of this association of bacteria to the plasma membrane and fluid secretion, it is probable that the mucosal cell surface may contain special anatomical structures (Gibbons and Van Houte, 1971), molecular configurations, or physical forces (Hattori, 1970) that facilitate binding of whole bacterial cells to the microvillus surface. Release of enterotoxin molecules during the course of bacterial cell division would then occur in immediate propinquity to the cell surface and the receptor binding sites for the enterotoxin. One is reminded of the data of Crane and Diedrich presented earlier in this volume in which, during transmucosal glucose transport, kinetic advantages were present for glucose molecules formed from brush border disaccharidase cleavage of lactose. Comparable conditions which would allow the release of enterotoxin close to its receptor binding site on the mucosal cell would result in a maximum net fluid secretory (diarrheal) response from small quantities of released enterotoxin.

A. Some General Characteristics of Labile and Heat Stable E.coli Toxin

LT has a high molecular weight (Table 2); an estimate of 5×10^6 is provided by Jacks, Wu, Braemer, and Bidlack (1973). In attempts to further purify this crude material these workers noted that endotoxin was linked to the enterotoxin and could not be separated after Sephadex G-200 column chromatography purification. Enterotoxin activity was acid labile, destroyed by pronase, but resistant to trypsin, a feature common to cholera and Shigella enterotoxins, as well.

TABLE 2. Characteristic features of heat stable (ST) and heat labile (LT) E. coli enterotoxin

	ST	LT
MW	$10^3–10^4$	$> 5 \times 10^6$
Dialyzability	slow	no
Antigenicity	?no	yes
pH	stable pH 1–10.0	acid labile pH < 3.0
Heat	stable after boiling for 30 min	inactivated by boiling
Inactivation by antibody	no	yes
Enterotoxicity after removal of toxin	no	yes
Resistance of pronase and trypsin	yes	yes
Plasmid control	yes	yes
Onset of secretion	rapid	delayed
Duration of secretion	short-lived	prolonged
Activation of adenylate cyclase	?no	yes

In spite of the differences in molecular weight and purity of *E. coli* LT and cholera toxin (MW estimated to be 84,000), several lines of evidence suggest that the two molecules have certain similar immunological determinants. Gyles and Barnum (1969) demonstrated that antisera against peptone dialysate LT, heterologous enterotoxin-producing *E. coli,* and *V. cholerae* neutralized porcine LT but was absent from antisera against heterologous enterotoxin-negative *E. coli*. Sack, Jacobs, and Mitra (1974) observed that antibodies to enterotoxin are regularly formed after infection with enterotoxigenic *E. coli* in man and that immunization with *E. coli* enterotoxin in rabbits (Sack, 1973) protected against homologous enterotoxin challenge, thereby suggesting a role for these agents in natural immunity to LT. Gyles (1974) was able to demonstrate identical precipitin lines against human and porcine *E. coli* LT using anti-LT serum. The antigen producing the precipitin line appeared to be identical in enterotoxin preparations from various serotypes of *E. coli,* and there were antigens common to *E. coli* LT and *V. cholerae* enterotoxins, which induced neutralizing antibodies against *E. coli* LT but not cholera enterotoxin.

ST has an estimated molecular weight of 1,000 to 10,000 (Bywater, 1972; Jacks and Wu, 1974). It is a slowly dialyzable nonantigenic protein which has only been partially purified. It is of interest that the toxin was resistant to acid, trypsin, and pronase, as well as heat stable; the purest preparation contained 15% protein and 2% carbohydrate.

B. Evidence for E.coli Enterotoxin Stimulation of an Active Fluid Secretory Process

Net fluid accumulation in isolated loops of small intestines exposed to *E. coli* enterotoxin has been found to be isotonic and of an electrolyte composition similar to that of intestinal fluid in the same region of the intestine (Pierce and Wallace, 1972; Sherr, Banwell, Rothfeld, and Hendrix, 1973). The fluid is low in protein content and free of cellular exudate (Moon, Whipp, and Baetz, 1971). Net fluid accumulation is independent of an osmotic driving force and any apparent alteration in transmucosal permeability, although this latter characteristic has not been experimentally proven as it has for cholera toxin.

Bidirectional fluxes for H_2O and Na *in vivo* indicate an increase in $Js \to m$ without significant change in $Jm \to s$ during net fluid secretion in response to both LT and ST (Bywater, 1973; Sherr et al., 1973). Al-Awquati, Wallace, and Greenough (1972) have examined the effects of crude broth culture filtrates of LT on rabbit mucosa using the Ussing *in vitro* chamber technique. In response to prior toxin exposure *in vivo,* net absorption of Na^+ was inhibited and secretion of Cl^- appeared as a new process, findings similar to those obtained by the same workers and others with crude and purified cholera toxin (Tables 3 and 4). The changes in short-circuit current and mucosal conductance that occurred were similar to those associated with cyclic AMP or theophylline addition to mucosa in the isolated chamber, providing evidence that LT exerts its effect through activation of the cyclic AMP–adenylate cyclase system.

Additional evidence for a role for the cyclic AMP–adenylate cyclase system in fluid secretion in response to *E. coli* toxin is provided by Evans and co-workers (Evans, Chen, Curlin, and Evans, 1972; Guerrant et al., 1973), who demonstrated increased cyclic AMP and adenylate cyclase activity in intestinal mucosa on exposure to LT. Guerrant et al. (1973) observed that the onset and recovery of enterotoxin-induced fluid secretion in the dog corresponded with changes in mucosal adenyl cyclase activation. However, although an immediate increase in adenylate cyclase corresponded with transient fluid secretion, adenylate cyclase activity remained elevated after net fluid secretion had reverted to net absorption. It would be desirable for this response to be defined in another animal species which responds to LT to provide conclusive evidence that adenyl cyclase activation was a prerequisite to fluid secretion in response to this enterotoxin. Adenyl cyclase activation in response to LT has been demonstrated in adrenal cell cultures (Donta,

TABLE 3. Short-circuit current (SCC), transmucosal resistance (R) and residual ion flux (J_v) in response to E. coli and V. cholerae enterotoxins

	SCC	R	J_v
Control	2.5 ± 0.2	36	2.2 ± 0.6
E. coli—crude	3.0 ± 0.3	45	2.7 ± 0.6
V. cholerae—crude	3.6 ± 0.2	58	1.4 ± 0.6
—pure	3.6 ± 0.2	50	1.6 ± 0.8

J_v = SCC—Na^+ and Cl^-.
All fluxes are expressed as $Eq/cm^{-2} hr^{-1}$.
After Al-Awquati, Wallace, and Greenough (1972) and Field, Fromm, Al-Awquati, and Greenough (1972).

Moon, and Whipp, 1974; Donta and Smith, 1974), hamster ovary cells, and rabbit intestinal cells (Kantor, Tao, and Borbach, 1974). In the adrenal and hamster ovary cell system (Guerrant, Brunton, Schnaitman, Rebhun, and Gilman, 1974) the response appears to be specific for LT. Kantor, Tao, and Gorbach (1974), however, showed that broth culture filtrates of a human E. coli strain, when concentrated (50 ×) after heat inactivation of LT, retained 17 to 26% of their stimulatory activity for cyclic AMP in rabbit intestinal cells. This raises a possibility that ST might also activate adenyl cyclase to some extent. The response of intestinal tissue to ST in the isolated chamber, as well as the adenyl cyclase response, needs to be defined with purer samples of ST free of all LT activity. LT did not inhibit phosphodiesterase activity or measurably alter guanyl cyclase levels. The stimulatory effect of LT was additive to that of prostaglandins and fluoride stimulation. Evidence for LT mediating its effect in a manner similar to cholera is, therefore, persuasive; but, most evidence is against ST exerting its fluid stimulatory effect through this system.

TABLE 4. Unidirectional and net ion fluxes across isolated mucosa of rabbit ileum in vitro

	Na^+			Cl^-		
	Ms	Sm	Net	Ms	Sm	Net
Control	13.9	12.3	+1.0 ± 0.3	9.4	8.1	+1.3 ± 0.5
E. coli—crude toxin	10.5	11.0	−0.6 ± 0.5[a]	5.9	6.7	−0.9 ± 0.4[a]
V. cholera—crude toxin	9.4	9.8	−0.4 ± 0.7[a]	5.8	8.3	−2.6 ± 0.5[a]
—pure	10.8	12.1	−1.3 ± 0.4[a]	6.0	7.9	−1.9 ± 0.2[a]

[a] Significantly different from control ($p < 0.05$).
Ms = Mucosa to serosal flux.
Sm = Serosa to mucosal flux.
Net = net flux.
After Al-Awquati, Wallace, and Greenough (1972) and Field, Fromm, Al-Awquati, and Greenough (1972).

C. Nature of Intestinal Mucosal Receptor Binding Sites for E. coli Enterotoxins

Pierce (1973) studied the inhibitory effect of cholera toxoids and crude ganglioside on *E. coli* LT and ST using the rabbit loop model. In this system, although ganglioside did inhibit *E. coli* enterotoxin activity, the mean amount of ganglioside producing a 50% decrease in secretory response to cholera enterotoxin was 18.9 ng, whereas, comparable reduction in the secretory response to the *E. coli* ST enterotoxin required 1,500 to 94,000 ng of ganglioside. This inhibition was, moreover, different from that observed with cholera enterotoxin: the slopes of the inhibition curves for *E. coli* being flatter and shallower. Holmgren (1973) made similar studies *in vitro* using a series of pure gangliosides and found that several orders more of ganglioside were required to achieve inhibition of LT than for cholera and that differences between the inhibitory effect of GM_1 ganglioside, now proposed as the tissue receptor binding site for cholera toxin (van Heyningen, Carpenter, Pierce, and Greenough, 1971; Cuatrecasas, 1973; Holmgren, Lonnroth, and Svennerholm, 1973; van Heyningen, 1974) and several other neutral sphingolipids and gangliosides, were less pronounced for *E. coli* LT. Holmgren (1973) was of the opinion that binding of *E. coli* toxin (LT) to GM_1 ganglioside was not pathogenetically significant and probably only a reflection of some structural similarities between *E. coli* LT and cholera toxin molecules. In support of this concept, choleragenoid, a pure toxoid of cholera toxin, was able to inhibit the ileal fluid secretory response to cholera toxin, but, it had no inhibitory effect on the secretory response to *E. coli* enterotoxin. This can be attributed to the fact that the intestinal receptor for *E. coli* toxin was not affected by the cholera toxoid molecule, and, therefore, must be different from the cholera toxin binding site.

There was no inhibition of *E. coli* ST by ganglioside (Pierce, 1973). The mechanism of ST interaction with the mucosa requires further study. The unusually small molecule size of ST raises the possibility that it could even enter the intestinal cell by pinocytosis or through the intercellular junctional zone (Yardley and Brown, 1973) and exert an effect in this manner rather than depending on interaction with a mucosal cell surface-receptor binding site.

D. In Vivo Fluid Secretory Response to E. coli Enterotoxins

The fluid secretory response in the dog (Pierce and Wallace, 1972) and the rabbit (Sherr et al. 1973) to a crude broth culture filtrate containing both human ST and LT have been described. Both studies demonstrated an early onset to the secretory response, occurring within 15 to 30 min of exposure in the dog and the rabbit and a more evanescent total duration of fluid secretion after exposure than found with cholera toxin. Glucose in a concentration of 60 mM was able to enhance sodium and water absorption to the same degree in the presence or absence of *E. coli* toxin. However, active transport of glucose and glycine after *E. coli* toxin exposure was decreased compared with that of the unstimulated intestine, suggesting that the *E. coli* enterotoxin or closely associated soluble products in the broth culture alter transport processes, as well as stimulate secretion. This effect on active glucose transport was not observed in the calf (Bywater, 1970), but could have remained undetected since higher concentrations (50 to 60 mM) of glucose were employed.

It has been known for some years, however, that porcine ST has a rapid onset of action and short duration and LT a slower onset and longer duration (Lariviere, Gyles, and Barnum 1972). Evans, Evans, and Pierce (1973) have recently analyzed the individual response to human ST and LT using isolated rabbit intestinal loops. The onset of net fluid accumulation in response to ST was immediate even at low doses. Onset of net fluid accumulation in response to LT was rapid at high doses but delayed at lower doses. Maximum fluid accumulation in response to ST occurred between 4 and 6 hr after injection of loops at all doses tested. Maximum loop response to LT, however, occurred 10 to 18 hr after injection and fluid accumulation to LT increased in duration with increasing doses.

Both LT and ST *in vivo* primarily enhanced transmucosal plasma to lumen flux of water and sodium in calves (Bywater, 1973) and rabbits (Sherr et al., 1973) without significantly altering lumen to plasma flux. These findings are similar to those made in human and experimental cholera. There is no information available concerning the influence of LT and ST on fluid transport in the colon, gallbladder, or other epithelia.

E. Influence of Age on Susceptibility to *E. coli* Enterotoxins

It is well known that human infants (South, 1971) and those of various animals (Stevens, Gyles, and Barnum, 1972) are especially predisposed to *E. coli*-induced diarrhea; resistance to infection increases with age. Stevens, Gyles, and Barnum (1972) have shown that resistance to porcine LT and ST toxin increases with age, and, although the resistance from day 18 to 38 of age could be accounted for solely by the increase in weight of the animal, the marked increase in resistance that occurred between birth and 18 days of age cannot be accounted for in the same manner. Antibodies in milk or colostrum may be responsible, in part, for the decrease in resistance after weaning, but the change in susceptibility to LT was the same as observed with ST, which is nonneutralizable, so that factors other than antibodies must also be involved. There may be factors, such as epithelial cell turnover, as well as changes in passive permeability of the mucosa (Orlic and Lev, 1973) which accompany development of the animal.

F. The Indirect Effect of *E.coli* Enterotoxins on Unexposed Intestinal Mucosa

ST and LT induce fluid secretion from the small intestine, and there is a cranial to caudal decrease in reactivity to both (Stevens, Gyles, and Barnum, 1972). *E. coli* toxin placed on one intestinal loop will cause secretion in an adjacent or unexposed loop in a manner similar to that observed following exposure to cholera toxin (Staley, Jones, and Smith-Staley, 1973). The mechanism of this effect is unknown. It now seems unnecessary to invoke a humoral messenger (or at least the release of endogenous prostaglandins) (Kimberg, Field, Gershon, and Henderson, 1974) in the link between direct binding of cholera toxin to the receptor and subsequent activation of intestinal mucosal adenyl cyclase. However, the unexposed loop effect, since it can be reproduced in cross circulation experiments (Vaughan and Dohadwalla, 1969), most probably depends on the humoral release from the intestinal wall of a circulating agent that causes intestinal secretion. Several "candidate" GI hormones are now recognized as capable of causing intestinal secretion, in particular, vasoactive polypeptide, gastric inhibitory polypeptide, gastrin, glucagon, cholecystokinin, pancreozymin, as well as prostaglandin release (Schultz, Frizzell, and Nellans, 1974). This unexposed loop phenomenon may have additional significance in relation to the intestinal secretion associated with other gastrointestinal diseases, such as ulcerative colitis and tropical sprue. Further definition of this interesting phenomenon will be dependent on the development of accurate assay techniques for detecting low concentrations of GI hormones, as well as enterotoxins.

II. SHIGELLA DYSENTERIAE ENTEROTOXIN

Keusch, Grady, Mata, and McIver (1972) have described the characteristics and obtained partial purification of this enterotoxin. It has a molecular weight of 55,000 to 60,000. Preliminary evidence from our laboratory indicates that the kinetics of the secretory process may be different from both cholera and *E. coli* enterotoxins. A delay of 100 min was observed after exposure to Shigella enterotoxin before the onset of fluid secretion (Steinberg, Banwell, Yardley, Keusch, and Hendrix, 1974). However, at maximum rates of fluid secretion, the secretory rate was not different from that of cholera toxin-induced secretion. There is, as yet, insufficient information available to state what pathogenetic mechanisms are involved in this secretory effect. Indeed, there is doubt whether this enterotoxin may be necessary for full expression of experimental bacillary dysentery and the diarrhea associated with it (Formal, Gemski, Giannella, and Austin, 1972). It may, however, be another useful stimulus to secretion by means of which fluid transport processes can be investigated.

III. ENTEROTOXINS OF STAPHYLOCOCCI, CLOSTRIDIA, AND PSEUDOMONAS

Staphylococcus (Sullivan, 1969; Sullivan and Asano, 1971), *Clostridium perfringens* (Duncan and Strong, 1969), and *Pseudomonas aeroginosa* (Kubota and Liu, 1971), all produce enterotoxins. Sullivan (1969) has demonstrated an acute reversible fluid secretory response in exposure to staphylococcal enterotoxin *in vitro*, but the mechanism of secretion remains to be clarified. Studies of Clostridial and Pseudomonas enterotoxins remain in an early phase and provide, as yet, no insight into problems of active fluid secretion.

In summary, a variety of enterotoxins, in addition to cholera toxin, cause net small intestinal fluid secretion. Several useful animal models are available for studying the characteristics of this secretory response. Enterotoxins of *E. coli* are the best defined and may prove to be of great interest in future studies of intestinal fluid secretion (Field, 1974).

ACKNOWLEDGMENT

Investigations carried out in the author's laboratory were supported by a research grant from the U.S. Public Health Service, National Institute of Arthritis, Metabolism, and Digestive Diseases.

REFERENCES

Al-Awquati, Q., Wallace, C. K., and Greenough, W. B., III (1972): Stimulation of intestinal secretion *in vitro* by culture filtrates of *Escherichia coli*. J. Infect. Dis. *125*:300–303.

Banwell, J. G., and Sherr, H. (1973): Effect of bacterial enterotoxins on the gastrointestinal tract. Gastroenterology *65*:467–497.

Bertschinger, H. U., Moon, H. W., and Whipp, S. C. (1972a): Association of *Escherichia coli* with the small intestinal epithelium. I. Comparison of enteropathogenic and nonenteropathogenic porcine strains in pigs. Infect. Immunity *5*:595–605.

Bertschinger, H. U., Moon, H. W., and Whipp, S. C. (1972b): Association of *Escherichia coli* with the small intestinal epithelium. II. Variations in association index and the relationship between association index and enterosorption in pigs. Infect. Immunity *5*:606–611.

Bywater, R. J. (1970): Some effects of *Escherichia coli* enterotoxin on net fluid, glucose and electrolyte transfer in calf small intestine. J. Comp. Path. *80*:565–567.

Bywater, R. J. (1972): Dialysis and ultrafiltration of a heat-stable enterotoxin from *Escherichia choli*. J. Med. Microbiol. *5*:337–343.

Bywater, R. J. (1973): Some effects of *Escherichia coli* enterotoxin on unidirectional fluxes of water and sodium in calf Thiry-Vella loops. Res. Vet. Sci. *14*:35–41.

Cuatrecasas, P. (1973): Interaction of *Vibrio cholerae* enterotoxin with cell membranes. Biochemistry *12*:3547–3581.

Donta, S. T., Moon, H. W., and Whipp, S. C. (1974): Detection of heat-labile *Escherichia coli* enterotoxin with the use of adrenal cells in tissue culture. Science *183*:334–5.

Donta, S. T., and Smith, D. M. (1974): Stimulation of steroidogenesis in tissue culture by enterotoxigenic *Escherichia coli* and its neutralization by specific antiserum. Infect. Immunity *9*:500–506.

Dupont, H. L., Formal, S. B., Hornick, R. B., et al. (1971): Pathogenesis of *Escherichia coli* diarrhea. New Eng. J. Med. *285:*1–9.

Duncan, C. L., and Strong, D. H. (1969): Ileal loop fluid accumulation and production of diarrhea in rabbits by cell-free products of *Clostridium perfringens*. J. Bacteriol. *100:*86–94.

Evans, Jr., D. J., Chen, L. C., Curlin, G. T., et al. (1972): Stimulation of adenyl cyclase by *Escherichia coli* enterotoxin. Nature New. Biol. *236:*137–138.

Evans, D. J., Jr., Evans, D. G., and Gorbach, S. L. (1973): Production of vascular permeability factor by enterotoxigenic *Escherichia coli* isolated from man. Infect. Immunity *8:*725–730.

Evans, D. G., Evans, D. J., Jr., and Pierce, N. F. (1973): Differences in the response of rabbit small intestine to heat-labile and heat-stable enterotoxins of *Escherichia coli*. Infect. Immunity *7:*873–880.

Field, M. (1974): Intestinal secretion. Gastroenterology *66:*1063–1084.

Field, M., Fromm, D., Al-Awquati, Q., et al. (1972): Effect of cholera enterotoxin on ion transport across isolated ileal mucosa. J. Clin. Invest. *51:*796–804.

Formal, S. B., Gemski, P., Giannella, R. A., et al. (1972): Mechanisms of *Shigella* pathogenesis. Am. J. Clin. Nutr. *25:*1427–1432.

Gibbons, R. J., and van Houte, J. (1971): Selective bacterial adherence to oral epithelial surfaces and its role as an ecological determinant. Infect. Immunity *3:*567–573.

Guerrant, R. L., Brunton, L. L., Schnaitman, T. C., et al. (1974): Cyclic AMP and alteration of Chinese hamster ovary cell morphology: A rapid, sensitive *in vitro* assay for the enterotoxins of *V. cholerae* and *E. coli*. Infect. Immunity., in press.

Guerrant, R. L., Ganguly, U., Casper, A. G. T., et al. (1973): Effect of *Escherichia coli* on fluid transport across canine small bowel. J. Clin. Invest. *52:*1707–1714.

Gyles, C. L. (1974): Immunological study of the heat-labile enterotoxins of *Escherichia coli* and *Vibrio cholerae*. Infect. Immunity *9:*564–570.

Gyles, C. L., and Barnum, D. A. (1969): A heat-labile enterotoxin from strains of *Escherichia coli* enteropathogenic for pigs. J. Infect. Dis. *120:*419–426.

Hattori, T. (1970): Adhesion between cells of *E. coli* and clay particles. J. Gen. Appl. Microbiol. *16:*351–359.

Holmgren, J. (1973): Comparison of the tissue receptors for *Vibrio cholerae* and *Escherichia coli* enterotoxins by means of gangliosides and natural cholera toxoid. Infect. Immunity *8:*851–859.

Holmgren, J., Lonnroth, I., and Svennerholm, L. (1973): Tissue receptor for cholera exotoxin: Postulated structure from studies with GM_1 ganglioside and related glycolipids. Infect. Immunity *8:*208–214.

Jacks, T. M., and Wu, B. J. (1974): Biochemical properties of *Escherichia coli* low-molecular-weight, heat-stable enterotoxin. Infect. Immunity *9:*342–347.

Jacks, T. M., Wu, B. J., Braemer, A. C., et al. (1973): Properties of the enterotoxic component in *Escherichia coli* enteropathogenic for swine. Infect. Immunity *7:*178–189.

Jones, G. W., and Rutter, J. M. (1972): Role of the K88 antigen in the pathogenesis of neonatal diarrhea caused by *Escherichia coli* in piglets. Infect. Immunity *6:*918–927.

Kantor, H. S., Tao, P., and Gorbach, S. L. (1974): Stimulation of intestinal adenyl cyclase by *Escherichia coli* enterotoxin: Comparison of strains from an infant and adult with diarrhea. J. Infect. Dis. *129:*1–9.

Keusch, G. T., Grady, G. F., Mata, L. J., et al. (1972): The pathogenesis of Shigella diarrhea. I. Enterotoxin production by *Shigella dysenteriae*. J. Clin. Invest. *51:*1212–1218.

Kimberg, D. V., Field, M., Gershon, E., et al. (1974): Effects of prostaglandins and cholera enterotoxin on intestinal mucosal cyclic AMP accumulation. Evidence against an essential role for prostaglandins in the action of toxin. J. Clin. Invest. *53:*941–949.

Kubota, Y., and Liu, P. V. (1971): An enterotoxin of *Pseudomonas aeroginosa*. J. Infect. Dis. *123:*97–98.

Lariviere, S., Gyles, C. L., and Barnum, D. A. (1972): A comparative study of the rabbit and pig gut loop systems for the assay of *Escherichia coli* enterotoxin. Can. J. Comp. Med. *36:*319–328.

Moon, H. W., Whipp, S. C., and Baetz, A. L. (1971): Comparative effects of enterotoxins from *Escherichia coli* and *Vibrio cholerae* on rabbit and swine small intestine. Lab. Invest. *25:*133–140.
Orlic, D., and Lev, R. (1973): Fetal rat intestinal absorption of horseradish peroxidase from swallowed amniotic fluid. J. Cell. Biol. *56:*106–119.
Pierce, N. F. (1972): Differential inhibitory effects of cholera toxoids and ganglioside on the enterotoxins of *Vibrio cholerae* and *Escherichia coli*. J. Exp. Med. *137:*1009–1023.
Pierce, N. F., and Wallace, C. K. (1972): Stimulation of jejunal secretion by a crude *Escherichia coli* enterotoxin. Gastroenterology *63:*439–448.
Rowe, B., Taylor, J., and Bettelheim, K. A. (1970): An investigation of traveller's diarrhoea. Lancet *1:*1–5.
Sack, R. B. (1973): Immunization with *Escherichia coli* enterotoxin protects against homologous enterotoxin challenge. Infect. Immunity *8:*641–644.
Sack, R. B., Jacobs, B., and Mitra, R. (1974): Antitoxin responses to infections with enterotoxigenic *Escherichia coli*. J. Infect. Dis. *129:*330–335.
Schultz, S. G., Frizzell, R. A., and Nellans, H. N. (1974): Ion transport by mammalian small intestine. Ann. Rev. Physiol. *36:*51–91.
Sherr, H. P., Banwell, J. G., Rothfeld, A., et al. (1973): Pathophysiological response of rabbit jejunum to *Escherichia coli* enterotoxin. Gastroenterology *65:*895–902.
Smith, H. W., and Gyles, C. L., (1969): The relationship between two apparently different enterotoxins produced by enteropathogenic strains of *Escherichia coli* of porcine origin. J. Med. Microbiol. *3:*387–401.
South, M. A., (1971): Enteropathogenic *Escherichia coli* disease: New developments and perspectives. J. Pediat. *79:*1–11.
Staley, T. E., Jones, E. W., and Smith-Staley, J. A. (1973): The effect of *Escherichia coli* enterotoxins on the small intestine with or without direct mucosal contact. Am. J. Dig. Dis. *18:*751–756.
Steinberg, S. E., Banwell, J. G., Yardley, J. H., et al. (1974): Comparison of secretory and histologic effects of Shigella and cholera enterotoxins in rabbit jejunum. Gastroenterology, in press.
Stevens, J. B., Gyles, C. L., and Barnum, D. A. (1972): Production of diarrhea in pigs in response to *Escherichia coli* enterotoxin. Am. J. Vet. Res. *33:*2511–2526.
Sullivan, R. (1969): Effects of enterotoxin B on intestinal transport *in vitro*. Proc. Soc. Exp. Biol. Med. *131:*1159–1162.
Sullivan, R., and Asano, T. (1971): Effects of staphylococcal enterotoxin B on intestinal transport in the rat. Am. J. Physiol. *220:*1793–1797.
Tennant, B. (1971): Neonatal enteric infections caused by *Escherichia coli* Ann. N.Y. Acad. Sci. *176:*1–401.
van Heyningen, S. (1973): Cholera toxin: Interaction of subunits with ganglioside GM_1. Science *183:*656–657.
van Heyningen, W. E., Carpenter, C. C. J., and Pierce, N. F. (1971): Deactivation of cholera toxin by ganglioside. J. Infect. Dis. *124:*415–418.
Vaughan, E. W. M., and Dohadwalla, A. N. (1969): The appearance of a choleragenic agent in the blood of infant rabbits infected intestinally with *Vibrio cholerae* demonstrated by cross circulation. J. Infect. Dis. *120:*658–663.
Yardley, J. H., and Brown, G. D. (1973): Horseradish peroxidase tracer studies in the intestine in experimental cholera. Lab. Invest. *28:*482–493.

DISCUSSION

Csáky remarked that the cholera vibrio produced "receptor-destroying enzyme" which interacts with the fuzzy coat of the intestinal cell and splits off a sialic acid, in addition to the typical cholera toxin. He wondered whether this enzyme had anything to do with the binding of the toxin to the effector cell and if it has any clinical role. Leach replied that the receptor-destroying enzyme is a sialidase, but in purified cholera toxin there is no sialidase activity. Sialidase produces some effect on the cell surface and also causes an increased cyclic AMP but this doesn't seem to be an essential part of the disease. PARSONS suggested that perhaps the cholera vibrio produces sialidase to increase the number of GM receptors, which then enable the toxin to latch on to a larger area on the effector cells. HENDRIX commented that there is evidence that the GM_1 ganglioside was resistant to sialidase; whereas, all others were not and, in fact, many gangliosides were indeed converted to GM_1 by sialidase.

Intestinal Absorption and Malabsorption,
edited by T. Z. Csáky.
Raven Press, New York © 1975

Recent Advances in Tropical Sprue

José J. Corcino

Tropical Malabsorption Unit, Departments of Medicine, Universities of Puerto Rico and Rochester, San Juan, Puerto Rico 00935

INTRODUCTION

Tropical sprue has been a subject of increasing interest and study in recent years. The application of new techniques for the study of intestinal transport and for the characterization of the intestinal microflora and its metabolic products has contributed significantly to a better understanding of its pathophysiology.

I. DEFINITION

Tropical sprue is an ill-defined syndrome, of unknown etiology, that occurs endemically and epidemically among residents, as well as among immigrants to the tropics (Klipstein, 1968). The wide spectra of clinical manifestations and marked fluctuations in absorptive function have generated considerable debate as to whether patients diagnosed as having tropical sprue in the various regions of the world suffer from the same disorder (Lindenbaum, 1973). Such debate will continue to exist until after the etiology of the syndrome is determined. It has been arbitrarily stated that all residents of or visitors to the tropics who have malabsorption of at least two unrelated substances, such as xylose and vitamin B_{12}, and in whom no specific cause can be found for the malabsorption be considered to have tropical sprue (Klipstein and Baker, 1970).

II. EPIDEMIOLOGY AND INCIDENCE

Tropical sprue has been conclusively shown to occur endemically in the West Indies, in the Indian subcontinent, and in Southeast Asia. It is of interest that although it is widely prevalent in the Caribbean, it has not been reported in Jamaica. Whether it occurs in other regions of the world remains undetermined, although several reports from North Africa suggest that the syndrome may exist there. A fascinating aspect of this syndrome is that its clinical manifestations may commence as long as 20 years after subjects migrate from the tropics to a temperate climate. It is well established that

Puerto Ricans who immigrate to the continental United States may develop "classical" tropical sprue several years afterward, even though they may not have returned to the island during this interval. The factors responsible for such a prolonged latent period are unknown.

The prevalence of tropical sprue among the indigenous population of endemic areas is unknown. Studies concerning intestinal function and structure as well as nutritional status in a randomly selected population from a rural community in Puerto Rico revealed abnormalities in two or more of the parameters of intestinal function measured in 12% of the subjects studied (Klipstein, Beauchamp, Corcino, Maldonado, Tomasini, Maldonado, Rubio; and Schenk, 1972). It is of interest that the dietary intake and nutritional status of such subjects can be considered adequate when compared to that of residents in temperate zones. It must be stressed that the significance of such subclinical abnormalities remains uncertain; whether they represent a mild form of tropical sprue cannot be ascertained until more is known about the etiology of this syndrome.

III. CLINICAL FEATURES

As stated in Sec. I, subjects with tropical sprue may present a wide spectra of clinical manifestations. The majority of the patients evaluated at our institution complain of diarrhea, anorexia, abdominal discomfort, weight loss, and weakness. Since the great majority of them have been symptomatic for over 4 months, they frequently show pallor, glossitis, and moderate to severe loss of muscle mass. Retinal hemorrhages, petechiae, ecchymoses, and mild icterus are present occasionally; the latter findings are more frequent in patients who have been symptomatic for longer periods of time. Edema of the lower extremities is rarely observed unless the patient has received some modality of therapy prior to hospitalization.

IV. STUDIES OF ABSORPTIVE FUNCTION

Several authors (Klipstein, 1970; Baker, 1972) have extensively reviewed the reported abnormalities of intestinal function in series of patients with tropical sprue from various parts of the world. In our experience, the assessment of xylose, vitamin B_{12}, and fat absorption is adequate for diagnostic purposes. Xylose and intrinsic-factor-bound vitamin B_{12} malabsorption are almost invariably present; steatorrhea is observed in 85% of our patients. For the sake of brevity, we will touch only on certain recent advances in the field.

A. Carbohydrate

The absorption of both monosaccharides and disaccharides is usually subnormal. Malabsorption of glucose (Sheehy, Anderson, and Baggs, 1966) and galactose (Jeejeebhoy, Desai, and Verghese, 1964) has been demonstrated.

We have recently performed studies directed at assessing the role that the intraluminal bacterial utilization of xylose may play in the malabsorption of this monosaccharide in tropical sprue (Corcino, Maldonado, and Klipstein, 1973). Utilizing a triple lumen perfusion technique, we have found an excellent correlation between the malabsorption present in such subjects, as determined by this technique, and the peak serum level attained as well as the urinary excretion of xylose after the administration of a 25-g dose of the pentose. Thus, the reported bacterial overgrowth (Gorbach, Mitra, Jacobs, Banwell, Chatterjee, and Guha Mazumder, 1969; Klipstein, Holdeman, Corcino, and Moore, 1973) present in the gastrointestinal tract of subjects with tropical sprue does not seem to play a significant role in the xylose malabsorption present in these subjects. Significant intraluminal bacterial utilization of xylose has been reported in the stagnant-loop syndrome (Goldstein, Karacadag, Wirts, and Kowlessar, 1970).

Levels of disaccharidase activity are subnormal in the jejunal mucosa of the majority of patients with untreated tropical sprue. Decreased levels of lactase, sucrase, maltase, and isomaltase have been reported (Bayless, Walter, and Barber, 1964). Impaired hydrolysis of all disaccharides tested in 11 patients has also been reported (Gray and Santiago, 1966).

B. Electrolyte and Water Transport

Limited attention has been given to electrolyte and water transport in tropical sprue. Banwell and colleagues (Banwell, Gorbach, Mitra, Cassells, Guha Mazumder, Thomas, and Yardley, 1970), utilizing a triple lumen tube perfusion technique, showed net secretion of water into the jejunum of six and into the ileum of seven of 13 patients with tropical sprue. Using a similar technique, our group has recently reported the results obtained in 10 patients with overt untreated tropical sprue and eight asymptomatic subjects (Corcino et al., 1973). Control subjects absorbed at a rate of 1.41 ± 0.23 ml/hr/cm of jejunum (mean $\pm$ SEM). Absorption of sodium and chloride was 141 and 129.9 μEq/hr/cm, respectively. The tropical sprue patients had a net secretion of water of 0.9 ± 0.2 ml/hr/cm and the secretion of sodium and chloride was 74.1 and 110.6 μEq/hr/cm, respectively. Differences concerning sodium, water, and chloride transport in tropical sprue as compared to control subjects were significant at the $p < 0.001$ level.

It is well established that glucose enhances the transport of both sodium and water in the small intestine of humans (Fordtran, Rector, and Carter, 1968). Figure 1 summarizes our findings concerning sodium, water, and chloride transport in 10 tropical sprue patients perfused with an isosmotic glucose (55.6 mM) saline solution when compared to that observed when the same subjects were perfused with a solution containing mannitol at the same concentration. A significant enhancement in sodium transport was observed

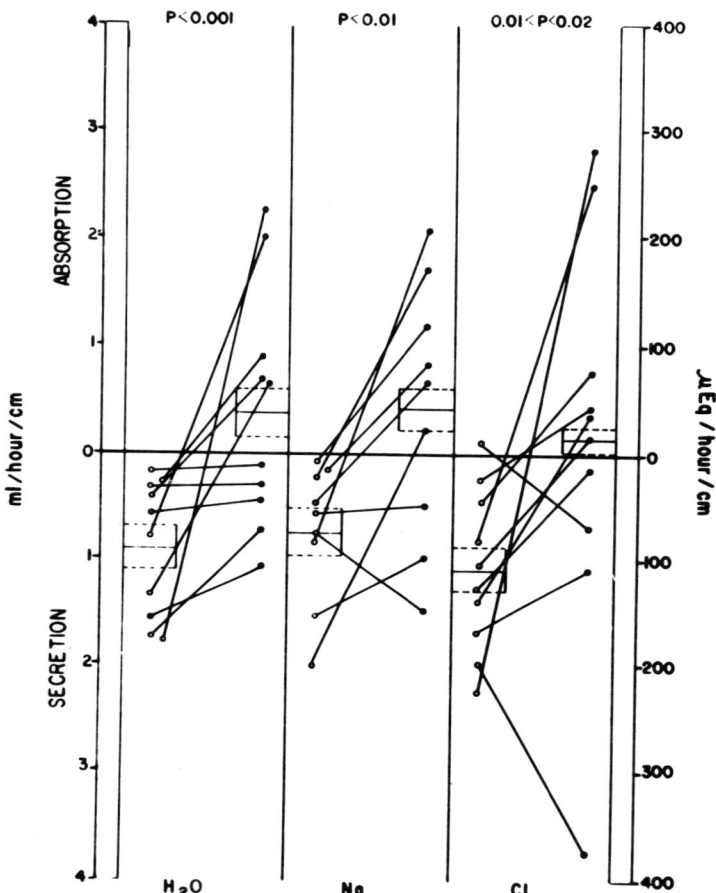

FIG. 1. Water, sodium, and chloride transport from an isosmotic mannitol saline solution (left side of each column) and from an isosmotic glucose saline solution (right side of each column) in tropical sprue subjects; mean ± SEM.

in seven out of the nine subjects studied; this was accompanied by a concomitant increase in water transport. Such an increase was, nevertheless, subnormal when compared to that observed in eight control subjects perfused under similar conditions (Fig. 2). Thus, in tropical, unlike in nontropical sprue (Fordtran, Rector, Locklear, and Eaton, 1967; Schmid, Phillips, and Summerskill, 1969) glucose enhancement of sodium and water transport is partially preserved. Whether these differences result from the variability of the jejunal mucosal lesion in tropical sprue or whether it has any relationship to the effect on electrolyte and water transport induced by the enterotoxins synthesized by the microorganisms present in the jejunum of such patients (Klipstein, et al., 1973) remains undetermined. No correlation was demon-

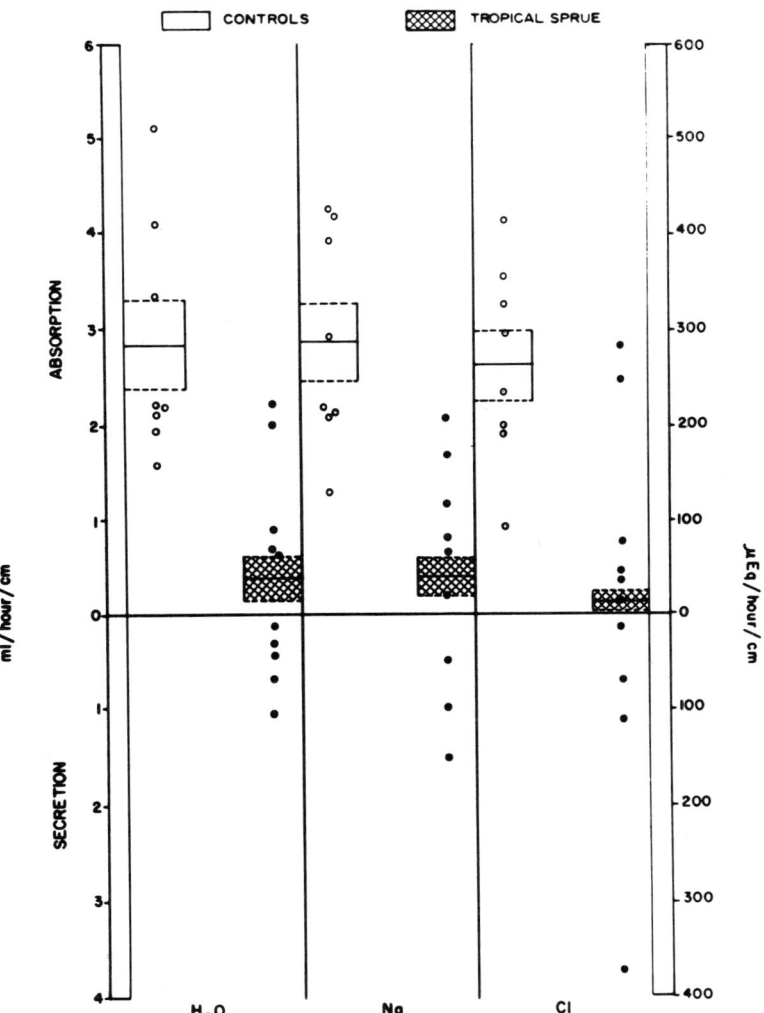

FIG. 2. Water, sodium, and chloride transport from an isosmotic glucose (55.6 mM) saline solution in controls and tropical sprue subjects; mean ± SEM.

strable between the severity of the jejunal lesion and the increase by glucose of sodium and water transport. It would seem logical to assume that, since glucose is malabsorbed in tropical sprue, its enhancement of sodium and water transport would be subnormal when compared to that observed in control subjects. Figure 3 shows that glucose malabsorption was, indeed, present in the tropical sprue subjects; although we were unable to obtain a significant correlation between the glucose absorbed by such subjects and the increase in sodium and water transport observed.

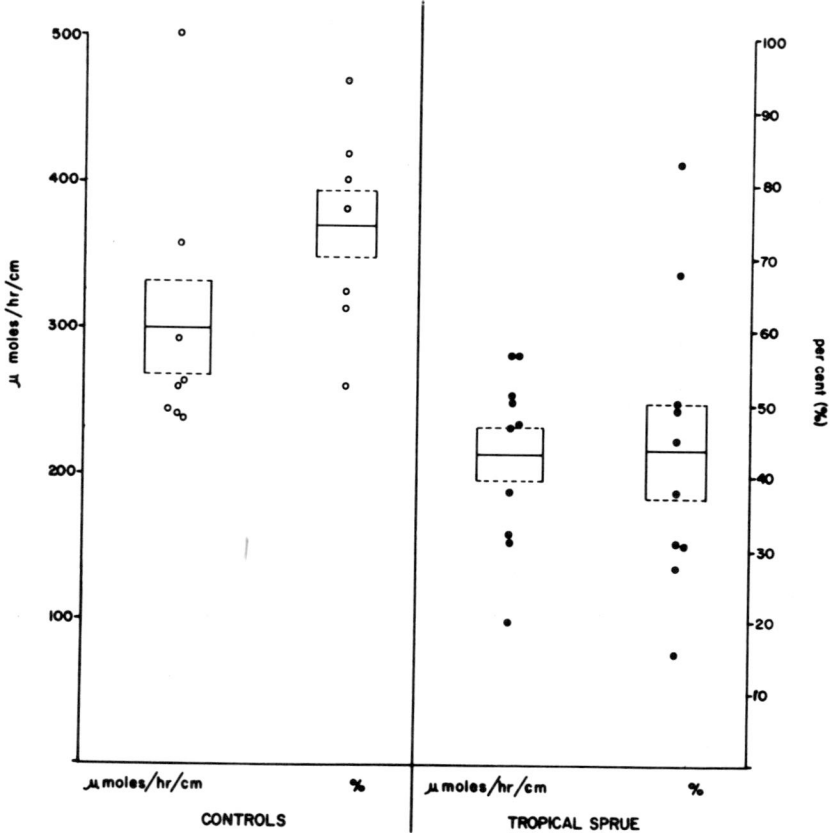

FIG. 3. Transport of glucose in controls and tropical sprue subjects; mean ± SEM.

C. Folate Absorption

Folate absorption in tropical sprue has been the subject of many investigations. Most of them have been performed with pharmacological doses of pteroylglutamic acid (PGA) administered orally (Girwood, 1953; Chanarin, Anderson, and Mollin, 1958); others have utilized physiological doses of labeled PGA. None of the techniques utilized heretofore has yielded consistent results concerning malabsorption of this vitamin in tropical sprue. We have recently applied a marker perfusion technique to assess the absorption of physiological concentrations of PGA (25 ng/ml) from an isosmotic glucose (55.6 mM) saline solution. The results, depicted in Fig. 4, show a highly significant difference in PGA absorption between the tropical sprue and the control subjects. These findings may be of limited significance from the digestive and nutritional standpoint since it is well known that most of

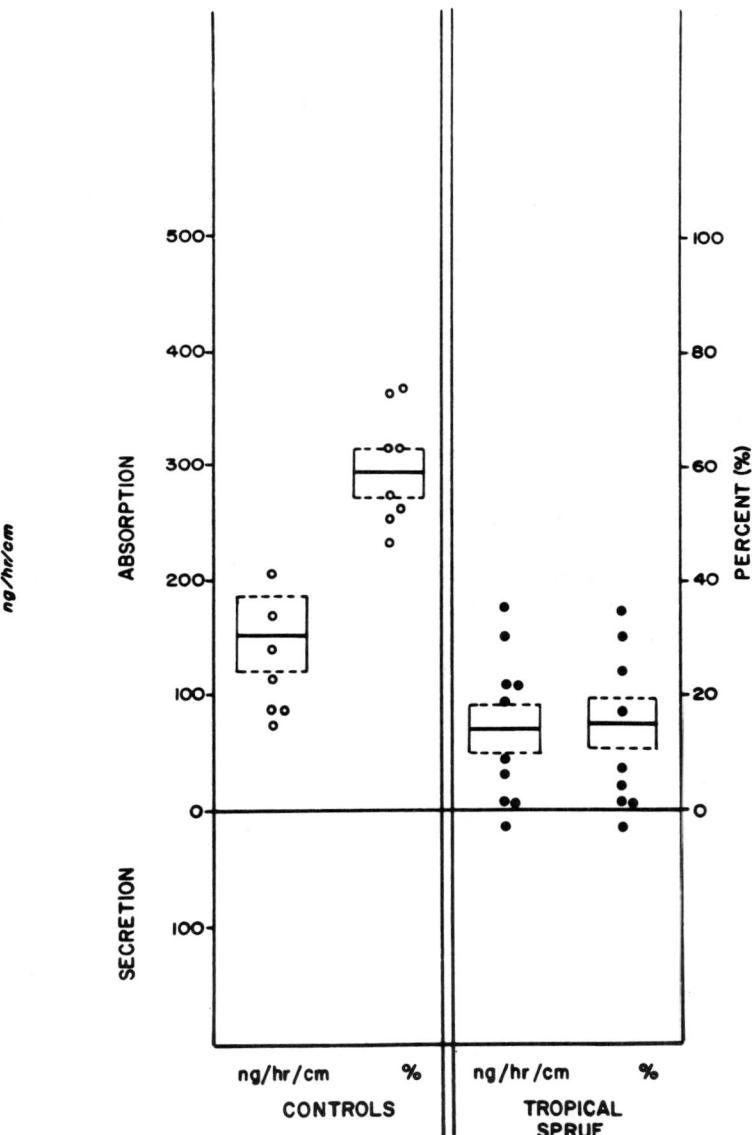

Fig. 4. Transport of pteroylglutamic acid from a glucose (55.6 mM) saline solution in controls and tropical sprue subjects; mean ± SEM.

the folates in foods are present in reduced, methyl or formyl-substituted polyglutamate forms.

A limited number of studies have been conducted utilizing polyglutamates obtained from various sources in an attempt to assess their absorption in tropical sprue (Hoffbrand, Necheles, Maldonado, Horta, and Santini, 1969). Impaired absorption has been reported in most of the patients studied. The small intestinal enzyme folate conjugase (gamma-glutamyl carboxypeptidase) converts folate polyglutamates to its mono-, di-, and triglutamate moieties during absorption. The possibility that the inability to absorb food folates in tropical sprue is due to decreased activity of this enzyme is unlikely since normal enzymatic activity has been found in both the succus entericus (Klipstein, 1967), as well as in jejunal biopsies of patients with this syndrome (Hoffbrand et al., 1969).

D. Vitamin B_{12} Absorption

Vitamin B_{12} malabsorption is almost invariably present in tropical sprue. In order to avoid the administration of pharmacological doses of this vitamin to patients during the performance of a Schilling test, we have recently applied the whole body counter technique for the assessment of the absorption of intrinsic-factor-bound vitamin B_{12}. With this technique one can perform serial B_{12} absorption studies without altering the patient's intestinal, hematological, or nutritional status. Patients with tropical sprue retain $9.6 \pm 13.4\%$ (mean $\pm$ 2 SD) of the administered radioactivity (0.5 μCi, as $^{57}CoB_{12}$, specific activity 1 μCi/μg) at the end of 7 days. Control subjects retain $55.7 \pm 29\%$ (mean $\pm$ 2 SD) during this same period of time (Corcino, Dietrich, and Lanaro, 1972). When patients with tropical sprue are treated with 1 g daily of oxytetracycline for 14 days, their absorption becomes normal; in contrast, patients who receive 3 mg of PGA orally for the same period of time show no significant improvement in their B_{12} absorption (Corcino and Dietrich, 1974). If one assumes that therapy with oxytetracycline but not with PGA suppresses or eradicates the bacterial overgrowth present in subjects with tropical sprue, one could hypothesize that both intraluminal (bacterial utilization) as well as ileal mucosal involvement may play a role in the vitamin B_{12} malabsorption observed in this syndrome. Preliminary *in vitro* studies utilizing both free and intrinsic-factor-bound B_{12} show that the coliforms more frequently isolated from the jejunum of patients with tropical sprue, *Klebsiella pneumoniae* and *Enterobacter cloacae,* have a strong avidity for the vitamin. Thus, as suggested by Lindenbaum (1973), certain similarities may exist between the stagnant-loop syndrome and tropical sprue. Final confirmation of the proposed mechanisms will require studies similar to those recently reported by Schjönsby (Schjönsby, Drasar, Tabaqchali, and Booth, 1973).

V. DEFICIENCIES

A. Folate and Vitamin B_{12}

Megaloblastic anemias due to combined folate and vitamin B_{12} deficiencies are observed in practically all the patients with tropical sprue seen in Puerto Rico. Although much emphasis has been given in the literature to the megaloblastic anemia found present in such patients, it must be emphasized that in areas where there is a high prevalence of parasitosis, concomitant iron deficiency may mask the bone marrow megaloblastic features. Iron deficiency is an infrequent finding in our patients. To our knowledge the only study directed at the assessment of inorganic iron absorption in tropical sprue yielded highly variable results (Wheby, 1969).

The usual cause of folate and vitamin B_{12} deficiency in tropical sprue is malabsorption. Besides the other possible mechanism mentioned under the section on studies of absorptive function (i.e., folate conjugase deficiency), it should be emphasized that most of the patients with tropical sprue are markedly anorectic. Thus, a suboptimal dietary intake may further aggravate pre-existing deficiencies, especially in the presence of malabsorption. Another factor that may accentuate or accelerate such deficiencies is the loss of both folates and B_{12} through bile and other gastrointestinal secretions; the small intestinal lesion present in such patients may result in an impairment of the enterohepatic circulation of these nutrients. A fourth, and thus far unproved mechanism, could be the increased loss of folates and B_{12} in the exfoliated epithelial intestinal cells. Studies performed by Swanson and co-workers (Swanson and Thomassen, 1965) suggest that in overt tropical sprue, jejunal epithelial cell turnover is decreased. Studies in progress utilizing an *in vitro* organ culture system (Browning and Trier, 1969) should shed some light into this problem.

B. Protein

Moderate to mild hypoalbuminemia is a common occurrence in tropical sprue in Puerto Rico. The mechanisms responsible for this finding may be manifold: poor protein intake due to severe anorexia, excessive loss of protein into the gastrointestinal tract (Rubini, Sheehy, Meroney, and Louro, 1961), decrease in albumin synthesis by the liver (Jeejeebhoy, Samuel, and Singh, 1969), and, last but not least, malabsorption of amino acids and oligopeptides.

We have recently performed studies utilizing marker perfusion techniques in nine tropical sprue and six control subjects in order to assess amino acid absorption from a mixture of eight essential amino acids (Adibi and Gray, 1967). The absorption of isoleucine, leucine, valine, and threonine was significantly lower in the subjects with tropical sprue (Corcino and Klipstein, 1974). Thus, an apparent selective malabsorption for the neutral amino acids, with the exception of methionine, seems to be present in this syndrome. In two out of the nine subjects treated for at least 6 months with oxytetracycline, folic acid, and vitamin B_{12}, perfusion with the same amino acid solution revealed that the absorption of all amino acids had returned to normal.

VI. INTESTINAL MORPHOLOGY

Morphological abnormalities in the jejunal mucosa of patients with tropical sprue are variable and, therefore, nondiagnostic. Figure 5 sumarizes the abnormalities found present in the jejunal biopsies of 50 subjects with tropi-

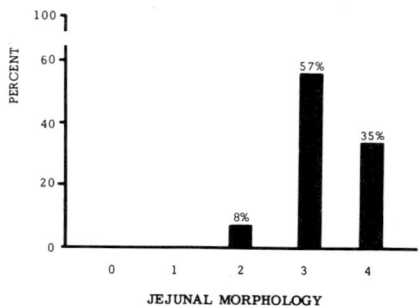

FIG. 5. Jejunal morphology in 50 patients with tropical sprue. The percent of patients with various morphological abnormalities are depicted above each bar.

cal sprue classified according to the criteria established in our laboratory (Schenk and Klipstein, 1972). Studies conducted in asymptomatic subjects from a rural community in Puerto Rico (Klipstein et al., 1972) also revealed variable abnormalities in jejunal morphology (Fig. 6). As shown, there is some overlapping between the abnormalities present in the patients with tropical sprue when compared to those found in asymptomatic subjects. The significance of these findings and its impact on the nutritional status of residents in the tropics remains undetermined.

Although more attention has been directed to the jejunal morphological derangements present in subjects with tropical sprue, ileal biopsies performed in several of these subjects have revealed morphological abnormalities almost identical to those described for the jejunum. Thus, the small intestine is uniformly involved in this syndrome in contrast to what has been reported in nontropical sprue.

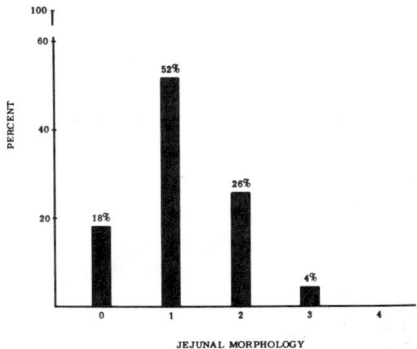

FIG. 6. Jejunal morphology in 93 randomly selected subjects from a rural community in Puerto Rico. The percent of patients with various morphological abnormalities are depicted above each bar.

VII. ETIOLOGY

Although dietary factors cannot be completely disregarded, the weight of the evidence currently available, although to a large extent circumstantial, favors an infectious etiology for this syndrome. It may be summarized as follows:

(a) The disease may be acquired by visitors to the tropics (Klipstein, 1968).

(b) Epidemics have been described among visitors (Avery, 1948) and local populations (Baker, Mathan, and Joseph, 1962).

(c) "Sprue" houses have been described in India (Mathan, Ignatius, and Baker, 1966).

(d) A seasonal incidence has been observed (Klipstein and Corcino, 1974).

(e) The disease responds to treatment with antibacterial agents (Guerra, Wheby, and Bayless, 1965; Maldonado, Horta, Guerra, and Pérez-Santiago, 1969).

Multiple bacteriological studies have been performed in subjects with tropical sprue in an attempt to characterize its intestinal microflora. Both aerobic and anaerobic organisms have been looked for in jejunal aspirates as well as in intestinal biopsies. Gorbach and colleagues (1969), while working in Calcutta, reported bacterial contamination by coliforms of the upper small bowel in patients with tropical sprue. More recently Klipstein and co-workers (Klipstein et al., 1973) have confirmed the previously reported coliform overgrowth found present in the jejunum of these patients and have demonstrated that *Klebsiella pneumoniae* and *Enterobacter cloacae* constitute the predominant organisms. They have demonstrated that these organisms synthesize an enterotoxin capable of producing a positive response in the rabbit ileal loop model and that ethanol is an important byproduct of their intermediary metabolism. The role that these recent findings play in the etiopathogenesis of the syndrome remains uncertain. Attempts to isolate mycoplasma (Lev, Alexander, Levenson, Hepner, Gerson, Corcino, Janowitz, and Herbert, 1969) or enteric viruses (Bayless, Guardiola-Rotger, and Wheby, 1966) from subjects with tropical sprue have been inconclusive. The role that the alga *Prototheca portoricensis* may play in the etiology of tropical sprue is also uncertain (Bernstein, Lepow, Wagle, Doran, and Brand, 1973). We have not been able to isolate this organism from the stools, jejunal aspirates, or jejunal biopsies of 10 patients recently studied (Corcino and Medina, 1974).

Thus, we can still quote the statement that Manson-Bahr made 21 years ago and conclude that "The true aetiology of tropical sprue remains one of the outstanding conundrums in tropical medicine."

VIII. TREATMENT

The effectiveness of therapy with folic acid and vitamin B_{12}, either singly or in combination, is well established (Klipstein et al., 1968). Follow-up studies of patients treated exclusively with these vitamins revealed the persistence of impaired intestinal function as well as of jejunal mucosal abnormalities.

Oral antibiotics have been reported effective in relieving diarrhea in tropical sprue since 1938 (Rogers, 1938). Short-term therapeutic trials with various antibacterials were used by French in 1956, by Sheehy and Pérez-Santiago in 1961, and by O'Brien and England in 1966. Guerra et al. (1965) were the first to report on the use of long-term (6 months) antibiotic therapy in the management of eight patients with tropical sprue. They obtained excellent results concerning the normalization of xylose, B_{12}, and fat absorption; jejunal morphology also returned to near normal in all eight. More recently, Maldonado and co-workers (1969) have demonstrated that 6-month courses with nonabsorbable sulfonamides are also effective in the treatment of tropical sprue.

The long-term results of prolonged antibiotic therapy in patients with tropical sprue who continue to reside in the tropics were recently evaluated (Rickles, Klipstein, Tomasini, Corcino, and Maldonado, 1972). Patients who had received long-term antibiotic therapy were reevaluated 5 or more years after the original treatment in order to be able to determine the long-term efficacy of such therapy. The majority had subnormal xylose and vitamin B_{12} absorption as well as an abnormal intestinal morphology. Whether such findings represent a relapse of the original disorder or a "reinfection" remains uncertain.

Although tropical sprue remains an ill-defined entity of unknown etiology, it has stimulated research on intestinal absorption and malabsorption in the tropics, as well as on the role that such malabsorption may play in the malnutrition observed in such regions.

ACKNOWLEDGMENTS

The author thanks Dr. F. A. Klipstein for invaluable cooperation and helpful discussions during much of this work; Dr. Rafael Santini, Miss G. Coll, Mrs. S. Millán, Mrs. A. Meléndez, Miss F. Rodríguez, Mr. J. Rodríguez, and Mr. W. Román for technical assistance; Miss M. Maldonado, R. N., and her staff at the Clinical Research Center for nursing care; and Mrs. A. Mejía for secretarial assistance.

This work was supported by a grant from Research Corporation, New York, New York; by U.S. Public Health Service Training Grant No. 5-TO-1-AMO 5177 (Gastroenterology) and Grant RR-63-12 from the General Clinical Research Center, Program of the Division of Research Resources, National Institutes of Health, Bethesda, Maryland. The author has an Academic Career Development Award (AM 70696) from the National Institute of Arthritis and Metabolic Diseases, National Institutes of Health, Bethesda, Maryland.

REFERENCES

Adibi, S. A. and Gray, S. J. (1967): Intestinal absorption of essential amino acids in man. Gastroenterology 52:837–845.
Avery, F. (1948): Outbreaks of sprue during the Burma campaign. Trans. Roy. Soc. Trop. Med. Hyg. 41:377–379.
Baker, S. J., Mathan, V. I., and Joseph, I. (1962): Epidemic tropical sprue. Am. J. Dig. Dis. 7:959–962.
Baker, S. J. (1972): Tropical sprue. Brit. Med. Bull. 28:87–92.
Banwell, J. G., Gorbach, S. L., Mitra, R., Cassells, J. S., Guha Mazumder, D. N., Thomas, J., and Yardley, J. H. (1970): Tropical sprue and malnutrition in West Bengal: II. Fluid and electrolyte transport in the small intestine. Am. J. Clin. Nutr. 23:1559–1568.
Bayless, T. M., Walter, W., and Barber, R. (1964): Disaccharidase deficiencies in tropical sprue. Clin. Res. 12:445.
Bayless, T. M., Guardiola-Rotger, A., and Wheby, M. S. (1966): Tropical sprue: Viral cultures of rectal swabs. Gastroenterology 51:32–35.
Bernstein, L. H., Lepow, H., Wagle, A., Doran, T., and Brand, B. (1973): Is tropical sprue and algal disease of man? Gastroenterology 64:697.
Browning, T. H. and Trier, J. S. (1969): Organ culture of mucosal biopsies of human small intestine. J. Clin. Invest. 48:1423–1432.
Chanarin, I., Anderson, B. B., and Mollin, D. L. (1958): The absorption of folic acid. Brit. J. Haemat. 4:156–166.
Corcino, J. J., Dietrich, R., and Lanaro, A. (1972): Assessment of vitamin B_{12} absorption in tropical sprue utilizing a whole body counter. Bol. Asoc. Med. P. R. 64:275.
Corcino, J. J., Maldonado, M., and Klipstein, F. A. (1973): Intestinal perfusion studies in tropical sprue: I. Transport of water, electrolytes and d-xylose. Gastroenterology 65:192–198.
Corcino, J. J., and Dietrich, R. (1974): Mechanisms of vitamin B_{12} malabsorption in tropical sprue. Clin. Res. 22:355.

Corcino, J. J., and Klipstein, F. A. (1974): Absorption of amino acids in tropical sprue. *Proceedings of the IV Western Hemisphere Nutrition Congress*, Miami Beach, Florida, in press.
Corcino, J. J., and Medina, M. (1974): *Unpublished observations.*
Fordtran, J. S., Rector, F. C., Locklear, T. W., and Ewton, M. F. (1967): Water and solute movement in the small intestine of patients with sprue. J. Clin. Invest. *73*:287–298.
Fordtran, J. S., Rector, F. C., and Carter, N. W. (1968): Mechanisms of sodium absorption in human small intestine. J. Clin. Invest. *47*:884–900.
French, J. M., Gaddie, R., and Smith, N. M. (1956): Tropical sprue: A study of seven cases and their response to combined chemotherapy. Quart. J. Med. *25*:333–351.
Girwood, R. H. (1953): A folic acid excretion test in the investigation of intestinal malabsorption. Lancet *2*:53–60.
Goldstein, F., Karacadag, S., Wirts, C. W., and Kowlessar, O. D. (1970): Intraluminal small intestinal utilization of d-xylose by bacteria. Gastroenterology *59*:380–386.
Gorbach, S. L., Mitra, R., Jacobs, B., Banwell, J. G., Chatterjee, B. D., Guha Mazumder, D. N. (1969): Bacterial contamination of the upper small bowel in tropical sprue. Lancet *1*:74–77.
Gray, G. M., and Santiago, N. A. (1966): Disaccharide absorption in normal and discased human intestine. Gastroenterology *51*:489–498.
Guerra, R., Wheby, M. S., and Bayless, T. M. (1965): Long-term antibiotic therapy in tropical sprue. Ann. Int. Med. *63*:619–634.
Hoffbrand, A. V., Necheles, T. F., Maldonado, N., Horta, E., and Santini, R. (1969): Malabsorption of folate polyglutamates in tropical sprue. Brit. Med. J. *2*:543–547.
Jeejeebhoy, K. N., Desai, H. G., and Verghese, R. V. (1964): Milk intolerance in tropical malabsorption syndrome. Lancet *2*:666–668.
Jeejeebhoy, K. N., Samuel, A. M., and Singh, B. (1969): Metabolism of albumin and fibrinogen in patients with tropical sprue. Gastroenterology *56*:252–267.
Klipstein, F. A. (1967): Intestinal folate conjugase activity in tropical sprue. Am. J. Clin. Nutr. *20*:1004–1009.
Klipstein, F. A. (1968): Tropical sprue. Gastroenterology *54*:275–293.
Klipstein, F. A. (1970): Recent advances in tropical malabsorption. Scand. J. Gastroenterol. Suppl. *6*:93–114.
Klipstein, F. A. and Baker, S. J. (1970): Regarding the definition of tropical sprue. Gastroenterology *58*:717–721.
Klipstein, F. A., Beauchamp, I., Corcino, J. J., Maldonado, M., Tomasini, J. T., Maldonado, N., Rubio, C., and Schenk, E. A. (1972): Nutritional status and intestinal function among rural populations in the West Indies: II. Barrio Nuevo, Puerto Rico. Gastroenterology *63*:758–767.
Klipstein, F. A., Holdeman, L. V., Corcino, J. J., and Moore, W. E. C. (1973): Enterotoxigenic intestinal bacterial in tropical sprue. Gastroenterology *79*:632–641.
Klipstein, F. A., and Corcino, J. J. (1974): Seasonal incidence of overt and subclinical malabsorption in Puerto Rico. Am. J. Trop. Med. Hyg., in press.
Lev, M., Alexander, L., Levenson, S., Hepner, G., Gerson, C., Corcino, J. J., Janowitz, H. D., and Herbert, V. (1969): Mycoplasma in the small intestine in tropical sprue. Clin. Res. *17*:595.
Lindenbaum, J. (1973): Tropical enteropathy. Gastroenterology *64*:637–642.
Maldonado, N., Horta, E., Guerra, R., and Pérez-Santiago, E. (1969): Poorly absorbed sulfonamides in the treatment of tropical sprue. Gastroenterology *57*:559–568.
Manson-Bahr, P. (1953): The causation of tropical sprue. Lancet *2*:389–391.
Mathan, V. I., Ignatius, M., and Baker, S. J. (1966): A household epidemic of tropical sprue. Gut *7*:490–494.
O'Brien, W., and England, N. W. J. (1966): Military tropical sprue from Southeast Asia. Brit. Med. J. *2*:1157–1162.
Rickles, F. R., Klipstein, F. A., Tomasini, J. T., Corcino, J. J., and Maldonado, N. (1972): Long-term follow up of antibiotic-treated tropical sprue. Ann. Int. Med. *73*:203–210.
Rogers, L. (1938): The use of Prontosil in sprue. Brit. Med. J. *2*:943–944.

Rubini, M. E., Sheehy, T. W., Meroney, W. H., and Louro, J. (1961): Exudative enteropathy: II. Observations in tropical sprue. J. Lab. Clin. Med. *58:*902–907.
Schenk, E. A., and Klipstein, F. A. (1972): A protocol for the evaluation of small bowel biopsies. Am. J. Clin. Nutr. *25:*1108–1117.
Schjönsby, H., Drasar, B. S., Tabaqchali, S., and Booth, C. C. (1973): Uptake of vitamin B_{12} by intestinal bacteria in the stagnant-loop syndrome. Scan. J. Gastroenterol. *8:*41–47.
Schmid, W. C., Phillips, S. F., and Summerskill, W. H. J. (1969): Jejunal secretion of electrolytes and water in non-tropical sprue. J. Lab. Clin. Med. *73:*772–783.
Sheehy, T. W. and Pérez-Santiago, E. (1961): Antibiotic therapy in tropical sprue. Gastroenterology *41:*208–214.
Sheehy, T. W., Anderson, P. R., and Baggs, B. E. (1966): Carbohydrate studies in tropical sprue. Am. J. Dig. Dis. *11:*461–473.
Swanson, V. L., and Thomassen, R. W. (1965): Pathology of the jejunal mucosa in tropical sprue. Am. J. Path. *46:*511–551.
Wheby, M. S. (1969): Iron absorption in tropical sprue. Am. J. Clin. Nutr. *22:*680.

DISCUSSION

The first comment quoted the known fact that young pigs show a greater sensitivity to bacterial toxins than older ones. It is also known that in non-tropical or celiac sprue there is an increase in the rate of jejunal epithelial cell turnover. What is the situation with the cell turnover in tropical sprue? CORCINO stated that little is known about this. Swanson measured crypt cell mytosis in Puerto Rican patients with tropical sprue and severe folate and B_{12} deficiencies and found a decreased mitotic index; this finding suggested to her that in tropical sprue there was a decrease in epithelial cell turnover.

DIETSCHY asked whether the organisms found in the small intestine of these patients or their enterotoxins are the etiologic agents in tropical sprue. CORCINO replied that he personally does not think that these organisms are the causal agents of tropical sprue. He feels that other factors or agents, as of yet undetermined, are responsible for the initial mucosal injury and that this in turn results in the bacterial overgrowth observed.

SUBJECT INDEX

A

Absorption
  acids and bases, 37
  ATP and, 9, 121-122
  in cholera, 255, 258-259
  energy expenditures for, 14-17
  energy source of, 9-12, 17-21, 23-28
  energy stores for, 13-14
  food ingestion rate and, 12-13
  intestinal flora and, 237-248
  of proteins, 95-96
  in tropical sprue, 286-290
  unloading and, 28-33, 36
  unstirred water and, 232-233
  of vitamins, 239
Adenyl cyclase
  cholera toxin and, 254, 262-264
  intestinal transport and, 41-43
Alanine transport
  binding and, 160, 162
  Na^+ effect, 114-116
Amino acids
  analogues and transport, 77-78
  binding affinity of, 79-84, 88-89, 175
  binding protein, 166-168
  brush border binding of, 159-163
  carrier sites for, 84-86
  cationic interactions of, 84-85
  D form uptake, 101
  as energy source, 13-14
  extrusion of, 67
  intestinal transport of, 48-54, 67, 77-91, 95-97, 171-172, 187-195
  K^+ extrusion and, 86, 93
  kinetic model for, 78-79
  mucosal membrane transport of, 78-89
  peptide uptake and, 98-99
  pyridoxine deficiency and, 102-103
  serosal membranes and, 89-90
  shunt pathway for, 90-91
  sodium and, 67, 77-78, 84-88
  sprue and, 293-294
  stereoisomers of, 83-84
  sugars and, 87, 93, 158-159
  sulfhydryl groups and, 85, 158-159
  translocation process of, 86-88
Antiabsorption drugs, 209-224
ATP
  absorption and, 9
  intestinal transport and, 40-43, 121-122, 136-137
  ionic gradients and, 23-26, 121-122
  membrane transport and, 22-23

ATP, contd.,
   Na^+ pump and, 136-137
   sources of, 17
   yield of, 17

B

Bacterial toxins (See also : Cholera)
   age of host and, 279, 299
   fluid transport and, 278-281
   immunology of, 275-276
   nature of, 273-276
Basolateral plasma membrane
   amino acid transport and, 89-90
   ATP and, 22
Bicarbamate effect
   on sugar transport, 195
Bisacodyl
   as hydragogue, 210-211, 213
Bowel, lower
   water absorption in, 240-244
Brush border
   absorption in, 156
   amino acid binding in, 156-157, 159-163, 166-169
   amino acid transport and, 78-79, 84-85, 93, 171-172
   cholera toxin and, 254
   cotransport in, 127-128, 141
   digestion in, 128-131
   enzymes of, 129-137
   fructose transport in, 128, 131
   functions of, 155
   β-glycosidase in, 144-145
   hexose transport in, 127-137
   hydrolase related transport and, 132-137, 142
   Li effect, 116-117
   Na^+ effect, 113-114, 127-130
   as organelle, 155-156, 171-172
   peptide absorption and, 105
   peptide hydrolysis by, 95
   sucrose metabolism in, 131, 137
   sugar binding in, 156
   sugar transport and, 73-74, 127-137
   sulfhydryl-reacting agents and, 158-159

C

Ca^{++}-activated ATPase
   in membrane, 22
Carbonic anhydrase
   intestinal transport and, 40-42
Carnosine
   intestinal transport of, 100
Chloride
   epithelial permeability and, 2
p-Chloromercuriphenyl sulfate
   amino acid transport and, 85, 124, 139
   Na^+ transport site and, 117-119
Cholera
   antibiotics and, 264-266
   absorptive functions in, 253
   cAMP in, 254-255, 262-264, 267, 270
   fluid composition of, 255
   fluid production in, 255-258
   glucose absorption in, 258-259
   intestinal secretion in, 259-262, 264-266
   prostaglandins and, 263-269
   secretion reversal, 264-266
   sialidase and, 283-284

Cholera, contd.,
  toxin
    cAMP and, 254-255, 262-264, 267, 270
    description of, 253-254, 263, 270
    epithelial cell effects, 254-255
    intestinal fluid and, 255-258
    receptor of, 254-255, 283-284
    secretion and, 259-266
Choline
  amino acid transport and, 114-117
Copper
  epithelial permeability and, 2
Coupled transport
  sugar and Na^+, 58-60, 62, 67, 127-128, 141
Cyclic AMP
  bacterial toxins and, 276-277
  cholera toxin and, 254-255, 262-264
  intestinal transport and, 41-42
Cystinuria
  peptide absorption in, 101-102

D

Deoxycholate
  action of, 210-212, 215-216, 219-224
  as antiabsorptive, 209-210
5,5-Dimethyl-2,4-oxazolidinedione
  intestinal transport of, 38-39
Diphenolic laxatives, 211-212

E

E. coli enterotoxin
  cAMP and, 276-277
  fluid transport and, 278-281
  nature of, 273-276
  receptor site of, 278
Electrical potential
  ion gradient hypothesis and, 120-121
Endoplasmic reticulum
  Na^+,K^+-ATPase and, 7
  sodium transport and, 4-5, 7
Enterocyte
  sugar pump of, 67-74
Epithelia
  cell organization of, 15-16
  cholera toxin and, 254-256
  energetics of, 9-17
  intercellular shunts in, 1-2
  multilayer effects, 2-4
  permeability of, 2
  sodium transport in, 4-5
  transcellular shunts in, 2
Extracellular space
  determination of, 75

F

Fatty acids
  as energy source, 13-14
Fluid transport
  in cholera, 255-258
  energy sources for, 18-19
  in germ-free animals, 240-244
  osmotic flow, 177-178

Folate absorption
  in tropical sprue, 291-293, 296
Frog skin
  cell coupling in, 2-4
Fructose
  absorption of, 229-230
  transport of, 128

G

Galactose
  absorption kinetics, 229-232
Germ-free animals
  absorption in, 237-248
  circulatory effects in, 245-249
  digestive enzymes in, 238-239
  muscle tone in, 244-245
  water absorption in, 240-244
Glucose
  absorption kinetics of, 229-231
  amino acid transport and, 93
  binding protein, 166-168
  brush border and, 131-133, 148-153, 157-159
  in cholera, 259
  as energy source, 11-12, 18-21
  intestinal transport and, 41-42, 48-54, 67-74, 144-145, 148-153, 183-185
  lactate and, 19-21
  sodium chloride and, 23-26
  sodium transport and, 7, 19-20, 58-60, 67, 171-172
  storage of, 13-14
D-Glucose binding
  intestinal absorption, 194-195
  Na^+-dependent, 163-168
  to brush borders, 157-159

Glycine
  intestinal transport of, 98-99
  Na^+ effect, 114-115
β-Glycosidase
  action of, 144-145
  active site of, 146-148
  of brush border, 144-145
  sugar transport and, 143-154

H

Hartnup disease
  peptide absorption in, 101-102
Histidine binding
  to brush border, 161-162
  Na^+-dependent, 165-166
  protein isolation, 166-168
Hydragogue drugs, 210-224

I

Intestinal flora
  absorption and, 237-248
Intestinal transport
  adenyl cyclase and, 41-43
  of amino acids, 48-54, 67, 77-91, 95-97, 171-172, 187-195
  ATP and, 16-17, 33-34
  cation effects, 113-122
  circulation and, 27-33
  of 5,5-dimethyl-2,4-oxazolidine-dione, 38-39
  electrical coupling of, 48-54, 62
  electrical properties of, 192-194
  energetics of, 9-34
  intercellular, 177-184
  ionic conductance and, 46-58

Intestinal transport, contd.,
  ionic gradients and, 23-26
  3-O-methyl glucose and, 29-33, 61-62, 67-75
  membrane potential and, 54-58, 235
  of monosaccharides, 67-74
  mucosal effects, 199-206
  Na^+ effect, 77-78, 84-88
  of peptides, 95-107
  pH gradients and, 39-40, 44, 180-181, 185
  of sodium, 45-62
  sodium chloride and, 23-26
  species differences, 70-71, 187-195
  of sugars, 48-54, 143-153, 171-172
  transcellular, 177-184
  unloading and, 28-33, 36
  water layer effects, 197-206
Ionic conductance
  intestinal transport and, 46-58
Ionic gradients
  electrical potential and, 121
  energy supply and, 23-26
Ion movement
  energy for, 11
  laxatives and, 213-216

J

Jejunum
  peptide absorption in, 97
  sugar transport in, 69-74

K

Ketone bodies
  as energy source, 14
K^+ extrusion
  amino acid uptake and, 86-88, 93
K^+ transport
  coupling of, 58-60

L

Laxative drugs, 211-212, 214-224
Lysine
  transport of, 89-90

M

Magnesium
  Na^+ substitution for, 232-233
Membrane potential
  intestinal transport and, 54-58
  osmolality and, 57-58
Mannitol
  Na^+ substitution and, 231-232
Mannose
  brush border binding, 157-159
Methionine
  absorption of, 102-103, 105
  transport of, 81
  uptake of, 97-98
3-O-Methyl glucose
  absorption of, 229-230
  in germ-free animals, 239-240
  intestinal transport and, 29-33, 36, 61-62, 69-75, 124, 234

3-O-Methyl glucose, contd.,
  Na^+ effect, 114, 118, 232, 234-235
  sugar transport and, 149
Mg-dependent ATPase
  Na-K-activated ATPase and, 22
Monosaccharides
  intestinal transport of, 67-74, 127-137
Mucosal membranes
  amino acid transport in, 78-89
  dimensions of, 207
  enterotoxins and, 274-275
  intestinal transport and, 202-206
  Na^+ and, 78-79

N

Na^+
  active transport and, 113-122
  amino acid transport and, 67, 77-78, 84-88, 114
  ATP and, 121-122
  brush border and, 127-128, 136-137
  choline and, 114-115
  D-glucose binding and, 163-168
  glucose and, 7, 19-20, 58-60, 67, 125-126, 179-180, 231-232
  histidine binding, 165-168
  intestinal transport and, 77-78, 84-88, 113-122
  ion concentration and, 119
  ion gradient hypothesis and, 120-121, 125
  laxatives and, 214-216
  Li substitution, 116-117
  magnesium substitution and, 232

mannitol and, 231-232
peptide transport and, 100
pump, 136-137
sugar transport, 125-126, 231-234
transport site of, 117-119
Na^+,K^+-ATPase
  deoxycholate and, 209-210
  in endoplasmic reticulum, 7
  in germ-free animals, 244
  membrane transport and, 22-23
  proton pump and, 40-41, 43

O

Oxyphenisatin
  action of, 214-224

P

Peptide transport
  absorption and, 105-107
  amino acid sequence in, 96-101
  amino acid transport and, 98-99
  brush border hydrolysis of, 95
  cystinurea and, 101-102
  Hartnup disease and, 101-102
  hydrolysis and, 99-100
  intestinal, 95-107
  mechanisms for, 105-107
  Na^+ dependence and, 100
  peptide hydrolysis and, 105-106, 111
  protein absorption and, 103-105
  pyridoxine deficiency and, 102-103
  rates of absorption, 96-97
  transport kinetics of, 97-98

Peptide transport, contd.,
  uptake systems for, 99
Peristalsis
  in germ-free animals, 244-245
Permeability
  chloride effects, 2
  in cholera, 257
  copper and, 2
  in mucosal membranes, 202-205
  in unstirred layers, 202-203
Phenethylamine
  transport of, 79-80
Phenylalanine
  analogues of, 79-80, 82-83
  transport of, 79-81
pH gradients
  adenyl cyclase and, 41-43
  carbonic anhydrase and, 40-41
  intestinal transport and, 39-40, 44
Phlorizin
  analogues of, 145-146
  glucose uptake and, 148-153
  mechanism of, 154
  structure of, 147-148
  sugar transport and, 143-144, 193
Proline
  transport of, 189-190
Proline binding
  to brush border, 161-162
Prostaglandins
  bacterial enterotoxins and, 276-277
  in cholera, 263-264
Protein absorption, 95, 103-105, 238-239

Proton pump
  intestinal transport and, 40-41, 43, 178

S

Serosal extracellular space
  determination of, 68-69
Serosal membrane
  amino acid transport in, 89-90
  structure of, 177
Serosal Na^+ pump
  intestinal transport and, 46-48
Shigella dysenteriae
  enterotoxin of, 280
Sodium chloride
  glucose absorption and, 23-25
Sodium transport
  amino acids and, 77-78, 84-88
  endoplasmic reticulum and, 4-5, 7
  glucose and, 19-20, 23-26, 58-60, 67
  site of, 117-119
  in small intestine, 45-62
Sprue, tropical
  absorption and, 286-297
  amino acid absorption and, 243-244
  clinical features of, 286, 295-296
  definition of, 285
  epidemiology of, 285-286
  etiology of, 295
  folate absorption in, 292-293, 296
  sugar absorption in, 286-290
  treatment of, 296-297
  vitamin B_{12} and, 292-293, 296
  water absorption in, 287-290

Sugars (See also: Specific sugar)
    amino acid transport and, 87, 93, 125-126, 158-159
    binding protein for, 166-172
    brush border and, 73-74, 127-137, 148-149
    intestinal absorption of, 229-234
    intestinal transport of, 48-54, 67-75
        glycosidase and, 143-153
        phlorizin and, 143-148
        species differences, 189
    pump for, 67-74
    uptake mechanism, 143-144

T

Translocation
    nature of, 86-88
Transmural potential difference
    amino acid transport and, 86-88
    in cholera, 261
    intestinal transport and, 45-48, 192-193
    osmolality and, 57-58
Tryptophan
    transport of, 188-192
Tyrosine
    transport of, 188-192

U

Unstirred layer effects, 197-206, 232-233

V

Vitamin B_{12}
    tropical sprue and, 292-293, 296

W

Water
    absorption of, 240-244, 287-290
    bacterial enterotoxins and, 273-281
    in cholera, 255-258
    hydragogue drugs and, 211-212, 214-224
    osmotic flow of, 177-178
    in tropical sprue, 287-290
    unstirred, 197-206, 232-233

X - Z

Xylose
    absorption of, 229-231
    intestinal transport of, 73-74

DATE DUE

APR 2 3 1982		
MAR 3 0 '82		
APR 0 1 1990		
MAR 2 9 1990		

DEMCO 38-297